Public Health in Developing Countries - Challenges and Opportunities

Edited by Edlyne Eze Anugwom and Niyi Awofeso

Published in London, United Kingdom

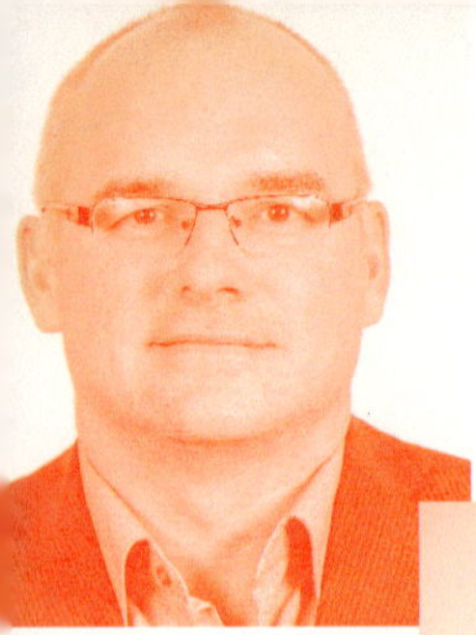
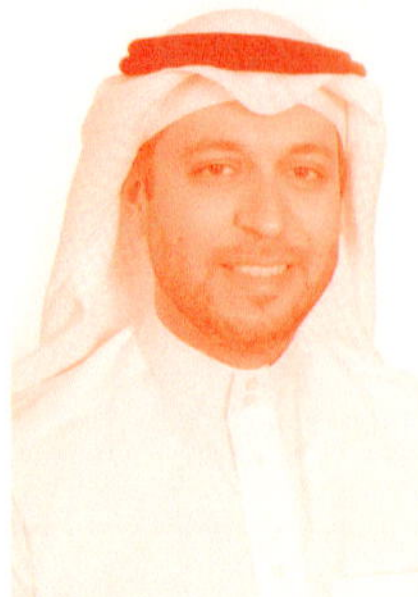
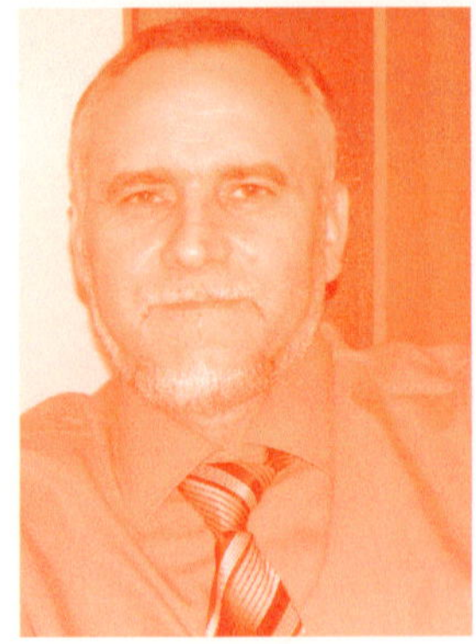
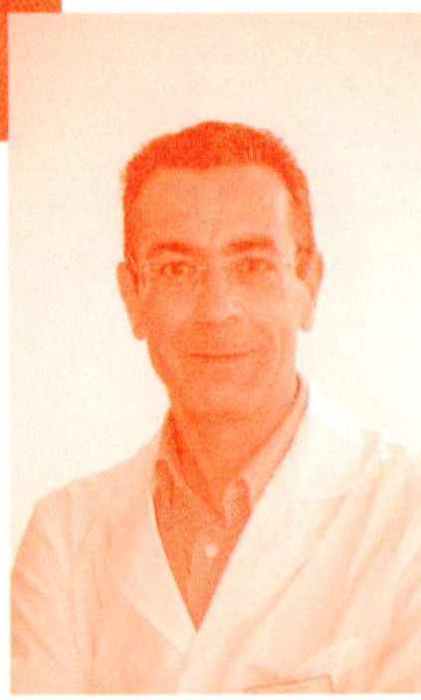
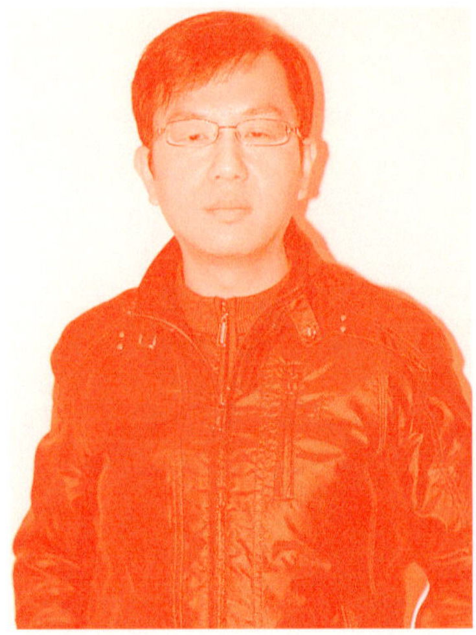
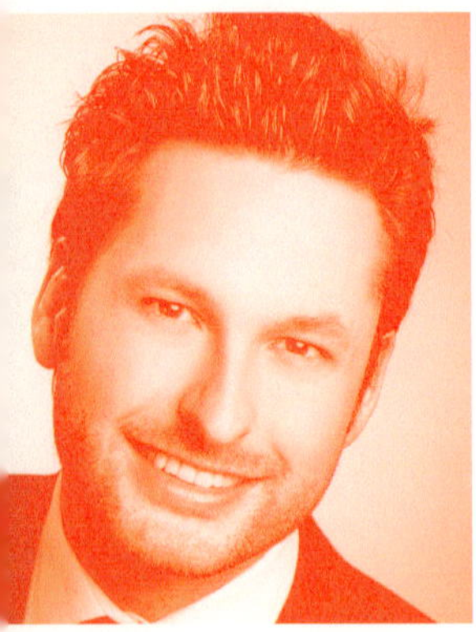
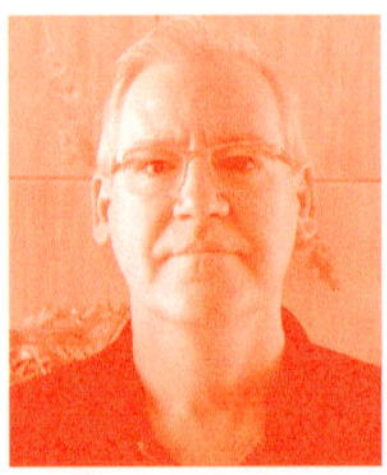

IntechOpen

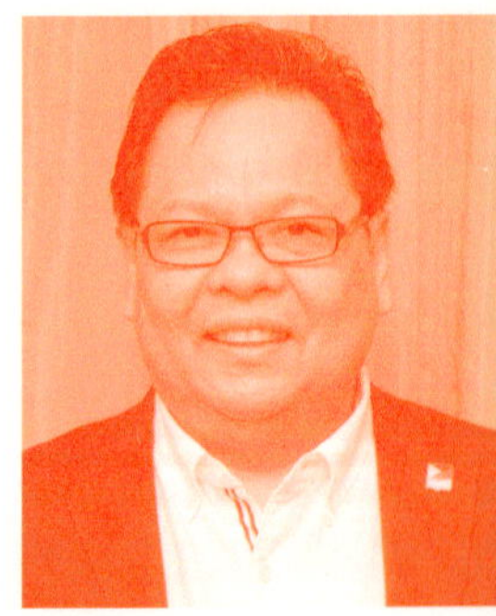
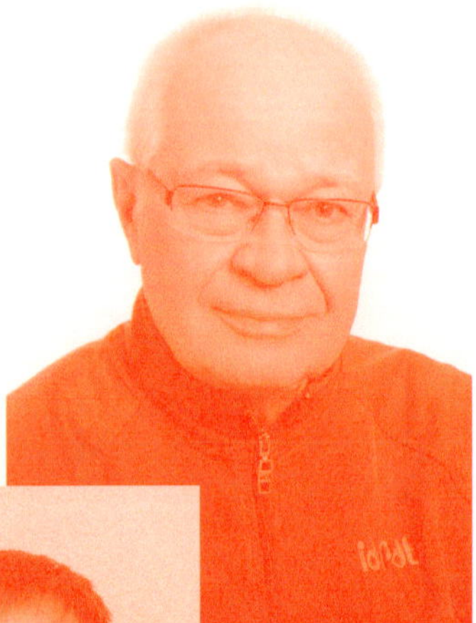
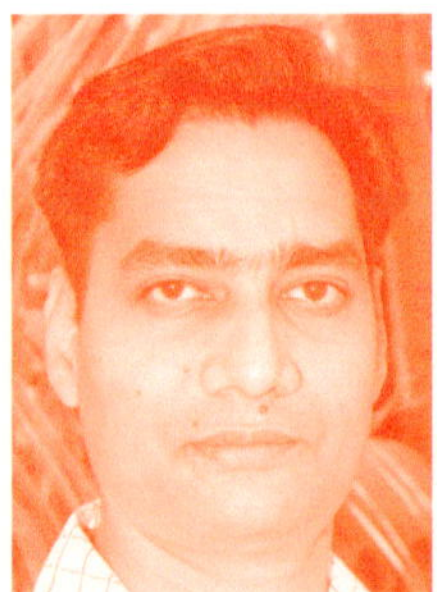
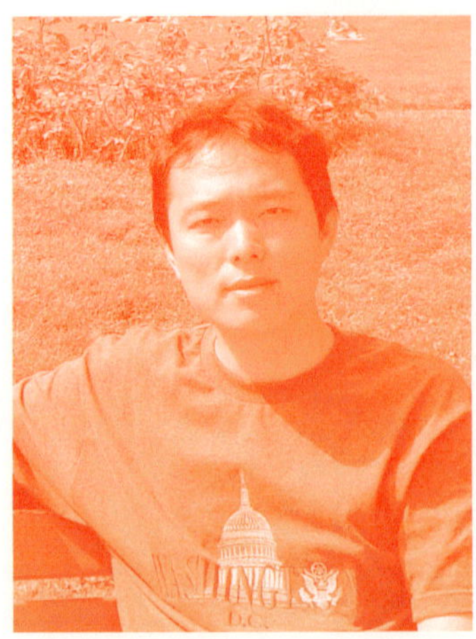
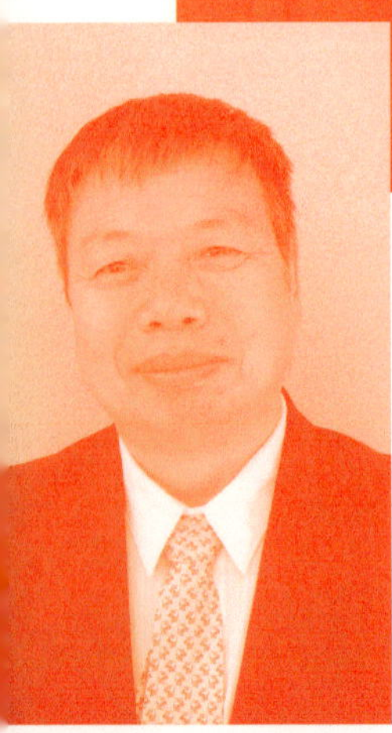
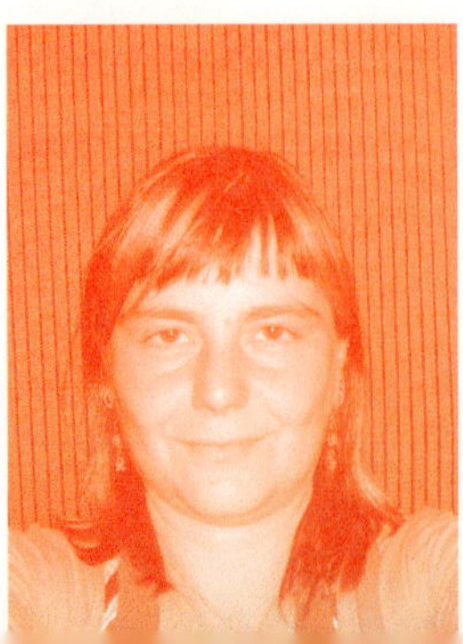

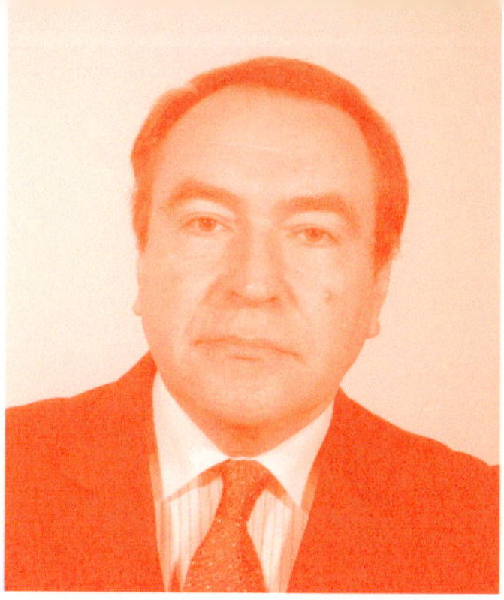
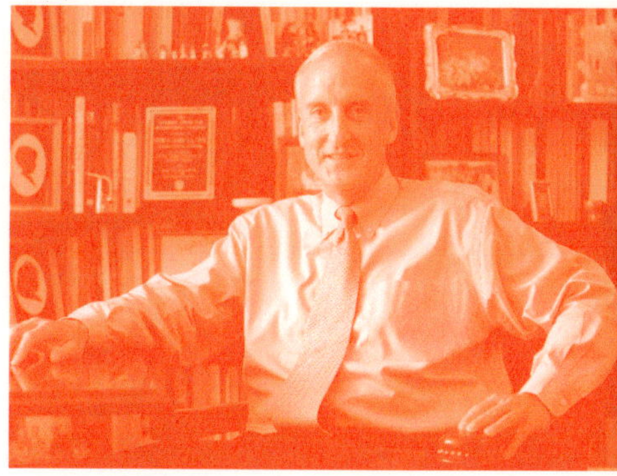
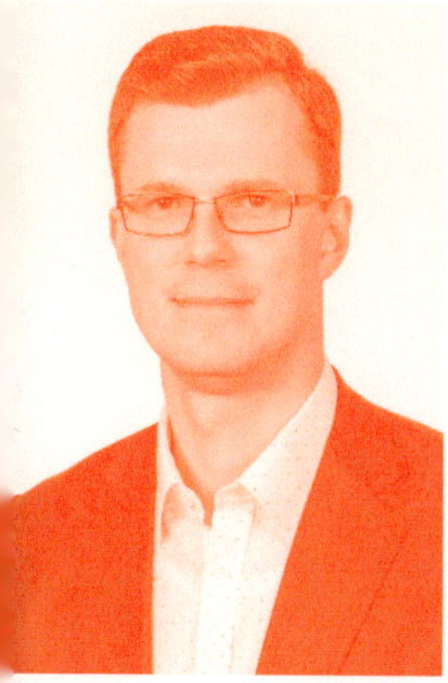
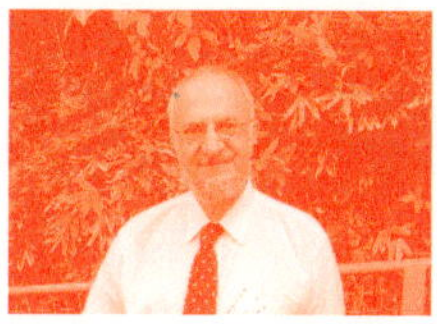
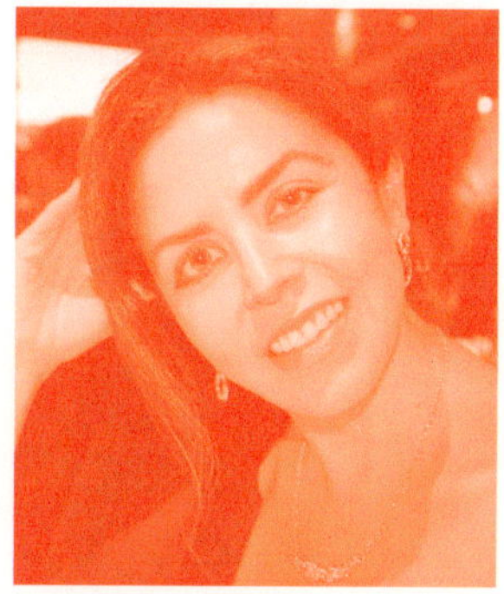

Supporting open minds since 2005

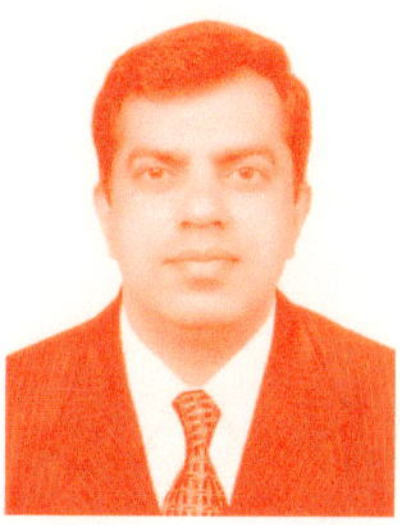
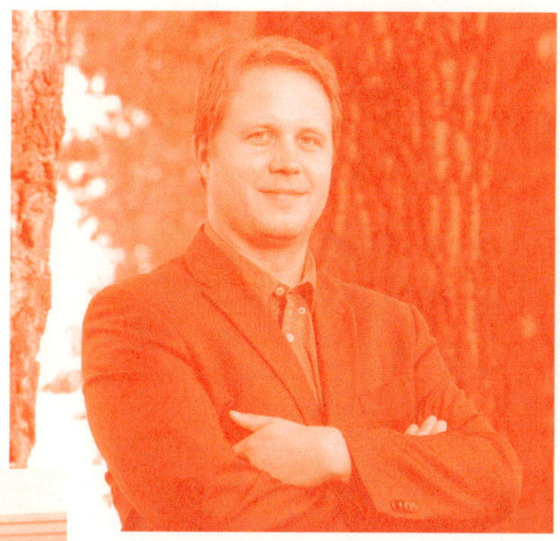
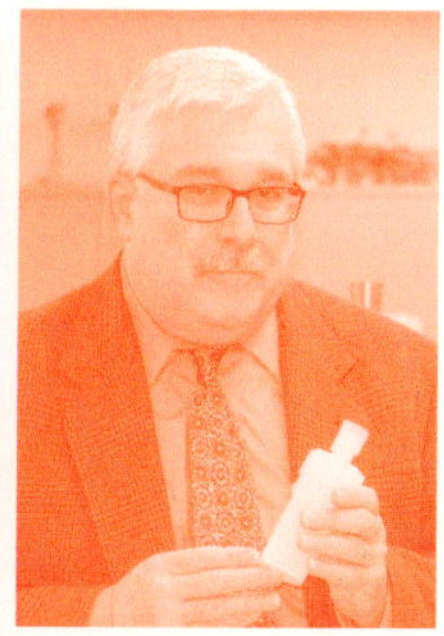
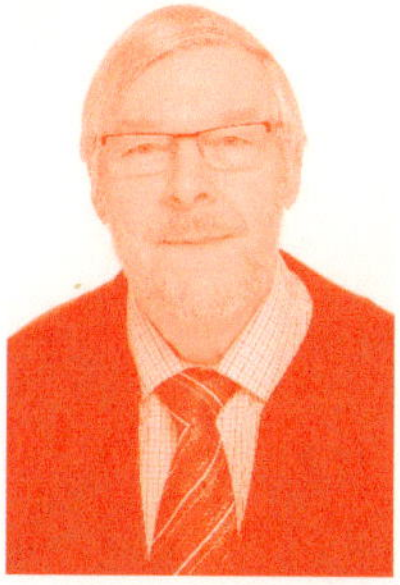
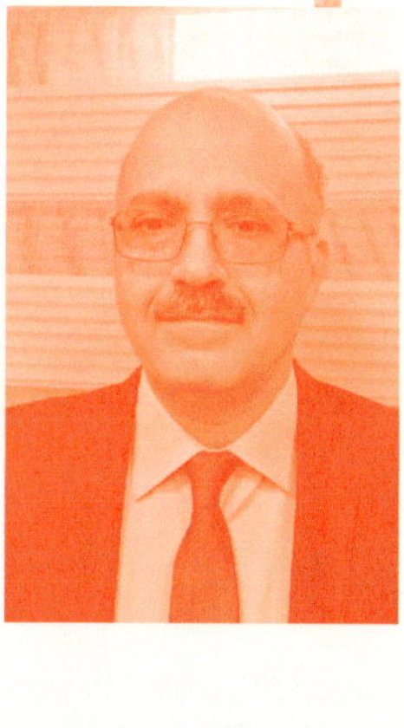
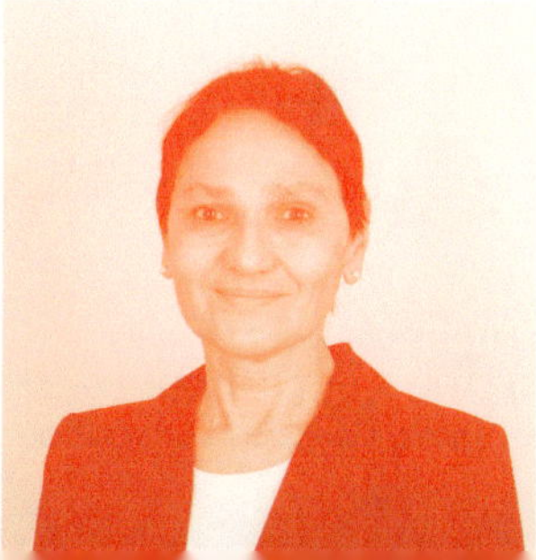
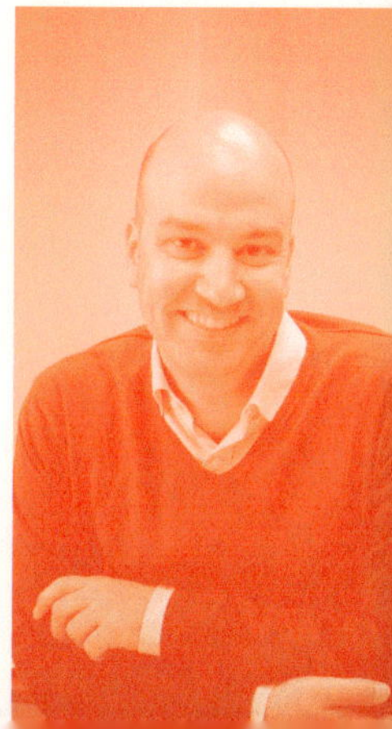

Public Health in Developing Countries - Challenges and Opportunities
http://dx.doi.org/10.5772/intechopen.83134
Edited by Edlyne Eze Anugwom and Niyi Awofeso

Contributors
Serge Mandiefe Piabuo, Janice Tieguhong Puatwoe, Radiance Ogundipe, Gina Alvarado, Jennifer Mueller, Stacey Scriver, Lila O'Brien-Milne, Ama Fenny, Nata Duvvury, Sura Jassim, Basant Kumar Panda, Kenechukwu Anugwom, Vaseem Anjum, Simon Nemutandani, Kenneth Juma, Gershim Asiki, Pamela Juma, Peter O Otieno, Constance Shumba, V K Sashindran, Puja Dudeja, Mary Ann Cooper, Ronald L. Holle, Richard Tushemereirwe, Susanta Ghosh, Chaitali Ghosh, Melkamu Kassa, Grace Jeanne, Edlyne Eze Anugwom, Ignatio Madanhire, Roy Mushonga, Loice Gudukeya, SJH Hendrick, FM Mulaudzi

First published in London, United Kingdom, 2020 by IntechOpen
IntechOpen is the global imprint of INTECHOPEN LIMITED, registered in England and Wales, registration number: 11086078, 7th floor, 10 Lower Thames Street, London, EC3R 6AF, United Kingdom
Printed in Croatia

British Library Cataloguing-in-Publication Data
A catalogue record for this book is available from the British Library

Additional hard and PDF copies can be obtained from orders@intechopen.com

Public Health in Developing Countries - Challenges and Opportunities
Edited by Edlyne Eze Anugwom and Niyi Awofeso
p. cm.
Print ISBN 978-1-78985-873-0
Online ISBN 978-1-78985-874-7
eBook (PDF) ISBN 978-1-83962-380-6

For EU product safety concerns:
IN TECH d.o.o., Prolaz Marije Krucifikse Kozulić 3, 51000 Rijeka, Croatia, info@intechopen.com or visit our website at intechopen.com.

Meet the editors

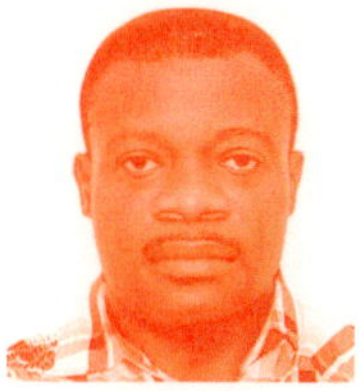

Edlyne Anugwom is a Professor of Sociology and Development at the University of Nigeria and until recently Georg Forster Senior Research Fellow of the Humboldt Foundation at the Institute of African Studies, Leipzig University. He has held teaching positions/fellowships in such diverse places as Leiden, Wassenaar, Birmingham, Bridgewater, Edinburgh, Mainz, Cape Town, and others. His research interests are in the areas of social research, public health, political sociology of development, social conflict and terrorism in Africa. Significant publications include: *Research Methods in Social Sciences* (2010, Fourth Dimension Pub); *The Boko Haram Insurgence in Nigeria: Perspectives from Within* (2019, Palgrave Macmillan); *From Biafra to the Niger Delta Conflict: Memory, Ethnicity and the State in Nigeria* (2019, Lexington Books); and *Development in Nigeria – Promise on Hold?* (2020, Routledge). In addition, he has published more than 100 peer-reviewed journal articles and as many book chapters.

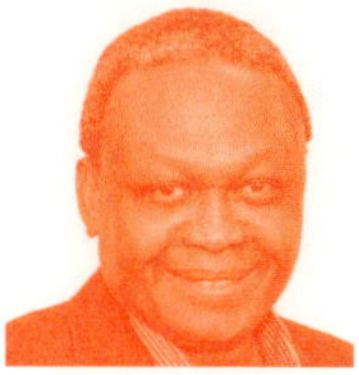

Niyi Awofeso is currently a professor at the School of Health and Environmental Studies Hamdan Bin Mohammed Smart University (HBMSU), Dubai. He commenced his public health career as an infectious disease physician and acting medical director at Nigeria's National Tuberculosis and Leprosy Training Centre in 1990. Prior to joining HBMSU in 2013 from the University of Western Australia where he worked as Professor of Health Management, he accumulated extensive research and professional experience at both middle and senior management levels in academia and the international health industry. He holds postgraduate qualifications in infectious diseases medicine, public health, business administration and health administration. He has so far published more than 120 peer-reviewed articles in well-regarded academic journals, authored five books and eight book chapters.

Contents

Preface

The current volume focuses on public health in developing societies with particular emphasis on the challenges of public health delivery. Public health, as the name suggests, is about the public sector ownership of health delivery and general access to health mediated by public institutions, agencies and concerted community action. In the developing world, public health seeks to close the gap between health needs of the populace and affordability/availability of clinical health. In other words, apart from its traditional concerns, public health with emphasis on generalised afflictions, epidemics, diseases and infections also seeks to make health services accessible to communities and societies. Incidentally, the crucial issue of equitable access to health services is a much more acute problem in the developing world and public health services are often seen as the last resort of common everyday people who otherwise might find it impossible to access health services. The above situation entails a public health system that is severely overburdened and mostly under-resourced.

Nevertheless, developing nations have demonstrated increasing strengths in their health systems, as illustrated by morbidity and mortality trends in Novel Coronavirus disease 2019 (COVID-19). To date, only about 22% of all COVID-19 deaths are from developing countries, yet these countries collectively account for 86% of the global population. Since the turn of the century, and as exemplified by achievements related to the Millennium Development Goals, developing countries have made significant progress in addressing social determinants of health and improving case management standards by taking deliberate, evidence-based and decisive steps.

While the focus on public health in the developing world here would seem intuitively topical and necessary, there is the need to equally appreciate that the health status of these societies ultimately relates to and affects general development. Thus, health and access to health services remain critical indicators of development and social improvement. As a result, the discourse of public health in these societies is also ultimately the discourse of development.

This book, even though it has a titular focus on the developing world, draws its case studies mainly from Sub-Saharan Africa and India. India, interestingly, straddles both the developed and developing world. However, with the second largest population in the world, it presents so much contrast between socio-economic and social groups that equally underlines another contrast in access to health: limited resources and burgeoning needs for public health delivery.

Without doubt, the developing world generally faces a perplexing mixture of inadequate health delivery and predilection towards diseases and infections resulting largely from nutritional challenges, economic status, unequal access to healthcare and epileptic institutional responses to health issues. In the above situation, these nations present formidable health delivery challenges that automatically call attention to the need for a robust and dynamic public health system. Evidently, diseases and afflictions ranging from SARS, coronaviruses,

HIV to the recurrent Ebola all make the imperative of good and effective public health systems unquestionable in these areas. While not necessarily re-echoing the nexus between health and development here, there is no argument that the improvement of health delivery in these nations would have salubrious impacts on development, economic improvements and longevity.

Therefore, in addition to the economics and politics of development in these nations, there is even more urgent need to continuously improve and reposition the public health systems of these nations not only to tackle old and familiar health foes but equally be equipped to proactively deal with new threats and the ever-increasing needs of a rapidly growing population. The above provides general context for the subjects dealt with in the various chapters of this book. While a broad conceptualization of the focus and issues under public health was favoured in this volume, there has also been attempts in some of the chapters to provide unique insights and lessons learnt in specific case studies from different parts of the developing world. Even though these chapters are not mutually reinforcing, they tackle different and critical aspects of public health ranging from health promotion, leprosy, and violence against women to indigenous health systems and breast cancer management.

Hence, the chapters in this volume present both theoretical insights and evidence-based knowledge that is useful to medical/public health practitioners, students, academics and general readers. The subjects treated are as diverse as they are informative and insightful. In addition, the case studies are derived mainly from West Africa (Ghana, Nigeria) and India. For ease of comprehension and flow, chapters are organized into two main parts including sixteen chapters as follows:

Part 1: "General and Crosscutting Issues in Public Health"

> Chapter 1: "Introductory Chapter: Public Health Afflictions and Challenges in the Developing World"
>
> Chapter 2: "The Global Burden and Perspectives on Non-Communicable Diseases (NCDs) and the Prevention, Data Availability and Systems Approach of NCDs in Low-resource Countries"
>
> Chapter 3: "Non-Communicable Diseases and Urbanization in African Cities: A Narrative Review"
>
> Chapter 4: "Health Promotion and Its Challenges to Public Health Delivery System in Africa"
>
> Chapter 5: "Understanding the Science of Indigenous Health System: Key to Sustainable Collaborations"
>
> Chapter 6: "Public Health Effects of Wood Fuel in Africa: Bioenergy from Tree Commodities as a Sustainable Remedy"
>
> Chapter 7: "Cultural Practices and Health Consequences: Health or Habits, the Choice Is Ours"
>
> Chapter 8: "Mitigating the Hazard of Lightning Injury and Death across Africa"

Chapter 9: "Leprosy: Prevention and Control

Chapter 10: "Laser Applications in Periodontology"

Chapter 11: "Development of a Rough Terrain Wheelchair Design"

Part 2: "Case Studies and Country-Specific Issues in Public Health"

Chapter 12: "Temporal Trend and Inequality in Immunization Coverage in India"

Chapter 13: "Social and Institutional Support in Breast Cancer Management among Elderly Women in Nigeria"

Chapter 14: "The Health and Economic Costs of Violence against Women and Girls on Survivors, Their Families, and Communities in Ghana"

Chapter 15: "Obesity in School Children in India"

Chapter 16: "Innovations in Vector-Borne Disease Control in India"

Public health is the art and science of optimising the health of people and their communities, mainly through promoting healthy lifestyles, researching disease and injury prevention, and detecting, preventing and responding to infectious diseases. Many developing countries are increasingly realigning health care, programs and services with the public interest, with significant benefits in terms of poverty reduction, infectious disease control, and improvements in maternal and child health, to mention but a few. There have also been noteworthy challenges along the way, particularly with regards to health system financing. This compendium showcases examples of progress and encumbrances of public health operations in developing nations.

Edlyne E. Anugwom, PhD
Professor of Sociology and Development,
Department of Sociology and Anthropology,
University of Nigeria,
Nsukka, Nigeria

Niyi Awofeso, PhD
Professor and Chair of Master of Public Health/Master of
Hospital Management Programs,
Hamdan Bin Mohammed Smart University,
Dubai, United Arab Emirates

Section 1

General and Crosscutting Issues in Public Health

Chapter 1

Introductory Chapter: Public Health Afflictions and Challenges in the Developing World

Edlyne Eze Anugwom

1. Conceptualizing public health

The most interesting definition of public health is probably that provided by Sir Donald Acheson and colleagues who in the influential report published in 1998 apprehended it as "the science and art of preventing disease, prolonging life and promoting, protecting and improving health through the organized efforts of society" [1]. Generally, and as the name implies, public health is concerned with the health of a given population or group which is pursued as part and parcel of the agenda of governments and public institutions to improve the lives of the people under their domains. In other words, it is health conceived as a critical element of regulations, policies, and support framework of the government or its agencies. Public health is as well a common domain between individuals, communities, groups, and government and/or its institutions and agencies. Even where there are formal and institutional provision of facilities and services, accessing these services and responding to guidelines and procedures of health are usually at the level of individuals and communities. The above is especially obvious in the area of infectious or contagious diseases where prevention and curtailment are deemed necessary. In other words, a good public health system depends as much on formal provision of facilities and services as it depends on a responsive public.

Therefore, health promotion is a key element and goal of public health. In doing this, public health strives to encourage healthy lifestyles and the prevention of diseases and epidemics through health education and intervention actions. There is no gainsaying the fact that public health interventions that are carefully tailored and conscientiously implemented would lead to reduced mortality in the general population and improved quality of life and life expectancy. These would in turn impact positively on socioeconomic development.

By definition, public health lays emphasis on social and environmental contexts of diseases and health problems. It, from this pedestal aspires to improve health through large-scale societal initiatives like vaccinations, fluoridation of drinking water, easy and affordable access to health facilities, and even such behavior modifying acts like prohibition of smoking and demonizing cigarettes as a way of curbing the spread of tobacco-related diseases in the population. In other words, public health while including the treatment of individuals or communities goes beyond this to focus on health promotion, disease prevention, recovery, rehabilitation, and broad health support for the community or society.

From the perspective of the present volume, the conceptualization of public health as both art and science is very instructive. In this sense, it provides a unique opportunity for a fusion or coming together of science and arts. Therefore, public health is neither all about biomedicine nor about the policies and programs on health from public institutions, communities, and government. It is in reality, comprehensive and demands concerted action from different actors. It is thus how disease is prevented, life prolonged, and health promoted through public instruments and policies systematically driven and coordinated or organized to achieve the goals of good health.

In view of the above, it has been posited that "the mission of public health is therefore to achieve an equitable distribution of health for the total population" ([2] p. 5). Equally of interest is that public health is a multidisciplinary domain and thus involves different professionals and practitioners working in concert. However, a critical skill set is knowledge of the principles of epidemiology which gives one the insights into disease patterns, risk factors, and outcome of treatments and even prevention initiatives. Also, a good social knowledge and environmental awareness are equally recommended. In more recent times, political savvy has equally come in handy in dealing with policy makers and governments that provide much of the funding for public health.

2. Major concerns and approaches

Public health as compared to clinical health approach focuses on the health of the population, i.e., group, community, and society, unlike clinical health that is concerned with the health of the individual alone. In other words, while the clinical health provider assists or helps an individual with her own healthcare issues, the public health approach is more broad-based and encompassing beyond the individual. Therefore, while the clinical health approach may focus on why a given individual confronts a particular health issue, public health would take a look at the given social group (neighborhood, community, society) to identify prevalence of a given health issue, risk factors associated with it, accessibility of healthcare for the issue by the members of the society, measures at prevention, and curtailment among the given group. As a result, "public health seeks to improve the health of the whole community with emphasis on protection, prevention of diseases, and promotion of well-being" ([2] p. 5).

The major areas or concerns of public health include hygiene and sanitation; epidemiology; environmental factors; disease prevention; and policies/regulations that address these concerns. Public health focuses on the prevention of diseases or ailments through health education; focused policies; and research and programmed intervention services. Also, public health in principle seeks to address inequity in health; accessibility of health services especially to the marginal or less privileged members of the society; and ensuring quality health provisioning both in public and private health facilities.

In terms of approach, public health takes the community or society as a whole as its focus rather than the individual. It therefore aims at improving the health of communities and societies through concerted efforts. Some of the prominent functions of public health include surveillance, analysis, and evaluation of the health status of the population; health promotion; development of policies and plans that engender health; disease prevention activities and campaigns; development of effective programs and facilities for health protection; evaluation and monitoring of public health policies; and strategies and facilities, among others.

Public health emphasizes a collective approach to health in the population. It usually privileges preventive efforts and health education of the general public aimed at both improving health and reducing risks to health ailments. This collective approach which nowadays entails systematic and public policy response to health issues is different from the provision of medical treatment to an individual or on the basis of one patient per time.

3. The developing world and public health challenges

The conceptualization of public health is generally very close to the comprehensive view that health goes beyond the mere absence of illness or disease. Thus, public health also mirrors a broad definition of health especially along the lines of the emblematic position of the World Health Organization that in 1946/1948 conceptualized health simply as "state of complete physical, mental and social well-being and not merely the absence of disease" ([3] p. 100). However, the reality of the structural challenges of the developing world has created a unique public health orientation that focuses essentially on the absence of diseases. Apart from a history of proliferating diseases and health challenges, the paucity of technical competence, funds, and good leadership have all made public health systems in these parts of the world overburdened and often inadequate to the needs of the people.

While public health concerns in the developing world are very encompassing and often include long list of health ailments and impediments, the core public health problems include such diseases and ailments with high mortality as malaria, infections, diarrhea, respiratory tract infections, HIV/AIDS, anemia and malnutrition, intestinal worms, and lately Ebola. These diseases are usually more prevalent among poor and marginal members of the population. In an ironic sense, those who are far away from necessary health support or lack the resources to access health services are much more affected and afflicted. The above is a core justification for the enthronement of responsive and expansive public health services and public health provisioning to tackle these diseases.

In a succinct take on the health system in sub-Saharan Africa, which is typical of the developing world, sometime in the past (a scenario that has hardly changed), it was postulated, "in spite of prolonged efforts in reforms, meetings, declarations, policy rhetoric as well as the massive input of financial and technical resources, the continent records some of the highest rates of infant deaths and maternal mortality in the world. Also, Africa represents about 10 percent of the global population but accounts for 63 percent of individuals living with HIV/AIDS and 90 percent of malaria infections worldwide" ([4] p. 7). The foregoing calls attention not only to the imperative of a robust public health sector in Africa, but the unending spate of health deficiencies challenge innovation and proactive response in different African countries where lessons have neither been learnt from the past nor experiences harnessed for improved health delivery.

Health delivery from the perspective and experience of the developing world goes beyond the orthodox and Western-defined purviews of medicine and science. In other words, indigenous knowledge as philosophy and ethos of practice affect healthcare decisions and choices in these areas.

The call for the exploitation of meaningful ways of integrating traditional medicine into the health system benefits from the undeniable easy availability and accessibility of traditional healers in most parts of the world especially Africa and India. In fact, Chatora [5] contends that the availability of traditional or unorthodox (non-Western) medical practitioners generally far outstrip that of conventional medical doctors in most parts of the African continent. Incidentally, these traditional healers are accessible both in terms of geographical proximity and finance. They also often initiate a one-on-one interaction with their patients in the process of healing that can hardly obtain within the formal health system.

Another fundamental issue in public health in most of the developing world revolves around the role of the private and informal sectors in public health provisioning. Organizations in these sectors especially the faith-based organizations (FBOs), i.e., churches, religious organizations, religious NGOs, etc., have featured prominently in the health decisions and choices of people overtime. In fact, FBOs, for instance, are seen as critical role players in health delivery and choice people make with regard to health [6–8]. While these private and informal sectors and their roles have been well-studied and even targeted in the guise of public private partnership in health, there is still an overwhelming number of things that happen in these sectors that are neither formally recognized nor regulated. In other words, there is need for not only the formal recognition of these sectors but crucially how synergies can be built to harness what is good in these sectors and expunge what is bad or counter-productive. A big selling point of these alternative health sectors is perhaps their affordability and easy access to a great majority of the people. Therefore, we need to begin conceptualizing public health systems that build also on the good aspects of the private and informal sectors and which also seek to recreate their general appeal within the context of formal health provisioning in the continent.

The three biggest infectious diseases in Africa from both prevalence and resources committed are HIV/AIDS, tuberculosis, and malaria. These are the three giants of public health interventions and efforts in the continent. However, there have been new challenges especially in the form of new and periodic diseases like Ebola which has emerged in the last decade as a major public health concern in some African countries. As has been aptly summarized, "nowhere are global public health challenges more acute than in Sub-Saharan Africa. With just 13 percent of the world population, the region carries 24 percent of the global burden of disease" ([9] p. 1). Even though, globally and continentally, good strides have been made in curtailing the ravages of HIV, there is still a huge disease burden arising from it especially in Africa. Thus, "antiretroviral treatment is being provided to many of those in need in Africa, in numbers greater than was thought possible at the beginning of the decade. Nonetheless, for most Africans living with HIV, such treatment remains out of reach" ([9] p. 4).

The above indicates that in spite of the recent improvements made in curtailing both the spread of HIV/AIDS and the mortality from it, there is still much work to be done in the public health system especially in sustaining the progress made and in scaling up general response. Incidentally, apart from donor/international support, there is a need for committed leadership, good governance, and policies backed by reasonable internal funding in African countries especially those heavily affected in terms of the disease burden. The situation is a little better in India, but acute population growth and dearth of potable water have meant that India confronts a fragile public health situation. Therefore, the need for concerted efforts as well as dynamic and proactive measures against diseases and afflictions cannot be overemphasized.

Without doubt, the most current global public health scourge in the form of the corona virus which caught the whole world by surprise underlines the need for robust public health systems. The fact that such developed nations of the world as the USA, the UK, France, Italy, Spain, Germany, etc. could be caught napping and severely devastated as a result by the new virus with origins in Wuhan, China, calls attention to the inescapable fact that public health delivery and the institutions involved in it are by nature dynamic and confront ever-changing and mutative human environments. That health systems in the developed nations of the world that are well-developed and heavily-resourced could be severely eroded by the corona virus simply underlines the huge challenges of public health in the developing parts of the world, where both structural and environmental forces function as ready impediments to effective health delivery.

There is therefore a need to interrogate prevailing health systems and health delivery in these parts of the world in relation to what appears to be a cyclic incapacity of public health. Perhaps, the contention of Kaseje that "the health system is neither robust nor flexible enough to respond to emerging scenarios that lead to reversal of gains. Traditional, faith, and other informal sources of care are used more because they are more available, accessible, affordable, and acceptable yet

DOI: http://dx.doi.org/10.5772/intechopen.93145

they are ignored and therefore unregulated and unsupported" ([4] p. 7) is really instructive. We need to confront the various problems or challenges bedeviling the system and reposition the system for improved quality of life and overall development.

In effect, the chapters in this volume deal with various and complementary issues in public health from the perspective of the developing world. While these chapters have discussed some of the most pressing and prominent issues in public health in the developing world, there is no doubt that some pertinent issues have gone untreated in it. Therefore, while the volume has sought to be comprehensive, it cannot claim to have treated all there is to know about public health in the developing world. However, the volume draws strength and relevance from the deep theoretical insights of some of the chapters and more crucially from the penetrating case studies from different parts of the developing world that some of the other chapters provide.

Author details

Edlyne Eze Anugwom
Department of Sociology and Anthropology, University of Nigeria, Nsukka, Nigeria

*Address all correspondence to: akommiri@gmail.com

References

[1] Acheson D. Independent Inquiry into Inequalities in Health Report. London, UK: Stationery Office; 1998

[2] Binns C, Low W-Y. What is public health. Asia-Pacific Journal of Public Health. 2015;**27**(1):5-6

[3] World Health Organization (WHO). Preamble to the Constitution of the World Health Organization. Geneva: WHO; 1946/48

[4] Kaseje D. Health care in Africa: Challenges, opportunities and an emerging model for improvement. In: Paper Presented at the Woodrow Wilson International Centre for Scholars (November 2); 2006

[5] Chatora R. An Overview of the Traditional Medicine Situation in the African Region. African Health Monitor, World Health Organization Africa Region (WHO-AFRO). 2003;**4**(1):4-7

[6] Anugwom EE. Beyond morality: Assessment of the capacity of faith-based organizations (FBOs) in responding to the HIV/AIDS challenge in southeastern Nigeria. Iranian Journal of Public Health. 2018;**47**(1):70-76

[7] Dilger H. Doing better? Religion, the virtue ethics of development, and the fragmentation of health policies in Tanzania. AFR Today. 2009;**56**:89110

[8] Chikwendu E. Faith-based organizations in anti-HIV/AIDS work among African youth and women. Dialectical Anthropology. 2004;**28**:307-327

[9] Cooke J. Public Health in Africa: A report of the CSIS Global Health Policy Centre. Washington, D.C: Center for Strategic and International Studies (CSIS); 2009

Chapter 2

The Global Burden and Perspectives on Non-Communicable Diseases (NCDs) and the Prevention, Data Availability and Systems Approach of NCDs in Low-resource Countries

Melkamu Kassa and Jeanne Grace

Abstract

The burden of non-communicable diseases (NCDs) is growing swiftly in low-resourced countries resulting in deleterious health resembling the NCDs burden in high-resourced countries. Despite the availability of information on the escalating adverse economic and health effects of NCDs globally, specific strategies designed to address the growing burden of NCDs in low-resourced countries remain substandard. Research engines like EBSCOhost, Science Citation Index, CINAHL database, PsycINFO, Cochrane Database of Systematic Reviews, published and unpublished abstracts and a hand search of reference lists and table of contents of relevant journals and books were searched from January 2011 to June 2019. In total, 84 studies met the inclusion criteria. Most studies confirm that low-resourced countries compared with high-resourced countries battle to implement NCDs prevention strategies; fail to record data on the risk factors of NCDs; medical records and surveillance data are unavailable. Due to a lack of knowledge and skill, low-resourced countries show no urgency to implement a systems approach for NCDs management. The findings confirm disparities between high-resourced and low-resourced countries regarding NCDs prevention, availability of quality data, and strategies to prevent and manage NCDs through a systems approach that can assist healthcare institutions in reducing the damaging effect of NCDs globally.

Keywords: changing environment, health information, low resourced countries, modernisation, NCDs data, system approach

1. Introduction

As with many high-resourced countries, low-resourced countries have not been spared the global challenges caused by non-communicable diseases (NCDs), such as cardiovascular diseases, coronary heart disease, hypertension, diabetes mellitus, and obesity [1, 2]. For countries with minimal health budgets, every effort needs to be made to reduce patients' reliance on costly medical solutions to health problems, including NCDs, for which drugs are often the first line of treatment to reduce the associated morbidity and premature mortality [3]. Prevention efforts within the healthcare system need to take a broader public health approach to motivate people to address their unhealthy lifestyles that result in the development of NCDs. To achieve this, however, Ministries of Health in low-resourced countries needs factual, timely, and reliable NCDs data that can build a comprehensive information system to provide evidence-based decision-making and to develop appropriate prevention strategies for the specific population affected by NCDs [4, 5].

All healthcare organisations, including governmental and non-governmental institutions, have their strategies to prevent and control diseases and to maintain the health of their community effectively and efficiently. Likewise, healthcare organisations have a strategy for disease prevention and control to maintain the health of the community. Most healthcare systems rely on accurate, timely, correct, and factual data to make political and administrative decisions [4–6]. Moreover, healthcare systems should have a balanced approach in preventing both infectious communicable disease and NCDs, which require factual data at the mega, macro, meso, and micro level of healthcare.

This chapter aims to create a better understanding of the growing global burden and perspectives on NCDs. It also aims to reflect on the prevention of NCDs, the global status and availability of NCDs data, and effective strategies to prevent the growing burden of NCDs in low-resourced countries.

1.1 The global burden of non-communicable disease

Non-communicable diseases (NCDs) are the leading public health challenges globally in the twenty-first century, resulting in ill health, economic loss, life loss, diminished quality of life, and poor social development equally in both high-resourced and low-resourced countries [7, 8]. According to the World Health Organisation Global Status Report (GSR) on non-communicable disease, from 38 million deaths due to NCDs each year, more than 40% were premature and were preventable [9]. Based on the projection of the WHO, by 2025 NCDs will account for over 70% of all deaths globally, with 85% of these occurring in developing countries [10]. Evidences show that if proper prevention approaches are not designed and applied, an estimated 41 million people in low-resourced countries will die from NCDs by 2025, mainly due to cardiovascular diseases (CVDs) (48%), cancers (21%), chronic respiratory diseases (12%), and diabetes (3%) [11].

Globally, more than 9 million deaths occurred due to NCDs in people under the age of 60, with most being preventable. Untimely losses from NCDs range from 22% amongst men and 35% amongst women in low-resourced countries to 8% amongst men and 10% amongst women in high-resourced countries [10]. According to current research, more than 80% of heart diseases, stroke, hypertension and type 2 diabetes, and over a third of cancers can be prevented by eradicating the common risk factors, mainly tobacco use, unhealthy diets, physical inactivity, and the harmful use of alcohol [12]. The effective prevention and management of common NCDs risk factors require the establishment of a strategic framework which can tackle health problems associated with the growing burden of morbidity and mortality of these diseases [13]. According to evidence by the WHO, globally, NCDs deaths will increase by 17% over the next 10 years, with the most considerable increase being in low-resourced countries such as Africa (27%) and the Eastern Mediterranean region (25%) [7, 8]. Current research indicates that cancer, diabetes, high blood pressure, cardiovascular diseases, and kidney diseases are no longer the illness of high-resourced countries, but also, non-communicable disease hampers the people and the economies of the deprived populations even more than communicable diseases, representing a public health emergency in slow motion [14, 15].

As illustrated in **Figure 1**, common NCDs account for most of the avoidable morbidity and preventable mortality, these being cardiovascular disease, coronary heart disease, high blood pressure, diabetes, and obesity. The percentage of mortality associated with the major NCDs across three regions of the world, such as high-resourced countries, low-resourced countries, and Africa varies. In high-income countries, the percentage of mortality related with NCDs such as cardiovascular disease, coronary heart disease, high blood pressure, diabetes, and obesity decreases, whilst in low-resourced countries and Africa, it continues to raise. For instance, the percentage of mortality due to cardiovascular disease is 38% in high-resourced countries [16] and 42% in low-resourced countries, from which 20% is the share of Africa [17–19].

In low-resourced countries, the largest percentage of mortality (70%) is due to coronary heart disease with Africa's share 10% [19]. In high-resourced countries, coronary heart disease accounts for 20% of mortality. The share of high blood pressure is 46% in Africa, exceeding the total percentage of deaths in low-resourced countries (40%) [20]. In high-resourced countries, high blood pressure accounts for a relatively lower 35% of mortality [21].

The percentage of mortality as a result of diabetes is 8, 12, and 14% in high-resourced, low-resourced countries, and Africa, respectively [22, 23]. The percentage of deaths due to obesity is 29.5% in high-resourced countries and 37.5% in low-resourced countries with the share of Africa 33% [24–27].

1.2 The global perspective on NCDs

In 2011, the United Nations High-Level Meeting presented and promised a unique opportunity for international communities to take action against the rising

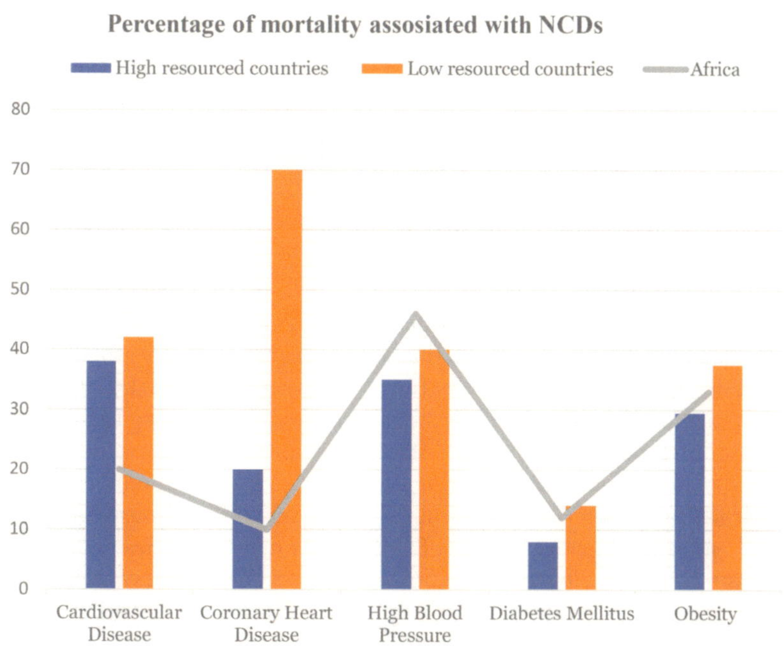

Figure 1.
Percentage of mortality associated with NCDs in Africa, high-resourced and low-resourced countries.

epidemic of NCDs. The WHO asserts that the world has reached a decisive point in the history of NCDs and has an unprecedented opportunity to alter its course. In an attempt to alter the damaging progression of NCDs, the WHO Member States agreed on a time-bound set on the following nine voluntary global targets to be attained by 2025 [9, 28]:

1. A 25% relative reduction in the overall mortality from cardiovascular diseases, cancer, diabetes, or chronic respiratory diseases.

2. At least 10% relative reduction in the harmful use of alcohol, as appropriate, within the national context.

3. A 10% relative decrease in pervasiveness of deficient physical action.

4. A 30% relative decrease in mean populace admission of salt/sodium.

5. A 30% relative decrease in the pervasiveness of current tobacco use in people matured 15+ years.

6. A 25% relative decrease in the pervasiveness of raised circulatory strain, or regulation of predominance of raised pulse, as indicated by national conditions.

7. Stop the rise in diabetes and fat.

8. At least 50% of eligible people receive drug therapy and counselling (including glycaemic control) to prevent heart attacks and strokes.

9. An 80% accessibility of the moderate fundamental innovations and essential drugs, including generics, required to treat major NCDs in both open and private offices.

Furthermore, the world health assembly set a target of a 25% reduction in overall mortality from four major NCDs, including cancer, diabetes, cardiovascular-, and chronic respiratory disease by 2025 [28]. The 25 × 25 strategy is today included in the World Health Organisations Global Action Plan 2013–2020. Amongst the nine voluntary national strategies, two are intended to reduce deaths due to the four illnesses mentioned earlier and to stop the increase in obesity and diabetes. The remaining national strategies focus specifically on incorporating decreased alcohol intake, promoting physical exercise, reducing nutritional salt and smoking, enhancing hypertension control, and improving the treatment of those at risk from the main NCDs. Countries need to make progress on all these targets to attain the overarching target of a 25% reduction of premature mortality from the four major NCDs by 2025 [29–32].

The action plan advocates a comprehensive vision, recognising the social, economic, and political determinants of diseases and the wide-ranging developmental healthcare scheme [29]. Conversely, it is uncertain, in low-resourced countries at a much lower economic level, how these declarations of commitment will be interpreted and implemented [33–35]. The prioritising of infectious communicable disease, a frail healthcare system, and poorly designed NCDs prevention policies prevent low-resourced countries not to implement these declarations of commitment [1, 4].

Moreover, to improve the prevention and control of NCDs, the United Nations High-Level Meeting presented four additional time-bound commitments in 2014 which incorporates: "*1) by 2015, consider setting national NCD targets for 2025, 2) by 2015, consider developing national multisector policies and plans to achieve the national targets by 2025; 3) by 2016, reduce risk factors for NCDs, building on guidance set out in the WHO Global NCD Action Plan, and 4) by 2016, strengthen health systems to address NCDs through people-centred primary health care and universal health coverage, building on guidance set out in WHO Global NCD Action Plan*" [28]. Despite the formulation of these four additional time-bound commitments by United Nations High-Level meeting, progress made by the majority of low-resourced countries is plodding and incomparable with that of high-resourced countries [1, 36].

The WHO argues that the global epidemic of NCDs can be reversed through modest investments in interventions that are so low in cost that countries' income levels need not be a significant barrier to successfully implement the nine voluntary global targets and the 25 × 25 strategy. However, what is needed, more importantly, is high levels of commitment, proper planning, community mobilisation, and an intensive focus on a small range of critical actions. The above will ensure quick gains to reduce the significant behavioural risk factors, namely tobacco use, harmful use of alcohol, an unhealthy diet, and physical inactivity, as well as biological risk factors, such as blood glucose [29, 37].

If the current trends continue, the probability of dying prematurely from the four main NCDs is projected to increase in Sub-Saharan Africa but will show a relative decrease in areas such as Europe, the western Pacific, Americas, eastern Mediterranean, and Southeast Asia [37]. It is believed that if the risk factor targets set by the WHO are achieved, the 25 × 25 target will be surpassed in Europe amongst both men and women. In the western Pacific, the target will be achieved in women and almost achieved in men, whist the Americas, Eastern Mediterranean, and Southeast Asia will approach the target with the rising trend in Africa be reversed. In most regions, a more striving 50% tobacco reduction instead of the agreed 30% by 2016 will contribute the most to reducing premature NCD mortality amongst men, followed by addressing raised blood pressure [29, 38]. For women, the highest contributing risk factor towards the premature NCD mortality target will be raised blood pressure in every region except Europe and the Americas, where the ambitious but not approved tobacco reduction would have the most substantial benefit [33, 35].

2. Factors influencing the quality of NCDs prevention

Different factors predict healthcare systems' capacity to prevent NCDs and its related risk factors. These predictors are determinants of NCDs prevention including the level of physical exercise, dietary choice, organised infrastructure, urbanisation and related policy, cultural norms, and accessibility of health information.

2.1 Level of physical exercise

Worldwide industrial expansion and an increased service sector have resulted in less work-related physical exercise, whilst at the same time, modern technology has also made it increasingly convenient to remain sedentary. Many people lead a life with little or no physical exercise, and their leisure time is often spent on sedentary activities such as live online chats, playing computer games, and watching television, with 60% of the world's population being estimated to lead a sedentary life [39, 40].

Research indicates that low-resourced countries are experiencing rapid nutritional transitions, lifestyle changes, and epidemiological transition following modernisation, westernisation, and increased reliance on technology. As a result, more time is available to pursue leisure activities, which leads to lifestyle diseases such as cardiovascular disease, diabetics, hypertension, overweight, and obesity [40, 41].

Naturally, the human body is designed for movement; however, planned strenuous physical exercise is not a part of the normal lifestyle. Furthermore, an individual cannot expect his/her body to function optimally and to remain healthy for extended periods if it is abused or is not used as intended [40]. In **Figure 2**, the diseases associated with a lack of physical exercise that contributes to a rise in NCDs are illustrated.

Research shows that physical inactivity is the most critical public health problem in the twenty-first century. For many years, scientists and health and fitness professionals have advocated regular physical exercise as the best defence against the development of many diseases, disorders, and illnesses [40]. Due to the recognised health benefits, it has, and the importance of maintaining a good quality of life, regular physical exercise received recognition in the first U.S. surgeon general's report on physical exercise and health. In this report, physical exercise was identified as a national health objective and recognised physical inactivity as a nationwide severe health problem; it provided clear-cut scientific evidence linking physical activity to numerous health benefits and presented demographic data describing physical exercise patterns and trends in the U.S. population. It also made physical exercise recommendations for improved health [42, 43].

2.2 Dietary choice

Consumption of high levels of trans fats, saturated fats, processed and refined foods, sugar, salt, and sugary drinks is associated with an increased risk of CVD and diabetes, whilst adequate consumption of fruit and vegetables is associated with a reduced risk of coronary heart disease and stroke. Unhealthy diets tend to follow a socio-economic gradient. Higher quality diets are associated with persons of greater affluence, whilst energy-dense nutrient-poor diets are associated with persons of more limited economic

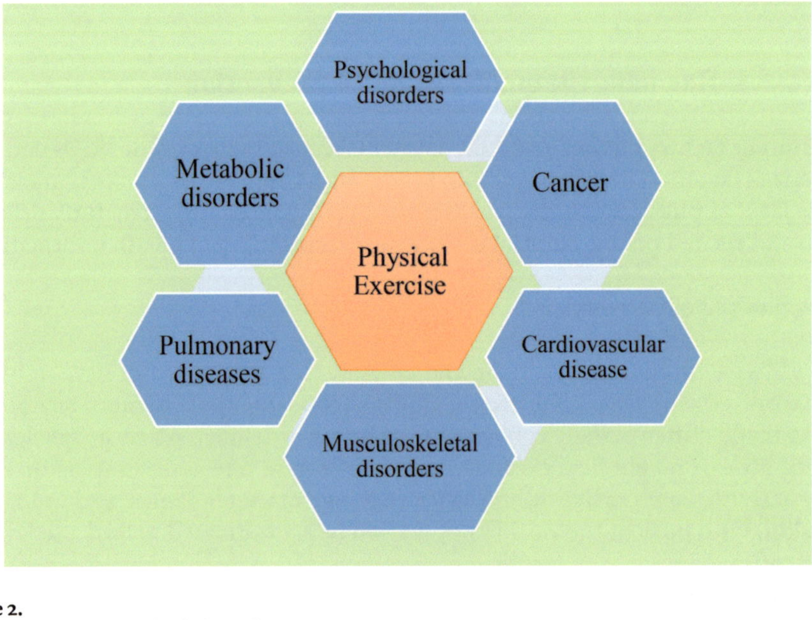

Figure 2.
NCDs associated with lack of physical exercise.

means [44, 45]. Education and gender also impact diet, with unhealthy eating habits associated with lower levels of education. Moreover, low fruit intake represented a 50% greater share of the disease burden amongst men than women [46, 47].

In low-resourced countries, the wrong perceptions about body image contribute to consume unhealthy dietary sources such as high level of trans fats, saturated fats, raw beef, goat meats, and fast foods [47]. In some Asian and the majority of African countries, having a big, fat stomach is considered as being charismatic, powerful, healthy, and perceived as a sign of wealthy [1, 48]. Following this perception, a more significant number (52%) of the public consumes high-fatty food substances which spontaneously results in acquiring NCDs [1, 49, 50]. **Figures 3a–c** depicts examples of red meats, such as raw beef meat called "Kurt Siga", red raw ground beef with spices and yoghurt called "Kitfo", and partially roasted meat respectively of which high levels of consumption and frequent consumption increased risk of NCDs due to high fat levels [1, 50]. This dietary practice is very customary amongst the diverse Ethiopian communities. Such unhealthy dietary practices are practised mainly amongst wealthy community groups and

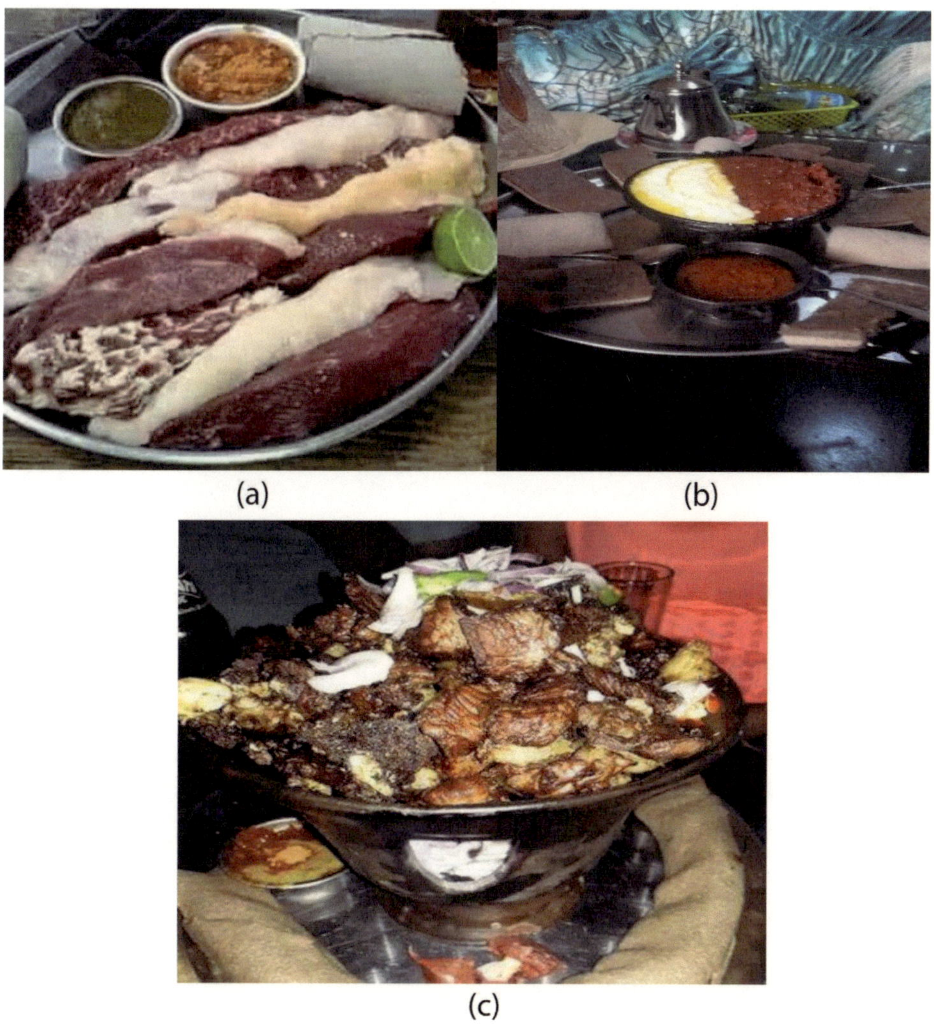

Figure 3.
(a) Raw fatty beef meat. (b) Raw grinded beef meat with spices and yoghurt. (c) Partially roasted beef meat for consumption.

high government officials [50]. Practising these dietary choices frequently result in overweight, obesity, high blood pressure, kidney disease, and premature ageing [51, 52]. Additionally, food cooking oil known as "Hayat" and "Palm oil" which is in use amongst the majority of the Ethiopian is full of high cholesterol, and this can easily harm the health of the users [1].

Another unhealthy dietary practice frequently practised amongst low-resourced populations, particularly in East Africa such as Ethiopia, Eritrean, Djibouti, Somalia, Kenya, Tanzania, and Sudan and Arab countries such as Saudi Arabia, United Arab Emirates, Yemen, Bahrain, Kuwait, and Oman, is "Khat chewing". Khat is a leafy plant with natural amphetamine content and chewed by 20 million people each day in Arabian peninsula and East African region mainly in Ethiopia (**Figure 4**) [53]. Khat chewing has incredible stimulation effects on chewers nervous system and predominantly addictive. The practice of Khat chewing is frequent amongst university students, shop keepers, drivers, and majority of the Muslim community, teachers, and some government officials [54]. Evidence shows that Khat chewing is associated with escalated degrees of cardiovascular complications, stroke, myocardial infections, cardiomyopathy, gastritis, poor oral hygiene, neurosis, poor academic performance, periodontal disease, and decreased quality of life [55, 56].

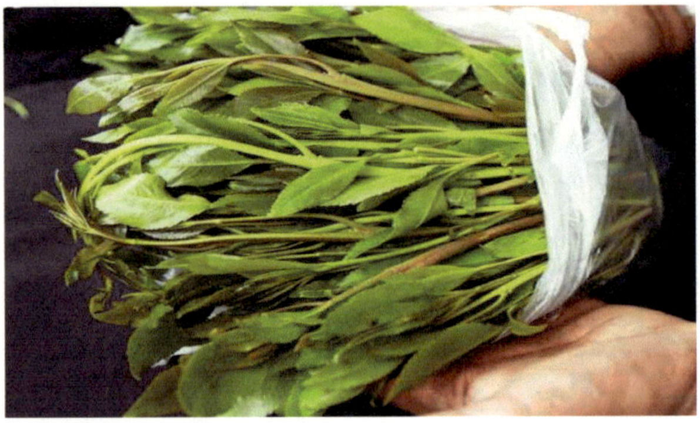

Figure 4.
Chewable leaves of Chat plant.

Khat dependence is associated with wasting of longer working hours and family time. Evidence in Yemen and Saudi Arabia shows that lousy mood, psychosomatic dependence, sleeplessness, and physical indicators were observed amongst Khat chewers, and they spend an aggregate of 6 hours a day and 5.7 days a week for Khat use [57, 58]. Similarly, Khat chewing is associated with diminished antioxidants of saliva Khat chewers [59]. Moreover, Khat chewing is associated with the development of type 2 diabetes. Evidence in Saudi Arabia indicates that Khat chewing increases the likelihoods of developing type 2 diabetic disease four times than non-chewers [60]. Evidence in East African countries such as Ethiopia, Kenya, Eretria, Somalia, Sudan, Rwanda, and Uganda indicates that Khat chewing is associated with the development of high blood pressure, type 2 diabetes, heart failure, mental health problems, group segregation, family cessation, and abandonment of public accountabilities [61, 62].

2.3 Organised infrastructure

Within the healthcare framework, the availability of interrelated material and infrastructure are other determinants of healthcare. For NCDs, neighbourhood environments broadly define the conditions in which people live and have a significant influence on the risk of NCDs [40, 63]. A randomised control study in which mothers and families were given the opportunity to move from a neighbourhood with a high level of poverty to one with a lower level found that moving to a better-off neighbourhood was associated with a reduction in NCDs. Multiple mechanisms have been proposed whereby the neighbourhood environment affects the risk of NCDs, including interrelated material mechanisms [64]. These material mechanisms include the nature of the built environment, such as proximity to food outlets selling processed foods, as well as psychosocial mechanisms, such as conforming to social norms of behaviour. Also, children living in unfavourable social conditions, unsafe surroundings, poor housing, and no access to sidewalks, parks, and recreation centres were 20–60% more likely to be overweight or obese compared with children not facing such conditions [2, 39, 64].

2.4 Urbanisation and urban development policy

Urbanisation is associated with an increased prevalence of NCD risk behaviours, which are increasing at a rapid rate. More than half of the global population lived in cities in 2010, a proportion expected to reach 60% in 2030 and 70% in 2050. In countries where rural-to-urban migration is commonplace, urban life may be less conducive to physical exercise than life in rural areas. As countries develop, the sprawling nature of urban expansion and increased disposable income encourages mechanised transport and discourages walking and cycling. The nature of work available in urban areas may require less energy expenditure than subsistence farming in rural areas [63, 64].

A study of physical activity concerning hypertension, obesity, and diabetes found that it was lower amongst rural than urban dwellers. The prevalence of obesity, diabetes, and hypertension was higher amongst the urban population, and physical inactivity amongst urban groups was associated with a higher BMI, blood pressure, and fasting blood glucose levels. NCD prevention and control may require that cities adopt models of urbanisation that address the health impacts and inequities associated with city living [65–67].

2.5 Cultural norms

Evidence indicated that beliefs and norms amongst some social groups might include preferences for foods high in animal fat, which is socially acceptable or perceived as a sign of good health but result in overweight, obesity, hypertension, and health problems. Ethnographic studies found that amongst blacks in South Africa, Arabs in Niger, groups in rural Jamaica, Puerto Ricans in Philadelphia, and members of a Fijian village, a big body size and fatness reflect wealth and prosperity, beauty, marriageability, attractiveness, fertility, and "closeness to God", as is the case of Habesha in Ethiopia [1, 48, 68]. In contrast, much of the industrial West associate fatness with ugliness, undesirability, and lack of self-control, whilst associating slimness with health, beauty, intelligence, wealth, self-discipline, and "goodness". There is some evidence that the Western slim-body ideal is becoming globalised, with thinness now being desired in many places where fatness was previously preferred. Moreover, the beliefs amongst those who idealise fatness may change when the associated health risks are explained [69].

2.6 Accessibility of health information

Health information is a tool that provides data to the healthcare system, which can be used to enhance, promote, improve, and create awareness about the health of a community. It is evidenced that health information systems are an essential tool for collecting data about the health conditions and indicators of a country to help with decision-making. It is documented that reliable health data that is collected, analysed, and interpreted can assist policymakers, health organisations, the healthcare system, and healthcare providers in formulating appropriate disease preventive strategies. It has also been demonstrated that health data can be made available to the public through various health information channels, such as healthcare providers, counselling, teaching, and advice; mass media, such as radio television, internet, social media; and telecommunication, such as mobile short message service (SMS) [4, 70].

Despite the wide-ranging health benefits of health information, the attention given to addressing NCDs-related risk factors, morbidity, mortality, the health burden, and preventive mechanisms using the various sources of health information is inadequate in low-resourced countries. Similarly, the attention devoted to the accessibility of health information coverage is deficient in the healthcare system of developing countries [4].

3. The global status and availability of NCDs data

The incidence of non-communicable diseases (NCDs) is increasing and resulted in the death of 38 million people in 2012, of which 28 million occurred in low- and middle-income countries, causing an estimated US$ 7 trillion economic loss [7, 9]. A significant number of NCDs, such as cardiovascular disease, diabetes, hypertension, and obesity, can be avoided by addressing the major behavioural and metabolic risk factors associated with such conditions. Their prevention and treatment require reliable, accurate, and timeous information on their symptoms and associated risk factors. The use of credible data has, therefore, become essential to identify current and potential NCDs morbidity, mortality, and related risk factors [4].

The availability of NCDs data at local, regional, and national levels is helpful for decision-makers to prioritise the prevention of NCDs and strengthen distribution and budget allocation in the healthcare system. It is demonstrated that strengthening the health system is a possible way to resist the growing burden of NCDs and ensure enhanced health results. An effective health system is built on a well-functioning information system that collects accurate, reliable, timeous, and relevant health data for optimal healthcare delivery and decision-making. The lack of data in the healthcare system is a hindrance to planning, allocating resources, and implementing appropriate NCDs intervention strategies [4, 71]. The effective prevention of NCDs is based on having consistent morbidity, mortality, and related risk factors data to plan, design, and implement evidence-based decision-making and its preventive strategies at regional and national levels. NCDs surveillance data can be best collected by establishing and implementing data collection standardised protocols in the healthcare system. Such standardised protocols are data collection forms used to obtain morbidity, mortality, and risk factor-related data [4, 72]. A study by Melkamu and Grace [4] indicated that collecting NCDs data alone is not enough to ensure effective prevention and intervention; what is needed is a well-organised healthcare system that periodically evaluates the data quality and is timeous and accurate on mortality, morbidity, and related NCDs risk factors to ensure effective decision-making. Whilst progress has been made to lead the development of national NCDs monitoring programmes, most low-resourced countries are still struggling to adequately establish robust information systems to help with their intervention, treatment, and related NCDs risk factors [4].

Health information systems store information that is obtained from patient records, surveys, health plans, and other data sources. Most first world and high-resourced countries, such as North America, Australia and Europe, have established standards and processes in their healthcare sector to obtain ongoing information on morbidity, mortality, NCDs risk factors, as well as determinants of their care services [73]. Middle-income countries, such as South Africa, and low-resourced countries, such as Ghana, Mozambique, Rwanda, Tanzania, and Zambia, conducted studies to investigate the capacity of their national health information systems, which resulted in them developing robust disease surveillance systems to understand the disease profiles of their population. The availability of health information in the healthcare system enabled these countries to exchange health-related data between healthcare providers, organisations, and health service consuming communities.

According to Diamantidis and Becker [74], the availability of NCDs-related public health data in the healthcare system enables timeous and appropriate healthcare decisions to be made, quick information retrieval, fast information sharing, improved data storage, improved information screening and reporting, all of which enhances the quality of healthcare. Furthermore, having NCDs mortality, morbidity, and risk factor data about a population can help policymakers and healthcare providers to establish relevant preventive strategies in their national healthcare system. In a healthcare system with accessible, accurate, reliable, timeous, and cleaned health information, it is possible to predict the future burden of NCDs in that country [4, 75]. Globally, various countries have established healthcare strategic plans in order to address the burden of NCDs by explicitly focusing on the four major lifestyle risk factors, these being an unhealthy diet, physical inactivity, tobacco use, and excessive alcohol consumption [76].

Low-resourced countries have made a concerted effort to improve the health status of its citizens, particularly regarding preventing and treating infectious communicable diseases, such as HIV/AIDS and tuberculosis [77]. However, little attention is devoted to preventing and treating NCDs in these countries, which resulted in an increased burden of such conditions on individuals, communities, and the healthcare system [4]. Despite the growing evidence of NCDs in this population, the operating healthcare system predominantly focuses on preventing and treating infectious communicable disease, with little evidence-based research that evaluates the availability of their morbidity, mortality, and associated risk factors data [78]. In low-resourced countries, the healthcare system must aim to establish the status of NCDs-related data, the presence of mechanisms to periodically evaluate NCDs data quality, reliability and timeliness, and the availability of standardised protocols for NCDs-related data collection.

Healthcare that has accurate data that serves as information for decision-making is imperative within the hastened speed of information-oriented universal environment. In the changing world, the desire of the community to obtain up-to-date health-related information has become crucial in both high-resourced and low-resourced countries. The accessibility of appropriate health-related information is associated with the availability of factual, accurate, timeous, and reliable data associated with NCDs [4].

4. Strategies to prevent the growing burden of NCDs

4.1 The system approach

The system approach (SA) was primarily established by Urie Bronfenbrenner in Russia as a human developmental approach in the 1970s. This approach explicates how diverse systems of the community impact the development of an individual. The approach involves the word "system" which refers to the relations of organisms within their setting. Moreover, from the sociological point of view, the system describes the way humans and the public interact with their natural and artificial atmosphere [79]. The term "approach" incorporates the way people are in constant relation with each other and the setting in which they live [80]. However, these chains could either have an encouraging or discouraging effect on an individual. The system approach is applied in social work as a meta-paradigm which is regularly referred to as "a person in the neighbourhoods". This meta-paradigm explains the way a person and different multifaceted settings interact and impact each other [81, 82]. The primary emphasis of the SA is that people are part of and continuously interact with other organisms in the setting. The system approach has been applied in healthcare to establish intercessions targeted at shifting the intrapersonal, interpersonal, organisational, community, and health policies levels [82].

The system approach has four stages or levels of impact known as M4, namely a micro-system, meso-system, macro-system, and mega-system [83]. The micro-system is the stage where the individual belongs, and it includes the impact relating to the person, which can come from the individuals' family, peer groups, and the neighbourhood collectively stated as social agents. Social agents interrelate directly with an individual and affect a persons' health behaviour either positively or negatively. For example, using networked communication such as sneezes, it will be easier for individuals to inform their families and friends about risk factors associated with NCDs and possible prevention mechanisms through verbal expression. Sneezes are imperative in NCDs prevention, and healthcare leading organisations need to ascertain who they are and give them incentives and motivations to blowout the conversation of the mouse. The meso-system is the level where the social representatives will be operating, and it is interrelated to the micro-system where the family experiences are associated to the peers' experiences and the peers' experiences to the neighbourhood experiences—for example, by using schmoozed messages such as hive, a community who has a common culture, religion, custom, rules, beliefs, and traditions can increase the spread information related to NCDs and its associated risk factors, so that awareness can be easily created [83, 84]. The macro-system is the stage where organisations are involved and demonstrate an individual's activities within it. An organisation can affect an individual's life by encouragement or discouragement and vice-versa. For example, by using diversified mediums and amplifiers such as posters, images, slogans or phrases, school mini-media, television and radio broadcasts, short message services (SMS), webpages, and the internet as a means of transmitting information related to NCDs can increase the strength of information as it gets passed across a broad audience. The mega-system level illustrates the state that reflects the culture in which individuals live. Also, the mega-system level incorporates advancement, industrialisation, urbanisation, socio-economic status, poverty, religion, and ethnicity. For example, by applying velocity and smoothness through high government officials involvement, NCDs-related messages can swiftly and efficiently reach a higher number of the public who can be reminded to abstain from behavioural practices that lead to NCDs. Likewise, working with multi sectors such as governmental and non-governmental organisations, developmental partners, religious institutions, and urban planners to increase access and availability to parks, public open spaces, and recreational facilities can lead to effective transfer of information related to NCDs to a large number of the community and its prevention [82–84].

4.2 The view of the systems approach

The system approach, as illustrated in **Figure 5,** is constructed on a supposition that when an individual, community, healthcare organisations, and the

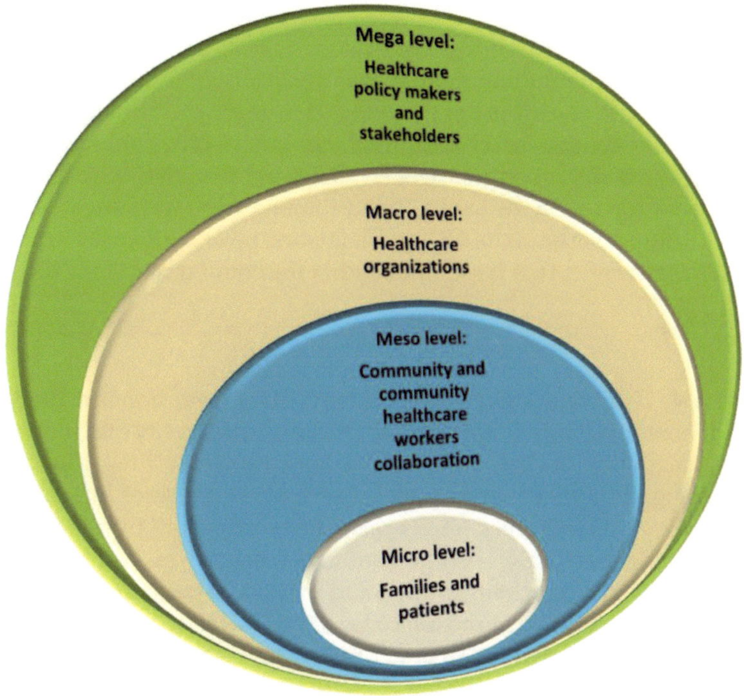

Figure 5.
Systems approach for NCDs prevention.

leading government authority are linked and operating together in a setting of a supportive system, the efficiency of preventing and controlling NCDs also increases.

4.2.1 Mega level

The mega-system level help to review and understand the existing NCDs prevention strategy, the practice of health information, the availability and status of data related to NCDs morbidity, mortality, and risk factors for decision-making at a national level. This level of the ecological system theory focuses on the status and availability of data related to NCDs at national level, so that plenty of information can be utilised in the healthcare system for effective decision-making for the prevention of NCDs. Availability of quality and timeous NCDs data and evaluating its status periodically help policymakers to redesign and strengthen the existing healthcare system to revert the growing burden of NCDs at national and international level [1, 4].

4.2.2 Macro level

The macro-level of the system approach explores and recognises strategies used by healthcare organisations such as health facilities, clinics, and hospital to prevent NCDs. The system approach at the macro level emphasises health professionals' perceptions of NCDs risk factors and how healthcare professionals use appropriate preventative strategies to prevent NCDs risk factors at the various healthcare organisations. Exploring the perceptions of healthcare professionals can help to understand the magnitude of the disease burden and help healthcare organisations to establish and implement local specific NCDs prevention strategies [1, 4].

4.2.3 Meso level

At the meso level, the community, community health counsellors, and stakeholders operate together to contribute to the prevention of NCDs. The emphasise of the meso level of the system approach is on creating awareness by community healthcare workers and community representatives on NCDs and related risk factors for the public in collaboration with the media. Telecommunication work together with the community to offer awareness on NCDs risk factors; promote a healthy diet and physical exercise benefits that is required within the community [1, 4, 40].

4.2.4 Micro level

The micro-healthcare system level is where NCDs prevention is managed and addressed at home and individual level. At this level, the family and the patients take full responsibility for their illness and self-manage their illness and diseases at home by using the advice they acquire from various sources of information and healthcare workers. At this level, NCDs-related education and preventative mechanisms can be thought at family level by family representatives, and home visiting healthcare professionals can help families and individual patients to practise self-management at their homes. At the micro level, NCDs-related data of the family in addition to detecting the challenges to self-management at this level, solutions to overcome the problem can be recorded [1, 4, 40].

5. Conclusion

The global burden of NCDs is increasing with devastating health consequences mounting swiftly in low- and middle-income countries (LMIC). The response and strategies used to prevent NCDs are inadequate in low-resourced countries due to the unavailability of timeous quality data at various stages of healthcare institutions. Data associated with the prevalence, morbidity, mortality, and risk factors of NCDs are required for evidence-based decision-making to ensure effective management of NCDs. Moreover, multi-sectoral response is required in low-resourced countries to urgently implement a systems approach at micro, meso, macro, and mega-level to prevent and control NCDs and its associated risk factors.

Acknowledgements

I wish to express my thanks to my family for their unconditional and unreservedly support and encouragement.

Conflict of interest

The authors declare no conflict of interest.

Author details

Melkamu Kassa* and Jeanne Grace
Discipline of Biokinetics, Exercise and Leisure Sciences, University of KwaZulu-Natal, Durban, South Africa

*Address all correspondence to: kassam@ukzn.ac.za

References

[1] Kassa MD, Grace J. Healthcare professionals' perceptions of non-communicable diseases risk factors and its regional distribution in Ethiopia. Global Journal of Health Science. 2018;**10**(1):88-97

[2] Juma K, Juma PA, Mohamed SF, Owuor J, Wanyoike A, Mulabi D, et al. First Africa non-communicable disease research conference 2017: Sharing evidence and identifying research priorities; on behalf of participants for the first Africa NCD research conference 2017 in Nairobi, Kenya. Journal of Global Health. 2019;**9**(1):1-13

[3] Justine F, Davies I, Wagner RG. Weighing up the costs of treating 'lifestyle' diseases in South Africa. University of the Witwatersrand. 2019;**24**(3):1-13

[4] Melkamu Dugassa Kassa JMG. A mixed-method study of quality, availability and timeliness of non-communicable disease (NCD) related data and its link to NCD prevention: Perceptions of health care workers in Ethiopia. Health Information Management Journal. 2018;**47**(4): 21-34

[5] Anwar MS, Id AGJ, Id NLM. Heart failure and healthcare informatics. PLoS Medicine. 2019;**16**(5):4-7

[6] WHO. WHO Methods and Data Sources for Country-Level Causes of Death 2000-2016. Vol. WHO/HIS/IE, Global Health Estimates; 2018

[7] WHO. Noncommunicable Diseases Progress Monitor. Vol. 46, World Health Organization. Geneva; 2017

[8] WHO. Noncommunicable Diseases Country Profiles; 2018

[9] WHO. Global Status Report on Noncommunicable Diseases. World Health Organization. Geneva 27, Switzerland; 2014

[10] WHO. Noncommunicable Diseases Progress Monitor. Geneva 27, Switzerland; 2015

[11] WHO. Global Status Report on Noncommunicable Diseases: "Attaining the Nine Global Noncommunicable Disease Targets; A Shared Responsibility." World Health Organization. 1211 Geneva 27, Switzerland; 2014

[12] WHO. Noncommunicable Diseases Key Facts: Who is at Risk of Such Diseases? Modifiable Behavioural Risk Factors; 2018

[13] Joshi R, Alim M, Kengne AP, Jan S, Maulik PK, Peiris D, et al. Task shifting for non-communicable disease management in low and middle income countries – A systematic review. PLoS One. 2014;**9**(8):1-9

[14] World Health Organization. Non-communicable Diseases Country Profiles. World Health Organization; 2014

[15] Siddharthan BT, Ramaiya K, Yonga G, Mutungi GN, Rabin TL, List JM, et al. Noncommunicable diseases in East Africa: Assessing the gaps in care and identifying opportunities for improvement. Health Affairs. 2015;**34**(9):1-8

[16] Barquera S, Pedroza-tobias A, Medina C. Cardiovascular diseases in mega-countries: The challenges of the nutrition, physical activity and epidemiologic transitions, and the double burden of disease. Current Opinion in Lipidology. 2016;**27**(10):329-344

[17] Allotey P, Davey T, Reidpath DD. NCDs in low and middle-income countries - assessing the capacity of health systems to respond to

population needs. MBC Public Health. 2014;**14**(Suppl. 2):2-4

[18] Peer N. The converging burdens of infectious and non-communicable diseases in rural-to-urban migrant Sub-Saharan African populations: A focus on HIV / AIDS, tuberculosis and cardio-metabolic diseases. Tropical Diseases, Travel Medicine and Vaccines [Internet]. 2015;**1**(6):1-8. DOI: 10.1186/s40794-015-0007-4

[19] Manuscript A, Countries I. Growing epidemic of coronary heart disease in low- and middle- income countries. NIH Public Access. 2011;**35**(2):1-34

[20] Nulu A, Wilbert S, William H. Hypertension in sub-Saharan Africa. Cardiology in Review. 2016;**24**(1):30-40

[21] Mills KT, Bundy JD, Kelly TN, Reed JE, Kearney PM, Reynolds K. Global disparities of hypertension prevalence and control. Circulation. 2016;**134**(August 9):441-450

[22] Cho NH, Shaw JE, Karuranga S, Huang Y, Rocha JD, Ohlrogge AW, et al. IDF diabetes Atlas: Global estimates of diabetes prevalence for 2017 and projections for 2045. Diabetes Research and Clinical Practice [Internet]. 2018;**138**(2018):271-281. DOI: 10.1016/j.diabres.2018.02.023

[23] Practice C. IDF diabetes Atlas estimates of 2014 global health expenditures on diabetes. Diabetes Research and Clinical Practice. 2016;**117**(July):48-54

[24] Ellulu M, Abed Y, Rahmat A, Ranneh Y, Ali F. Epidemiology of obesity in developing countries: Challenges and prevention. Global Epidemic Obesity. 2014;**43**(1):1-6

[25] Ford ND, Patel SA, Narayan KMV. Obesity in low- and middle-income countries: Burden, drivers, and emerging challenges. Annual Review of Public Health. 2016;**38**(10):145-165

[26] Agyemang C, Boatemaa S, Agyemang G. Obesity in sub-Saharan Africa. Metabolic Syndrome. 2016;**10**(5):41-53

[27] WHO. Second Joint Mission of the United Nations Interagency Task Force on the Prevention and Control of Noncommunicable Diseases Sri Lanka; 2018

[28] WHO. Time to Deliver: Third UN High-level Meeting on Non-communicable Diseases. World Health Organization; 2018

[29] WHO. Global Action Plan for the Prevention and Control of Noncommunicable Diseases 2013-2020; 2013

[30] Target G, Facts F. Global NCD Target Reduce Premature. World Heal Organ. 2018;138(WHO/NMH/NMA/16.189):1-2

[31] Wickramasinghe K, Wilkins E, Foster C, Fadhil I, Hammerich A, Slama S, et al. The development of national multisectoral action plans for the prevention and control of noncommunicable diseases: Experiences of national-level stakeholders in four countries. Global Health Action [Internet]. 2018;**11**(1):1-9. DOI: 10.1080/16549716.2018.1532632

[32] Pearce N, Ebrahim S, Mckee M, Lamptey P, Barreto ML, Matheson D, et al. Global prevention and control of NCDs: Limitations of the standard approach. Journal of Public Health Policy. 2015;**36**(4):408-425

[33] Palma AM, Rabkin M, Nuwagaba-biribonwoha H, Bongomin P, Lukhele N, Dlamini X, et al. Can the success of HIV scale-up advance the global chronic NCD agenda? Global Heart [Internet].

2016;**11**(4):403-408. DOI: 10.1016/j.gheart.2016.10.012

[34] Collins T, Mikkelsen B, Adams J, Chestnov O, Evans T, Feigl A. Addressing NCDs: A unifying agenda for sustainable development. International Journal for Research, Policy and Practice. 2017;**13**(9):1157

[35] Nyaaba GN, Stronks K, Aikins A, Kengne AP, Agyemang C. Tracing Africa's progress towards implementing the non-communicable diseases global action plan 2013-2020: A synthesis of WHO country profile reports. MBC Public Health. 2017;**17**(297):1-13

[36] WHO. Report of the WHO Independent High-Level Commission on Noncommunicable Diseases; 2018

[37] Naik R, Kaneda T. Noncommunicable diseases in Africa: Youth are key to curbing the epidemic and achieving sustainable development. Policy Brief Population Reference Bureau. 2015;**2014**(April):1-12

[38] Alvarado M, Murphy MM, Guell C. Barriers and facilitators to physical activity amongst overweight and obese women in an afro-Caribbean population: A qualitative study. International Journal of Behavioral Nutrition and Physical Activity [Internet]. 2015;**12**(79):1-12. DOI: 10.1186/s12966-015-0258-5

[39] Kassa MD, Grace J. Barriers to integrate physical exercise into the Ethiopian healthcare system to treat non-communicable diseases. Global Journal of Health Science. 2018;**10**(10):123-135

[40] Lear SA, Hu W, Rangarajan S, Gasevic D, Leong D, Iqbal R, et al. The effect of physical activity on mortality and cardiovascular disease in 130 000 people low-income countries: The PURE study. Lancet. 2017;**390**(10113):2643-2654

[41] Piercy KL, Troiano RP, Ballard RM, Carlson SA, Fulton JE, Galuska DA, et al. The physical activity guidelines for Americans. Special Communication. 2018;**320**(19):2020-2028

[42] Arem H, Moore SC, Patel A, Hartge P, Gonzalez AB De, Visvanathan K, et al. Leisure time physical activity and mortality a detailed pooled analysis of the dose-response relationship. Journal of the American Medical Association 2015;**175**(6):959-967

[43] Cm NC, Sauvé M, Facp F. Reducing deaths by diet: A call for public policy to prevent chronic disease. Canadian Journal of General Internal Medicine. 2016;**11**(1):7-9

[44] Itoh H, Kanayama N. Nutritional conditions in early life and risk of non-communicable diseases (NCDs) from the perspective of preemptive medicine in perinatal care. Hypertension Research in Pregnancy. 2015;**3**(1):1-12

[45] Oggioni C, Cena H, Wells JCK, Lara J, Celis-Morales C, Siervo M. Association between worldwide dietary and lifestyle patterns with total cholesterol concentrations and DALYs for infectious and cardiovascular diseases: An ecological analysis. Journal of Epidemiology and Global Health [Internet]. 2015;**5**(4):315-325. DOI: 10.1016/j.jegh.2015.02.002

[46] Misra A, Tandon N, Ebrahim S, Sattar N, Alam D, Shrivastava U, et al. Diabetes, cardiovascular disease, and chronic kidney disease in South Asia: Current status and future directions. BMJ. 2017;**357**(j1420):1-4

[47] Alisson-silva F, Kawanishi K, Varki A, Jolla L. Human risk of diseases associated with red meat intake: Analysis of current theories and proposed role for metabolic incorporation of a non-human Sialic acid. HHS Public Access. 2017;**15**(858):16-30

[48] Gorski I, Chung W, Herr K, Mehta K. Nyama Choma culture: Implications of increased red meat and alcohol consumption in East Africa Nyama Choma culture: Implications of increased red meat and alcohol consumption in East Africa. Journal of Sustainable Development. 2016;**9**(6):96-102

[49] Aurino E, Fernandes M, Penny ME. The nutrition transition and adolescents ' diets in low- and middle-income countries: A cross-cohort comparison. Public Health Nutrition. 2016;**20**(1):72-81

[50] Lijalem T, Beyan M, Banerjee S. Meat consumption patterns in Hawassa City, Southern Ethiopia. American Scientific Research Journal for Engineering, Technology, and Sciences. 2013;**3**(1):56-65

[51] Machovina B, Feeley KJ, Ripple WJ. Science of the Total environment biodiversity conservation: The key is reducing meat consumption. Science of the Total Environment [Internet]. 2015;**536**(2015):419-431. DOI: 10.1016/j.scitotenv.2015.07.022

[52] Domingo L, Nadal M. Carcinogenicity of consumption of red meat and processed meat: A review of scienti fic news since the IARC decision. Food and Chemical Toxicology. 2017;**114**(2017):256-261

[53] Astatkie A, Demissie M, Berhane Y, Worku A. Prevalence of and factors associated with regular khat chewing among university students in Ethiopia. Substance Abuse and Rehabilitation. 2015;**6**:41-50

[54] Teklie H, Gonfa G, Getachew T, Defar A, Bekele A, Bekele A. Prevalence of Khat chewing and associated factors in Ethiopia: Findings from the 2015 national non- communicable diseases STEPS survey. The Ethiopian Journal of Health Development. 2017;**31**(Special Issue):321-329

[55] Alemu WG, Zeleke TA, Takele WW. Prevalence and associated factors of khat chewing among students in Ethiopia: A protocol for systematic review and meta-analysis. MBJ. 2018;**8**(e021157):13-16

[56] Ayano G, Yohannis K, Abraha M. Epidemiology of khat (*Catha edulis*) consumption among university students: A. MBC Public Health. 2019;**19**(150):1-13

[57] Nakajima M, Hoffman R. Level of khat dependence, use patterns, and psychosocial correlates in Yemen: A cross-sectional investigation. Eastern Mediterranean Health Journal. 2017;**23**(3):161-167

[58] El-setouhy M, Alsanosy RM, Alsharqi A, Ismail AA. Khat dependency and psychophysical symptoms among chewers in Jazan region, Kingdom of Saudi Arabia. BioMed Research International. 2016;**2016**(4):1-7

[59] Masoud A, Al-qaisy A, Al-faqeeh A, Al-makhadri A, Al-awsh D, Al-madhagi H, et al. Decreased antioxidants in the saliva of Khat chewers. Saudi Journal of Oral and Dental Research [Internet]. 2016;**7**(1):18-23. DOI: 10.1016/j.sjdr.2015.02.004

[60] Al-hadrani AM, Hummadi A, Al-hoot MA. An association between chronic Khat chewing and the development of type 2 diabetes. Life Science Journal. 2018;**15**(1):56-59

[61] Omar YS, Jenkins A, Altena MVR, Tuck H, Hynan C, Tohow A, et al. Khat use: What is the problem and what can Be done? BioMed Research International. 2015;**2015**(2015):1-8

[62] El-menyar A, Mekkodathil A, Al-thani H. Khat use: History and

heart failure. Oman Medical Journal. 2015;**30**(2):77-82

[63] Cerin E, Sit CHP, Zhang CJP, Barnett A, Cheung MMC, Lai PC, et al. Neighbourhood environment, physical activity, quality of life and depressive symptoms in Hong Kong older adults: A protocol for an observational study. BMJ Open. 2016;**6**(1):1-19

[64] Kelly S, Martin S, Kuhn I, Cowan A, Brayne C, Lafortune L. Barriers and facilitators to the uptake and maintenance of healthy behaviours by people at mid-life: A rapid systematic review. PLoS One. 2016;**11**(1):1-26

[65] Pereiro AC, Gold S. Building an innovative Chagas disease program for primary care units, in an urban non- endemic city. MBC Public Health. 2019;**19**(904):1-9

[66] Oyebode O, Pape UJ, Laverty AA, Lee JT, Bhan N, Millett C. Rural, urban and migrant differences in non-communicable disease risk-factors in middle income countries:A cross-sectional study of WHO-SAGE data. PLoS One. 2015;**10**(4):1-14

[67] Angkurawaranon C, Jiraporncharoen W, Chenthanakij B, Doyle P, Nitsch D. Urbanization and non-communicable disease in Southeast Asia: A review of current evidence. Public Health [Internet]. 2014;**128**(10):886-895. DOI: 10.1016/j.puhe.2014.08.003

[68] Angkurawaranon C, Lerssrimonkol C, Jakkaew N, Philalai T, Doyle P, Nitsch D. Living in an urban environment and non-communicable disease risk in Thailand: Does timing matter? Health & Place [Internet]. 2015;**33**(5):37-47. DOI: 10.1016/j.healthplace.2015.02.005

[69] Ajayi IO, Adebamowo C, Adami H, Dalal S, Diamond MB, Bajunirwe F, et al. Urban – Rural and geographic differences in overweight and obesity in four sub-Saharan African adult populations: A multi-country cross-sectional study. BMC Public Health [Internet]. 2016;**166**(1126):1-13. DOI: 10.1186/s12889-016-3789-z

[70] Gitau TM, Micklesfield LK, Pettifor JM, Norris SA. Ethnic differences in eating attitudes, body image and self-esteem among adolescent females living in urban South Africa. Journal of Psychiatry. 2014;**17**(January):468-474

[71] Oung MT, Richter K, Prasartkul P, Aung Y, Soe KT, Tin TC. Reliable mortality statistics in Myanmar: A qualitative assessment of challenges in two townships. MBC Public Health. 2019;**19**(356):1-10

[72] Cresswell KM, Sheikh A. Health information technology in hospitals: Current issues and future trends. Future Hospital Journal. 2015;**2**(1):50-56

[73] Aziz HA. A review of the role of public health informatics in healthcare. Journal of Taibah University Medical Sciences [Internet]. 2017;**12**(1):78-81. DOI: 10.1016/j.jtumed.2016.08.011

[74] Taylor SL. Harnessing data science through healthcare IT interoperability. Online Journal of Public Health Informatics. 2019;**11**(1):3-4

[75] Diamantidis CJ, Becker S. Health information technology (IT) to improve the care of patients with chronic kidney disease (CKD). BMC Nephrology. 2014;**15**(7):1-6

[76] Tsolekile LP, Puoane T, Schneider H, Levitt NS, Steyn K, Africa S, et al. The roles of community health workers in management of non-communicable diseases in an urban township. African Journal of Primary Health Care & Family Medicine. 2014;**6**(1):1-8

[77] Letebo M, Shiferaw F. Adapting HIV patient and program monitoring

tools for chronic non-communicable diseases in Ethiopia. Globalization and Health. 2016;**12**(26):1-8

[78] Eyler AA, Valko C, Ramadas R, Macchi M, Fershteyn Z, Brownson RC. Administrative evidence-based practices in state chronic disease practitioners. American Journal of Preventive Medicine [Internet]. 2018;**54**(2):275-283. DOI: 10.1016/j.amepre.2017.09.006

[79] Scholarship O. Systems thinking as a framework for analyzing commercial determinants of health. The Milbank Quarterly. 2018;**96**(3):472-498

[80] Joly M, Rond HC, Sp P. The future of computational biomedicine : Complex systems thinking. Mathematics and Computers in Simulation . Elsevier. 2017;**132**:1-27

[81] Littlejohns LB, Wilson A. Strengthening complex systems for chronic disease prevention: A systematic review. BMC Public Health. 2019;**9**(729):1-13

[82] Wutzke S, Roberts N, Willis C, Best A, Wilson A, Trochim W. Setting strategy for system change: Using concept mapping to prioritise national action for chronic disease prevention. Health Research Policy and Systems. 2017;**15**(69):1-13

[83] Vogt H. The new holism: P4 systems medicine and the medicalization of health and life itself. Medicine, Health Care and Philosophy. 2016;**19**(2):307-323

[84] Sharma SR, Matheson A. Systems thinking in 21st century: A call to health promoters. Journal of Public Health. 2016;**15**(2):24-25

Chapter 3

Non-Communicable Diseases and Urbanization in African Cities: A Narrative Review

Kenneth Juma, Pamela A. Juma, Constance Shumba, Peter Otieno and Gershim Asiki

Abstract

Rapid urbanization in Africa has been linked to the growing burden of non-communicable diseases (NCDs). Urbanization processes have amplified lifestyle risk factors for NCDs (including unhealthy diets, tobacco use, harmful alcohol intake, and physical inactivity), especially among individuals of low and middle social economic status. Nevertheless, African countries are not keeping pace with the ever increasing need for population-level interventions such as health promotion through education, screening, diagnosis, and treatment, as well as structural measures such as policies and legislation to prevent and control the upstream factors driving the NCD epidemic. This chapter highlights the NCD burden in urban Africa, along with the social determinants and existing interventions against NCDs. The chapter concludes by offering insights into policy and legislative opportunities and recommends stronger efforts to apply multisectoral and intersectoral approaches in policy formulation, implementation, and monitoring at multiple levels to address the NCD epidemic in African cities.

Keywords: NCDs, risk factors, urbanization, African cities, Africa

1. Introduction

Over the last few decades, the proportion of the world's population living in urban areas has grown to 55%, and is expected to increase to 68% by 2050 [1]. Africa's urban growth is unfolding more rapidly than anywhere in the world, with the share of urban dwellers projected to exceed 50% by 2035 [1]. However this growth has been characterized as "rapid, unplanned and unmanaged" because 62% of the urban population in Africa lives in informal settlements characterized by conditions of squalor, overcrowding, and small make-shift structures mostly made of sub-standard housing materials such as mud and scraps of wood or corrugated metal [2]. Unplanned settlement in cities is associated with increased inequality, urban poverty, social deprivation and lifestyle changes that could lead to an increased burden of non-communicable diseases (NCDs) [3]. Thus, changes in physical and social environment in the urban space favor the adoption of behaviors that promote unhealthy lifestyles such as physical inactivity, unhealthy diets, tobacco consumption and harmful alcohol consumption that predispose individuals living in the slums to NCDs [4, 5]. Even so, there is generally lack of consensus as to whether there exists any NCDs health advantages in urban area.

NCDs represent a leading threat to human health and development [6]. In 2015 alone, four major NCDs-cardiovascular diseases (CVDs), cancers, diabetes, and chronic respiratory diseases accounted for 72% of all deaths globally; 85% of these were from low and middle income countries (LMICs) [7]. In urban areas of SSA, NCDs are rising faster than anywhere else in the world [8]. The economic consequences of NCDs are enormous across the globe, and are felt at the individual, household, community and health systems levels. Bloom et al. (2011) [9], estimated that economic losses due to NCDs could amount to approximately 75% of the global GDP. While there is wider recognition of the increasing burden of NCDs across Africa [5], scanty literature exists on the link between urban environments and NCD risks in Africa, as well as the associated health and social consequences, and access to health services. Considering that future population growth will take place predominantly in African cities, there is need for a deeper understanding of urban health and the context of NCDs in African cities to identify tailored interventions to curb the epidemic. Urbanization in sub-Saharan Africa provides a unique opportunity to explore the mechanisms by which urban environment influences NCD epidemiology.

This chapter describes both the health determinants and outcomes in African cities with special attention to low-income urban areas. It further highlights the burden, impact and possible interventions for NCDs in African cities. The chapter draws on insights from relevant peer-reviewed and gray literature on NCDs, and the authors' own experiences on the subject in Africa.

2. Increasing urbanization and health consequences in Africa

While the African continent remains largely rural, it is one of the fastest urbanizing regions in the world [1]. Africa's transition into the 'urban age' is seen in the prolific growth of megacities as well as smaller towns [10]. The urban population increased from 14 to 32% between 1950 and 1990 and is projected to rise to 54.1% by the year 2025 [11]. In absolute terms, the urban population will rise from 395 million in 2010 to 1.339 billion in 2050 [12]. Currently, the continent has seven megacities (cities with populations over 10 million): Cairo, Kinshasa, Lagos, Accra, Johannesburg, –Pretoria and Khartoum with cities such as Lagos having an average annual growth rate of 5.8% (**Table 1**).

Other big cities expected to join the megacity list include Nairobi, Luanda, Dar es Salaam and Addis Ababa [13]. Urbanization trends in most of African

	Urban population as a percentage of total population*			**Urban population average annual growth rate**		
	1970	**1991**	**2000**	**1970–1980**	**1980–1990**	**1991–2000**
Low-income countries	28	39 (3127)	–3686	3.7	5	2.4
Kenya	10	24 (25)	32 (34)	8.5	7.8	7
Zimbabwe	17	28 (10)	35 (12)	5.6	5.8	5.4
Nigeria	20	36 (99)	43 (128)	6.1	5.8	5.4

**Figures in parenthesis are estimates of total population in millions.*

Table 1.
Urbanization of low-income countries in sub-Saharan Africa.

countries are mainly demographically driven without commensurate socioeconomic development [14]. With no massive social, economic and infrastructural transformations in place, growing cities and towns in Africa experience high rates of poverty, unemployment, low wages and inequality [15, 16]. Urbanization in African is rather chaotic and is dogged with complex urban health crises arising from inadequate safe water supply, squalor and shanty settlements (**Figure 1**), poor sanitation, poor solid waste and toxins disposal that contaminates food and water [3]. These living conditions drive a high incidence of infectious diseases [17].

Injuries are also common because of inefficient, congested, and risky transport system [18]. It is estimated that up to 62 percent of SSA's urban population live in informal settlements characterized by pervasive poverty and overcrowding [19]. While the poor in the cities continue to suffer marginalization and experience excess social and economic vulnerability from unstable employment, external shocks such as natural disasters, the affluent section of cities are much more planned and with significant policy attention, and development that ensures healthy living such as presence of walk ways, parks and playing fields (**Figure 2**) [20, 21]. Therefore, the divide between the rich and poor urban dwellers remains wide in African cities, and the extent of inequality reduces access to healthy living as well as essential and quality health services particularly for the poor. Young people face several challenges when transitioning to adulthood within such settings.

There is substantial evidence from studies conducted in Nairobi slums, indicating an increase of smoking along decreasing social economic status (SES) gradient, and within overcrowded settings, thereby elevating the risks of second hand smoking [22]. While urban poverty remains a critical trigger of NCD risks, the existing obesogenic environments and weak health systems in most of urban Africa portend a bleak future for NCD prevention and control. Studies in Kenya, Ghana and South Africa have also shown that living in a city is associated with higher odds of obesity and cardio-metabolic risk factors [23–25]. Similarly, Peer et al., (2013) [26], in South Africa found that urban environments are associated with an increase in prevalence of the traditional risk factors for NCDs including smoking, harmful alcohol consumption, inadequate physical activity, and inadequate fruit/vegetable consumption. In addition, early life exposure to urban environment has been linked to an increased risk of obesity and impaired fasting glucose in later adulthood [27].

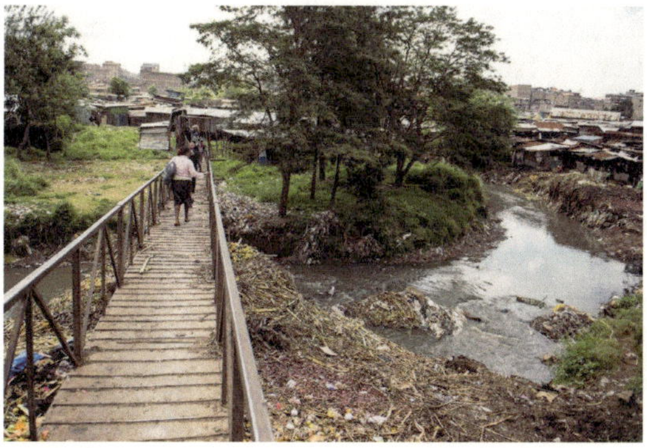

Figure 1.
Korogocho slums in Nairobi. Credit: APHRC.

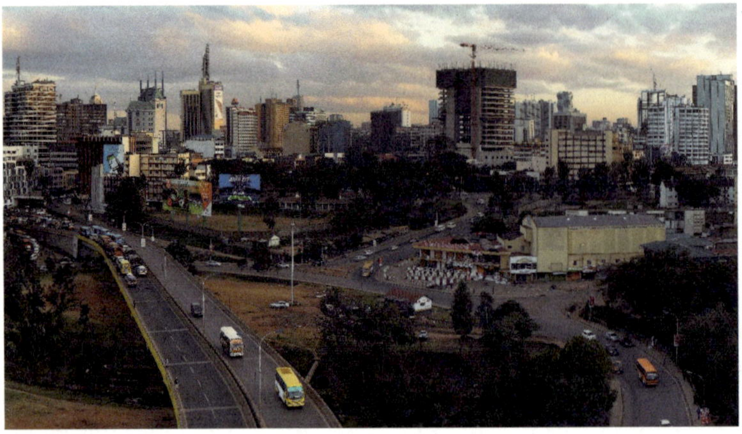

Figure 2.
A section of the Nairobi Central Business District (CBD).

3. Burden and trends of NCDs in Africa

The world health organization (WHO), defines NCDs as any medical condition or disease that is non-infectious and non-transmissible among people. The four main NCDs include cardiovascular diseases, chronic respiratory diseases, diabetes, and cancers which share a set of four key behavioral risk factors: tobacco use, harmful alcohol use, physical inactivity, and unhealthy diet [28]. These behaviors mediate biological risk factors such as obesity, raised blood pressure, and increased blood glucose, elevated blood lipids which ultimately progress to more advanced disease [29]. Other examples of NCDs include mental illnesses, injuries, and chronic kidney diseases. From 1990 to 2015, NCDs related deaths in SSA increased from 25% (1.7 million) to 34% (2.7 million). During the same period, the total NCD burden expressed as disability adjusted life years (DALYs) increased by 45% [7]. Cardiovascular diseases (CVDs) are the leading cause of NCD deaths. In 2013, CVDs caused nearly 1 million deaths in SSA, constituting 38.3% of non-communicable disease deaths and 11.3% of deaths from all causes in the region [30]. Cancers come second causing 12% NCDs deaths with wide variations across regions in SSA. Among males in SSA, leading cancer cases (in age-standardized incidence rate (ASIR) per 100,000 population) included, prostate cancer (27.9), liver cancer (10.2), Kaposi sarcoma (7.2), oesophageal cancer (6.8) and colorectal cancer (6.4). While among females, cervical cancer (34.8), breast cancer (33.8), liver cancer (5.4), colorectal cancer (5.4), ovarian (4.6) [31], are the most common causes of death. Tragically, survival from cancer is worse than in the rest of the world. For many cancers, the risk of getting cancer and the risk of dying from it are nearly the same in SSA [32]. Chronic respiratory diseases and diabetes are each responsible for about 10% and 5% of total deaths in SSA respectively [7]. The NCD risk factors such as high blood pressure, poor diets, air pollution, high body-mass index, tobacco smoking, alcohol and drug use, high fasting plasma glucose, high total cholesterol, and low physical activity are the top 10 global risk factors for death [7].

Other forms of NCDs such as injuries are responsible for a significant proportion of DALYS. Injuries resulting from road accidents (motor vehicles and motor bikes) have increasingly taken a growing toll on human health [33]. Mental disorders, including depression and anxiety, or severe forms like psychosis, schizophrenia and bipolar, as well as alcohol and substance dependence are common. Over the next decade, it is projected that NCD associated DALYs will surpass that contributed by infectious diseases, perinatal and maternal conditions combined (**Figure 3**).

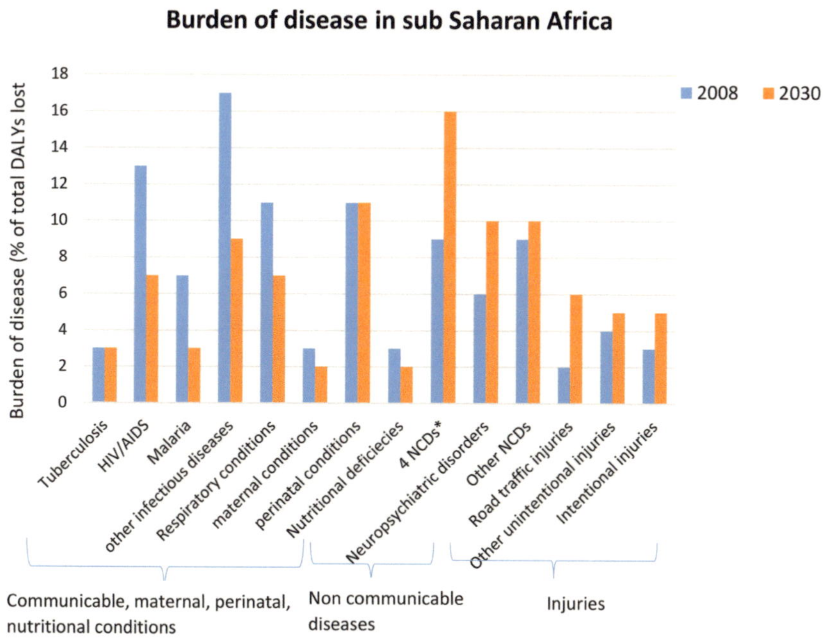

Figure 3.
Projected burden of disease in SSA, 2008 and 2030. Source of data: Authors from (World Health Organization, 2008). NCDS: Cardiovascular diseases, cancer, diabetes, chronic respiratory diseases.*

4. Hypertension in African cities

Hypertension is a leading risk factor for mortality, and is the prime risk factor for the CVD epidemic in Africa [34]. Hypertension is defined as an average systolic blood pressure ≥140 mmHg and/or average diastolic blood pressure ≥90 mmHg among adults aged at least 18 years. Data available on hypertension prevalence are from a wide range of studies [35, 36], majority of which are not age-standardized, and this limits the opportunity for reliable comparison between different African countries and cities. Nevertheless, several WHO STEPwise surveys reported a hypertension prevalence of 19.3–39.6% in Africa [35, 37]. Additional data from epidemiological modeling project suggest that 216.8 million people will have hypertension by 2030. Urban settings consistently have a higher prevalence of hypertension compared to rural areas [38, 39] (**Figure 4**).

Of great concern, is the proportion of individuals with hypertension who remain underdiagnosed, lack access to treatment and are prone to severe complications and increased risk of premature deaths [40]. Evidence from a review of hypertension in 23 African countries, shows that less than half of those with hypertension are aware of their diseases and only one third of those who are aware start treatment, and less than 10% of those on treatment have their blood pressure controlled [41]. It is thus crucial to understand the risk factors driving the rise of hypertension in urban areas to inform preventive interventions. Several factors have been cited as responsible for the rise of hypertension among urban populations in Africa.

Early studies by Donnison et al. (1929) in an African rural community established the role of civilization and urbanization on the development of hypertension [42]. Later, Poulter et al. (1990) established social-behavioral origins with sedentary lifestyles and increased consumption of unhealthy diets among rural–urban migrants in Kenya as major factors driving elevated blood pressure [43]. Researchers also observed that mean diastolic blood pressure of migrants (aged 15–34 years) who moved to the cities increased markedly over time, compared to

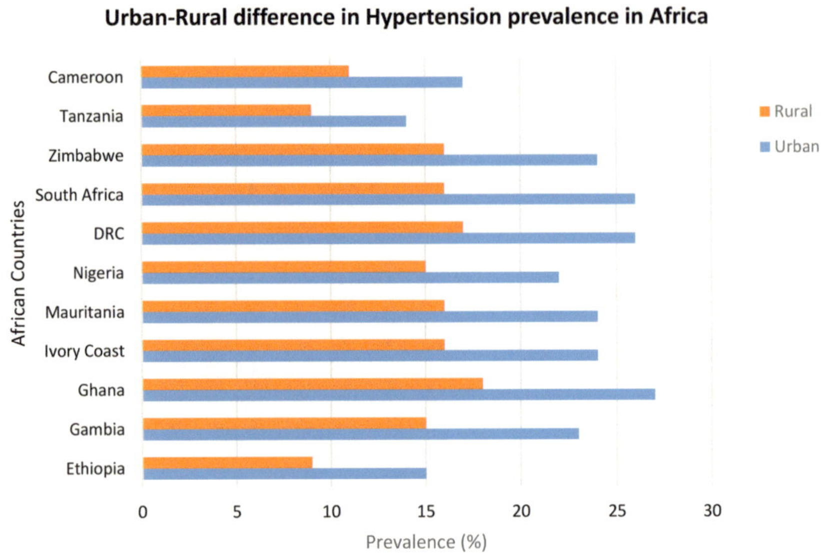

Figure 4.
Prevalence of hypertension by rural–urban residence in selected African countries. Source of data: World Health Survey (2003).

their controls in the rural areas. In addition, migrants' mean urinary sodium: potassium ratio, weight and pulse rate were higher than for controls [43]. Cooper et al., also hypothesized that environmental and behavioral changes that occur when individuals move from rural to urban settings all coalesce to increase predisposition to hypertension [44].

Urban poverty which is common in African cities, is also known to mediate deleterious risks factors for hypertension among urban residents [45]. In LMICs, poverty exposes people to behavioral risk factors for NCDs and in turn, resulting NCDs become an important driver for poverty. The urban poor experience increased vulnerability to unhealthy diets and physical inactivity. Evans et al., (2010) found that informal settlements within cities in South Africa had unhealthy diets and inadequate physical activity because they lacked access to organized markets for healthy foods, and had inadequate resources for physical activity [46].

Urban living in South Africa, Tanzania and Cameroon was also reported to be associated with increased exposure to tobacco use, excessive alcohol intake, unhealthy diets (high in salt, and sugar and less in fiber) and also physical inactivity [47, 48]. In the next section, we review how urban environment modifies NCD risk factors.

5. How urban environment determines the rise of NCD risk factors in African cities

5.1 Unhealthy diets in African cities

There is evidence alluding to the link between diet and development of overweight, obesity and occurrence of NCDs [49]. However, the understanding of the nexus between urbanization and changes in dietary patterns and nutrient intakes in Africa remains limited. As African cities grow, the rise in urban population's increases pressure on arable land for farming, and coupled with rural urban migration, this reduces the ratio of food producers to food consumers [16]. This consequently leads to severe disruptions in healthy food availability, distribution, access and affordability [50, 51]. As healthy foods such as fresh vegetables and fruits, cereals and plant proteins diminish in urban settings, populations resort to the readily available which often unhealthy. A survey in major cities of Cape Verde, Ghana and Senegal reported an increased consumption of energy-dense foods such as candies, ice cream and sweetened beverages up to seven times as frequently as fruit and vegetables [50]. This finding affirms previous studies that showed rapid rise in fat intake across low income countries, including in Africa [52]. Proliferation of fast-food outlets, supermarkets, food vendors, and restaurants in cities have facilitated increased access to unhealthy diets, thus transforming urban settlements into highly obesogenic environments. Nevertheless, for individuals of higher socio-economic status, these changes may offer improved access to nutritious foods since they can afford more healthy foods [53]. While for the urban poor, choices for healthy foods are restricted and they easily resort to the most easily available and affordable diets that are largely unhealthy [54]. In the cities, there are aggressive powerful commercial and emotional advertisements and marketing through various media outlets, which greatly influence preferences and choices of fast-foods and sugary drinks, especially among children and young adults [55, 56].

5.2 Physical inactivity and sedentary lifestyles in cities

Physical activity (PA) has many health-promoting effects and is associated with reduced risk of cardiovascular and metabolic diseases, obesity, and some cancers [57]. Insufficient physical activity is a leading risk factor for NCDs and has a negative effect on mental health and quality of life. Levels of physical activity in many African countries vary widely across geographic regions and population subgroups. For instance, country level prevalence of PA ranged from 46.8% in Mali to 96.0% in Mozambique [58]. While current data shows that SSA has the least prevalence of insufficient physical activity compared to the rest of the world [59], trend data shows decreasing levels of physical activity and increasing levels of sedentary lifestyles across all age groups [60]. Country-specific population-based data on physical activity prevalence show lower levels of PA in urban environments attributed to built-up environment leaving no green spaces for physical activity [61]. In addition, congestion in cities, availability of motorized transport and absence of paved walk-ways makes it impractical for physical activity to happen in African cities. In low income informal settlements in African cities, several physical barriers and insecurity limit physical activity [46]. In Kenya for instance, young adults in rural areas were found to be more physically active compared to those in urban areas. A study conducted by Mashili et al. (2018) in Tanzania also found that being employed, higher education and wealth status (mainly among urban residents) were associated with less physically activity [62].

5.3 Tobacco and alcohol use in African cities

The WHO considers tobacco use as the single leading cause of avoidable death and ill health, contributing to lung cancer, chronic respiratory disease and cardiovascular disease [63]. While the use of cigarette and other tobacco products has declined in high-income countries [64], cigarette use in LMICs including in SSA is rising [65]. Demographic Health Surveys (DHS) conducted in 16 African countries revealed that cigarette use was highest among urban dwellers, less educated, and lower socioeconomic status individuals [66]. Consistent with previous studies in Africa, urban residents are most at risk for cigarette use [67], and start smoking at a younger age [68]. A study by Williams et al., (2008) in Cape Town concluded that urbanicity was associated with smoking attitudes among women [69]. Notably, increased marketing of tobacco products target women and youths in urban SSA [66]. Young adults in African cities, for example in Nairobi, Kigali and Dar-es-salaam, have taken into trendier smoking habits such as *"shisha" (pipe smoking)* [70–72]. In addition, since informal settlements in the cities are overcrowded, there is increased the risk of second hand smoking and indoor pollution from cooking–all linked to cardiovascular and respiratory complications [73].

Comparative literature about alcohol use in urban and rural settings is rare. Some studies have linked urban living to the rise of psychological distress and alcohol-related problems. However, there is paucity of research that investigates the link between urbanization stress and alcoholism in SSA [74]. Similarly, harmful use of alcohol is often associated with injuries, violence, crime, suicide and risky sexual behaviors [75].

5.4 Obesity and overweight

The link between obesity, poor health outcomes and all-cause mortality is well established. Obesity is known to increase the likelihood of diabetes, hypertension, coronary heart disease, and stroke, certain cancers, obstructive sleep apnoea and osteoarthritis. It also negatively affects reproductive performance [24, 27, 76]. Research evidence now characterizes the rapid rise in obesity levels in urban parts of Africa over the last 25 years as an epidemic. A study in Nairobi informal settlements found three times higher obesity prevalence than that rural areas in Kenya [77]. An analysis of demographic and health survey data from 24 African countries over the past 25 years revealed a consistent increase in obesity levels in all study countries. Obesity more than doubled or tripled in 12 of the 24 countries including Kenya, Benin, Niger, Rwanda, Ivory Coast and Uganda, Zambia, Burkina Faso, Mali, and Malawi, while Tanzania experienced a three-fold increase over the same period [78]. Substantial differences were observed between countries: Egypt and Ghana had the highest prevalence of obesity in the survey estimated at 39 and 22%respectively [79]. Obesity was higher among women aged between 15 and 49 years and those living in urban areas [80]-see **Figure 5**.

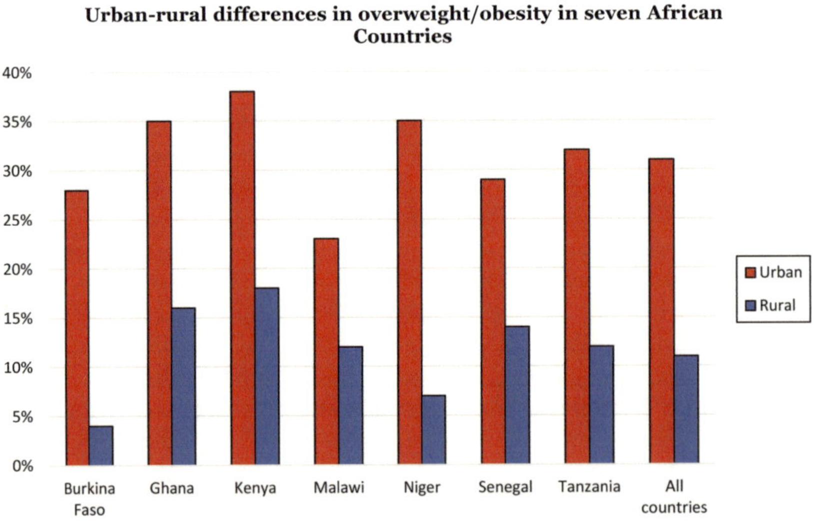

Figure 5.
Differences in urban and rural overweight and obesity prevalence in Africa. Source of data: Demographic Health Surveys (DHS).

Several studies have described the role of urbanization in the rising obesity epidemic in the African continent [79–81]. Urbanization along with socioeconomic transformation lead to increased access to high energy-dense foods and more sedentary lifestyles resulting in a positive energy balance leading to obesity. Access to cheap foods, high in fat and sugar content among the urban poor is easier than in rural communities, thus the higher prevalence of obesity in urban areas [82]. In an analysis of data from seven African countries including Malawi, Senegal, Kenya, Ghana, Tanzania, Niger and Burkina Faso, Ziraba et al., found that the greatest increase in prevalence of overweight and obesity over a ten-year was among the poorest people living in the cities [83].

6. Control of NCDs in Africa cities

Many interventions for prevention and control of NCDs exist but because most African countries have limited resources, choices have to be made about which of the interventions are prioritized [84]. WHO proposed several NCD "best-buy" strategies - proven and cost-effective approaches for addressing NCDs- within LMICs through tacking of the modifiable risk factors for NCDs [85]. Examples of the "best buys" include increasing taxes on tobacco and alcohol, legislation to restrict smoking zones, bans on advertising, reducing salt and sugar in food and raising public awareness on dangers of all risk factors for NCD and promoting healthy behaviors. A number of African governments made commitments in domesticating and implementing NCD related international commitments, such as the Global NCD Action Plan 2013–2020 with targets and indicators to accelerate NCD control [86]. Nevertheless, progress has been slow, and in some cases off-track in achieving the NCDs indicators by the set deadlines [87]. Scarcity of resources and several competing priorities in the health sectors across African countries limits the ability of countries to achieve their targets. A recent WHO NCD Progress Monitor report revealed that less than half of WHO Member States have set NCD targets/indicators to track progress of implementing NCD "best buys" [88]. Some of the "best-buys" that have been implemented by African countries include; taxes and legislations to create a protective environment that limits exposure to harmful behaviors especially for the most vulnerable.

Both excise and sales tax on tobacco products in Kenya and South Africa were increased [89]. Similarly, several countries including Botswana, Kenya, The Gambia, Ghana, South Africa, Tanzania, and Zimbabwe have imposed taxes on alcoholic beverages [90]. While the enforcement of the alcohol and tobacco policies may be lacking the needed regulatory teeth, there is some evidence suggesting higher levels of alcohol and tobacco abstinence in countries implementing these interventions compared to countries without any regulations [90]. Between 1993 and 2009, cigarettes sales declined by 30% in South Africa, and the rate of smoking among adults dropped by 25%, even as government revenues from tobacco taxes increased by 800% [91, 92]. South Africa imposed taxes on sugary drinks in 2017, becoming the first African country to do so, in an attempt to reduce excessive consumption of sugary drinks [93], the effect of this is yet to be seen. South Africa also passed a legislation to enforce salt reductions in the food industry by establishing maximum sodium content limits to be achieved by 2019 [94]. Some countries are now pushing for bans on alcohol advertising. In Gambia, alcohol advertising is banned on national television and radio.

Some African cities have chosen a more positive and interactive approach through health promotion such as raising awareness about NCDs and encouraging disease screening through campaigns (e.g. for hypertension and diabetes). Most of these health promotion approaches are aimed at achieving positive health behaviors at individual and community levels [95]. For example in Kigali, Rwanda physical activity is promoted among city residents by encouraging people to leave work early once in a week to engage in physical activity [96]. Such preventive approaches to NCD control targeting the behavioral risk factors are more cost-effective than treating the NCDs. A more concerted, strategic, and multi-sectorial policy approach is essential to help reverse the negative trends of NCDs in urban Africa.

7. Challenges of NCD control in urban Africa

Several challenges hinder efforts to address the NCD burden in cities. The main challenges include lack of data needed to inform primary prevention, care and treatment, low community awareness on NCDs and risk factors, weak policies and poverty in the informal settlements.

7.1 Dearth of NCD data

Limited availability of representative data on the burden of NCDs in Africa [97], leads to a gross underestimation of burden, thus the inability to lobby for investment in NCD care service delivery. Some countries have collected national NCD data through the NCD WHO STEPwise surveys. Up to 33 countries in WHO African Region have conducted at least one round of STEPwise survey which draws a nationally representative sample and about 19 countries have conducted the global school-based student health surveys (GSHS) [98]. Routine data captured by health facilities on morbidity and mortality could be a potential sources of data, but these data are limited by non-representativeness due to differential use of health services, inaccuracies from paper-based data capture systems, thus the data are largely regarded as of poor quality [99]. Insurance firms also provide important morbidity data, but these have limited value since a small proportion of the population access health insurance. The Global Burden of Disease study combines several datasets to model national NCD morbidity and mortality estimates, but rarely reports NCD burden by rural versus urban locations. Data challenges such as the variation in methodologies used to capture data, the rigor of instruments, sampled populations, design used as well as the variations in how the indicators are defined continue to hamper the comparability and learning across countries [100]. Planning of NCD services without reliable data is almost impossible.

7.2 Lack of community awareness

Lack of knowledge and awareness on risk factors at community level hinders healthy behavior change and uptake of early NCD screening and treatment services [101]. A study in Abuja reported a high prevalence of hypertension among the elderly populations, and majority of whom were unaware about their conditions [102]. Other studies have suggested that low levels of knowledge and awareness of hypertension are associated with undiagnosed, severe or complicated, and uncontrolled hypertension [103], lack of patients' adherence to lifestyle modifications and to medications [104, 105]. Certainly raising awareness particularly on uptake of screening services for most NCDs could be beneficial at both individual and population-levels. And in the context of urban Africa, such efforts could leverage on wide spread mass-media for health promotion. Low levels of NCD awareness or knowledge levels among health workers is also associated with reduced ability for case-finding, treatment and referrals [106].

7.3 Weak policies

Urban populations in Africa tend to be very diverse by education, religion, socioeconomic status and culture [5]. As a result, NCD prevention and control policies and programs need to be tailored to cater for variations at population levels [107]. In a review CVD policies in Kenya Asiki et al. (2018) found no standalone policies for CVD management and care but some aspects of CVD policy were covered in general NCD policy document [108]. NCD policies in most African countries suffer the same deficiencies as they do not reflect the typical realities of urban living –pervasive food marketing and complex urban food environments that may offer diversity as well as greater exposure to unhealthy foods [8]. These policies are also not well integrated with policies in other sectors such as spatial planning, infrastructure and housing, transport planning, education policy, access to energy, and water and sanitation policies and interventions [53]. As such minimum intersectoral and multisectoral engagements in policy formulation lead to standalone NCD policies that are not coherent with other policies [90]. Furthermore, national policies and plans for the prevention and control of NCDs often suffer from underfunding [109], and are thus not implemented. In addition, interference from commercial and economic interests of industry for tobacco, alcohol, and food industries makes it difficult to regulate these NCD risk factors as policy makers and law enforcers are often bribed or threatened not to formulate and or implement such policies [110].

7.4 Slow health system response

Health systems in SSA are characteristically weak and overburdened by the rapidly increasing double burden of communicable diseases and NCDs [17]. With more focus and investment on infectious diseases such as malaria, TB and HIV, very little attention is given to the rising NCD burden in cities [111]. As a consequence, several gaps and missed opportunities exist to offer services for patients and many miss diagnosis, and treatment to when they present to hospitals with other diseases [112]. Inadequate staff and as well as capacity of health staff in most countries, negatively affects NCD prevention and treatment at facilities. For instance, nurses at primary healthcare facilities should have skills to use simple point-of-care equipment such as glucometers for early screening, treatment and referral of individuals with abnormal blood glucose [113]. Frequent stock-outs of medicines and supplies remains a critical barrier to prompt treatment and adherence to these treatments. In Nairobi, Kenya medicines for NCDs are hardly available in public hospitals, and there is lack of integration of NCD services with other chronic diseases such as HIV or TB services [114]. Knowing that interventions targeted against one of the disease burdens will impact the other, it is critical that interventions are conducted jointly instead of competing for limited resources. A study in Malawi reported that the full cost of NCD care is often borne directly by patients through out-of-pocket (OOP) payments individuals [115]. Similarly, a study by Mwai and Muriithi (2016) in Kenya reported that NCDs reduce household income by almost 30%, compared to other general ailments that reduce household income by 13.6%. As a consequence, many people suffering from NCDs in Africa face risks of experiencing catastrophic health expenditures, impoverishment and may be deterred from seeking the care they need [116].

7.5 Poverty in informal settlements

Poverty is common among urban residents in Africa and this plays a fundamental role in the onset, progress and mortality of NCD patients [117]. Studies have suggested that the groups most at risk of NCDs in the next decade will be the urban poor [118]. While NCD epidemiology in high income countries is largely driven by explosion of traditional risk factors in Rwanda, increasing evidence points to a greater contribution of malnutrition, infections, and toxic environments - all exacerbated by poverty [119]. Poverty also limits access to quality NCD care. Majority of the urban poor lack access to health insurance and therefore resort to out-of-pocket payments, consequently leading to catastrophic spending [120]. Research on social and economic implications of NCDs remain scarce in most SSA countries yet such information is important for prioritization of NCDs by all relevant sectors [121].

8. Conclusion

The rapid urbanization in Africa continues to drive the NCD epidemic, increasing vulnerability of individuals, threatening development and sustainability of African cities. To mitigate this rising threat - effective evidence-informed multi-sectoral policies are needed to address prevention and control of NCD focusing on the major NCD risk factors. While several countries have developed national strategies for NCD prevention following the global WHO NCD prevention strategies, implementation of these policies is still inadequate. Thus there is need for governments to put more effort in strengthening implementation of these policies including allocation of financial and other resources to support implementation. NCD policies need to be integrated into urban planning to address air pollution as well as physical inactivity by designing and developing parks and recreational facilities including pedestrian and cycling tracks, zoning walk-ways where motorized vehicles are not allowed and providing incentives for the non-use of motorized vehicles. Fiscal policies and regulatory measures to restrict unhealthy food environment in urban areas of Africa are also needed to curtail the ever growing food marketing by a burgeoning food industry.

There is need to strengthen health care systems to make them more responsive to NCD prevention and control. This include building capacity of health workforce on prevention and control of NCDs, strengthening infrastructure, providing essential commodities and supplies and strengthen surveillance systems to be able to plan, monitor, and assess the effects of NCDs on population health and monitor the performance of interventions. A good balance of investment is required for the delivery and coordination of both curative and preventive and promotive services to avert the NCD disease burden. Countries need to explore various models of partnership with private sector partners aimed at scaling up their contributions to addressing NCDs directly or indirectly through various multi-sectoral strategies.

There is need to strengthen primary prevention interventions at community-levels. These interventions include early detection, active screening, case finding, referral and treatment and working with at-risk individuals to reduce high risk behavior. Expanding opportunities for early detection at the community and in primary health facilities could yield positive outcomes, especially through deliberate implementation of task shifting and task sharing models, involving community health workers (CHWs), while consistently mentoring and evaluating performance of such a model. Further community interventions include health education and promotion focusing on NCD risk factors including importance of reduced alcohol and tobacco consumption, physical activity and decreased consumption of high-calorie foods and highly processed foods while increasing consumption of fruits and vegetables. Some evidence exist on the potential positive results of such small-scale healthy food interventions utilizing platforms such as school feeding programs and workplaces. While documented community interventions addressing alcohol and tobacco consumption are scarce, interventions to enhance awareness and engagement in physical activity in major cities such as in Rwanda and Cameroon have been shown to work. Above all pro-poor primary health care programs targeting vulnerable and disadvantaged groups in African cities are needed to reduce the equity gap in NCD services.

Author details

Kenneth Juma[1*], Pamela A. Juma[2], Constance Shumba[3], Peter Otieno[1] and Gershim Asiki[1]

1 African Population and Health Research Center, Nairobi, Kenya

2 London School of Economics and Political Science, London, UK

3 Aga Khan Foundation and Aga Khan University, SONAM-EA, Nairobi, Kenya

*Address all correspondence to: kjuma@aphrc.org

References

[1] United Nations. 2018 Revision of World Urbanization Prospects. New York: United Nation Department of Economic and Social Affairs; 2018

[2] UN-Habitat. The State of African Cities, 2014. Re-Imagining Sustainable Urban Transitions. Nairobi: United Nations Human Settlements Programme 2014, UN-Habitat;

[3] Eckert S, Kohler S. Urbanization and health in developing countries: A systematic review. World Health & Population. 2014;**15**:7-20

[4] Smit W et al. Making unhealthy places: The built environment and non-communicable diseases in Khayelitsha, Cape Town. Health & Place. 2016;**39**:196-203

[5] The Lancet Diabetes Endocrinology. Urbanisation, inequality, and non-communicable disease risk. The Lancet Diabetes & Endocrinology. 2017;**5**(5):313

[6] Benziger CP, Roth GA, Moran AE. The global burden of disease study and the preventable burden of NCD. Global Heart. 2016;**11**(4):393-397

[7] Forouzanfar MH et al. Global, regional, and national comparative risk assessment of 79 behavioural, environmental and occupational, and metabolic risks or clusters of risks, 1990-2015: A systematic analysis for the global burden of disease study 2015. The Lancet. 2016;**388**(10053):1659-1724

[8] Hunter-Adams J et al. How to address non-communicable diseases in urban Africa. The Lancet Diabetes & Endocrinology. 2017;5(12):932-934

[9] Bloom DE et al. The Global Economic Burden of Non-communicable Diseases. Geneva: World Economic Forum; 2011

[10] Njoh A. Urbanization and development in sub-Saharan Africa. Cities. 2003;**20**:167-174

[11] Antoine P. Population and urbanization in Africa. Chron CEPED. 1995;**17**:1-4

[12] Burak G et al. Urbanization in Africa: Challenges and opportunities for conservation. Environmental Research Letters. 2017;**13**(1):015002

[13] Mariama S. Foresight Africa 2016: Urbanization in the African context. In: Africa in Focus. Herald House: The Brookings Institution; 2015

[14] Tabutin D, Schoumaker B. The demography of sub-Saharan Africa from the 1950s to the 2000s [a survey of changes and a statistical assessment]. Population. 2004:457-555

[15] Satterthwaite D. The impact of urban development on risk in sub-Saharan Africa's cities with a focus on small and intermediate urban centres. International Journal of Disaster Risk Reduction. 2017;**26**:16-23

[16] Satterthwaite D, McGranahan G, Tacoli C. Urbanization and its implications for food and farming. Philosophical Transactions of the Royal Society, B: Biological Sciences. 2010;**365**(1554):2809-2820

[17] Peer N. The converging burdens of infectious and non-communicable diseases in rural-to-urban migrant sub-Saharan African populations: A focus on HIV/AIDS, tuberculosis and cardio-metabolic diseases. Tropical diseases. Travel Medicine and Vaccines. 2015;**1**(1):6

[18] Adeloye D et al. The burden of road traffic crashes, injuries and deaths in Africa: A systematic review and meta-analysis. Bulletin

of the World Health Organization. 2016;**94**(7):510-521A

[19] African Population and Health Research Center (APHRC). Population and Health Dynamics in Nairobi's Informal Settlements: Report of the Nairobi Cross-Sectional Slums Survey (NCSS) 2012. Nairobi: African Population and Health Research Center; 2014

[20] Kjendseth TW. Social Exclusion, Urban Poverty and the Vulnerability to Forced Evictions: A Case Study of Kibera, Nairobi, in Department of Political Science. Reprosentralen: University of Oslo; 2014. p. 99

[21] Salami RO, von Meding JK, Giggins H. Urban settlements' vulnerability to flood risks in African cities: A conceptual framework. Jamba: Journal of Disaster Risk Studies. 2017;**9**(1):9

[22] Ndugwa RP et al. Adolescent problem behavior in Nairobi's informal settlements: Applying problem behavior theory in sub-Saharan Africa. Journal of Urban Health: Bulletin of the New York Academy of Medicine. 2011;**88**(Suppl 2): 298-317

[23] Haregu TN et al. Co-occurrence of behavioral risk factors of common non-communicable diseases among urban slum dwellers in Nairobi, Kenya. Global Health Action. 2015;**8**:28697

[24] Obirikorang C et al. Obesity and cardio-metabolic risk factors in an urban and rural population in the Ashanti region-Ghana: A comparative cross-sectional study. PLoS One. 2015;**10**(6):e0129494

[25] Oyebode O et al. Rural, urban and migrant differences in non-communicable disease risk-factors in middle income countries: A cross-sectional study of WHO-SAGE data. PLoS One. 2015;**10**(4):e0122747

[26] Peer N et al. Urban–rural and gender differences in tobacco and alcohol use, diet and physical activity among young black south Africans between 1998 and 2003. Global Health Action. 2013;**6**:297-305. DOI: 10.3402/gha.v6i0.19216

[27] Angkurawaranon C et al. Early life urban exposure as a risk factor for developing obesity and impaired fasting glucose in later adulthood: Results from two cohorts in Thailand. BMC Public Health. 2015;**15**:902

[28] Christopher M, Allan L. The Global Burden of Disease: A Comprehensive Assessment of Mortality and Disability from Diseases, Injuries, and Risk Factors in 1990 and Projected to 2020. USA: Harvard School of Public Health on behalf of the World Health Organization and the World Bank; 1996

[29] World Health Organization. Noncommunicable diseases. 2018 [cited 2018 23 September, 2018]

[30] Mensah GA et al. Mortality from cardiovascular diseases in sub-Saharan Africa, 1990-2013: A systematic analysis of data from the global burden of disease study 2013. Cardiovascular Journal of Africa. 2015;**26**(2 H3Africa Suppl):S6-S10

[31] Ferlay J, et al. GLOBOCAN 2012 v1.0, Cancer Incidence and Mortality Worldwide: IARC CancerBase No. 11. 2013

[32] Sankaranarayanan R et al. An overview of cancer survival in Africa, Asia, the Caribbean and Central America: The case for investment in cancer health services. IARC Scientific Publications. 2011;**162**:257-291

[33] Vissoci JRN et al. Road traffic injury in sub-Saharan African countries: A systematic review and summary of observational studies. Traffic Injury Prevention. 2017;**18**(7):767-773

[34] WHO. Global Status Report on Noncommunicable Diseases 2014. Geneva: WHO; 2014. p. 298

[35] Addo J, Smeeth L, Leon DA. Hypertension in sub-saharan Africa: A systematic review. Hypertension. 2007;**50**(6):1012-1018

[36] Hendriks ME et al. Hypertension in sub-Saharan Africa: Cross-sectional surveys in four rural and urban communities. PLoS One. 2012;**7**(3):e32638

[37] Opie LH, Seedat YK. Hypertension in sub-Saharan African populations. Circulation. 2005;**112**(23):3562-3568

[38] Agyemang C. Rural and urban differences in blood pressure and hypertension in Ghana, West Africa. Public Health. 2006;**120**(6):525-533

[39] Seedat YK. Hypertension in developing nations in sub-Saharan Africa. Journal of Human Hypertension. 2000;**14**(10-11):739-747

[40] Seedat YK. Why is control of hypertension in sub-Saharan Africa poor? Cardiovascular Journal of Africa. 2015;**26**(4):193-195

[41] Kayima J et al. Hypertension awareness, treatment and control in Africa: A systematic review. BMC Cardiovascular Disorders. 2013;**13**:54-54

[42] Donnison CP. Blood pressure in the African native. Its bearing upon the aetiology of hyperpiesia and Arterio-sclerosis. Lancet. 1929:6-7

[43] Poulter NR et al. The Kenyan Luo migration study: Observations on the initiation of a rise in blood pressure. BMJ. 1990;**300**(6730):967-972

[44] Cooper R et al. The prevalence of hypertension in seven populations of west African origin. American Journal of Public Health. 1997;**87**(2):160-168

[45] Montgomery MR, Hewett PC. Urban poverty and health in developing countries: Household and neighborhood effects. Demography. 2005;**42**(3):397-425

[46] Evans WD et al. Social marketing as a childhood obesity prevention strategy. Obesity (Silver Spring). 2010;**18**(Suppl 1):S23-S26

[47] Maletnlema TN. A Tanzanian perspective on the nutrition transition and its implications for health. Public Health Nutrition. 2002;**5**(1a):163-168

[48] Sobngwi E et al. Exposure over the life course to an urban environment and its relation with obesity, diabetes, and hypertension in rural and urban Cameroon. International Journal of Epidemiology. 2004;**33**(4):769-776

[49] Mu M et al. Dietary patterns and overweight/obesity: A review article. Iranian Journal of Public Health. 2017;**46**(7):869-876

[50] Bosu WK. An overview of the nutrition transition in West Africa: Implications for non-communicable diseases. The Proceedings of the Nutrition Society. 2015;**74**(4): 466-477

[51] Crush J, Frayne B, McLachlan M. "Rapid Urbanization and the Nutrition Transition in Southern Africa": Urban Food Security Series No. 7. Cape Town: African Food Security Urban Network (AFSUN); 2011

[52] Popkin BM. Global nutrition dynamics: The world is shifting rapidly toward a diet linked with noncommunicable diseases. The American Journal of Clinical Nutrition. 2006;**84**(2):289-298

[53] Smit W. Urban governance and urban food systems in Africa: Examining the linkages. Cities. 2016;**58**:80-86

[54] Nyandika O. Food Accessibility among the Urban Poor under Conditions of Structural Adjustment Programmes; A Case Study of Soweto/Kayole Nairobi, Kenya in Department of Urban and Regional Planning. Nairobi: University of Nairobi: ADD Library, Nairobi; 1995

[55] Harris JL, Graff SK. Protecting young people from junk food advertising: Implications of psychological research for first amendment law. American Journal of Public Health. 2012;**102**(2):214-222

[56] Laraia BA et al. Biobehavioral factors that shape nutrition in low-income populations: A narrative review. American Journal of Preventive Medicine. 2017;**52**(2, Supplement 2): S118-S126

[57] Adamu B, Sani MU, Abdu A. Physical exercise and health: A review. Nigerian Journal of Medicine. 2006;**15**(3):190-196

[58] Guthold R et al. Physical activity in 22 African countries: Results from the World Health Organization STEPwise approach to chronic disease risk factor surveillance. American Journal of Preventive Medicine. 2011;**41**(1):52-60

[59] Guthold R et al. Worldwide trends in insufficient physical activity from 2001 to 2016: A pooled analysis of 358 population-based surveys with 1-9 million participants. The Lancet Global Health. 2018;**6**(10):e1077-e1086

[60] Oyeyemi AL et al. Patterns and associated factors of physical activity among adolescents in Nigeria. PLoS One. 2016;**11**(2):e0150142

[61] Ojiambo RM et al. Effect of urbanization on objectively measured physical activity levels, sedentary time, and indices of adiposity in Kenyan adolescents. Journal of Physical Activity & Health. 2012;**9**(1):115-123

[62] Mashili FL et al. Physical activity and associated socioeconomic determinants in rural and urban Tanzania: Results from the 2012 WHO-STEPS survey. International Journal of Population Research. 2018;**2018**:10

[63] U.S. Department of Health and Human Services. The Health Consequences of Smoking—50 Years of Progress: A Report of the Surgeon General. Atlanta, GA: U.S. Department of Health and Human Services, Centers for Disease Control and Prevention, National Center for Chronic Disease Prevention and Health Promotion, Office on Smoking and Health; 2014

[64] Islami F et al. Global and regional patterns of tobacco smoking and tobacco control policies. European Urology Focus. 2015;**1**(1):3-16

[65] Brathwaite R et al. A systematic review of tobacco smoking prevalence and description of tobacco control strategies in sub-Saharan African countries; 2007 to 2014. PLoS One. 2015;**10**(7):e0132401

[66] Pampel F. Tobacco use in sub-Sahara Africa: Estimates from the demographic health surveys. Social Science & Medicine (1982). 2008;**66**(8):1772-1783

[67] Pampel FC. Patterns of tobacco use in the early epidemic stages: Malawi and Zambia, 2000-2002. American Journal of Public Health. 2005;**95**(6): 1009-1015

[68] Townsend L et al. A systematic review of tobacco use among sub-Saharan African youth. Journal of Substance Use. 2006;**11**(4):245-269

[69] Williams CT, Grier SA, Marks AS. "Coming to town": The impact of Urbanicity, cigarette advertising, and network norms on the smoking attitudes of black women in Cape Town, South Africa. Journal of Urban Health:

Bulletin of the New York Academy of Medicine. 2008;**85**(4):472-485

[70] Kimiyu H. Rwanda Bans Shisha Smoking Following Tanzania's Lead. Business Daily. Nairobi; 2017

[71] Omotehinwa OJ et al. Shisha use among students in a private university in Kigali city, Rwanda: Prevalence and associated factors. BMC Public Health. 2018;**18**(1):713

[72] Wanja M, Amuli L. Board Says Rise in Shisha Smoking by Women Worrying, in Daily Nation. Nairobi: Nation Media Group; 2017

[73] Ezeh A et al. The history, geography, and sociology of slums and the health problems of people who live in slums. Lancet. 2017;**389**(10068):547-558

[74] Walt LC, Kinoti E, Jason LA. Industrialization stresses, Alcohol Abuse & Substance Dependence: Differential gender effects in a Kenyan rural farming community. International Journal of Mental Health and Addiction. 2013;**11**(3):369-380

[75] Choudhry V et al. Patterns of alcohol consumption and risky sexual behavior: A cross-sectional study among Ugandan university students. BMC Public Health. 2014;**14**(1):128

[76] Bloomfield GS et al. Hypertension and obesity as cardiovascular risk factors among HIV seropositive patients in Western Kenya. PLoS One. 2011;**6**(7):e22288

[77] Asiki G et al. Sociodemographic and behavioural factors associated with body mass index among men and women in Nairobi slums: AWI-gen project. Global Health Action. 2018;**11**(Suppl. 2):1470738

[78] Amugsi DA et al. Prevalence and time trends in overweight and obesity among urban women: An analysis of demographic and health surveys data from 24 African countries, 1991-2014. BMJ Open. 2017;7(10):e017344

[79] Ajayi IO et al. Urban–rural and geographic differences in overweight and obesity in four sub-Saharan African adult populations: A multi-country cross-sectional study. BMC Public Health. 2016;**16**(1):1126

[80] Kandala N-B, Stranges S. Geographic variation of overweight and obesity among women in Nigeria: A case for nutritional transition in sub-Saharan Africa. PLoS One. 2014;**9**(6):e101103

[81] Kirunda BE et al. Population-based survey of overweight and obesity and the associated factors in peri-urban and rural eastern Uganda. BMC Public Health. 2015;**15**(1):1168

[82] Global Panel. Urban Diets and Nutrition: Trends, Challenges and Opportunities for Policy Action. London: Global Panel on Agriculture and Food Systems for Nutrition; 2017

[83] Ziraba AK, Fotso JC, Ochako R. Overweight and obesity in urban Africa: A problem of the rich or the poor? BMC Public Health. 2009;**9**(1):465

[84] Juma K et al. First Africa non-communicable disease research conference 2017: Sharing evidence and identifying research priorities. Journal of Global Health. 2019;**8**(2):020301-020301

[85] WHO. From Burden to "Best Buys": Reducing the Economic Impact of Non-Communicable Diseases in Low- and Middle-Income Countries. Geneva: World Economic Forum; 2011

[86] WHO. Global Action Plan for the Prevention and Control of NCDs 2013-2020. Geneva: WHO; 2013

[87] Nyaaba GN et al. Tracing Africa's progress towards implementing the

non-communicable diseases global action plan 2013-2020: A synthesis of WHO country profile reports. BMC Public Health. 2017;**17**:297

[88] WHO. Non Communicable Diseases Progress Monitor, 2017. Geneva: World Health Organization; 2017

[89] Vellios N, Ross H, Perucic A-M. Trends in cigarette demand and supply in Africa. PLoS One. 2018;**13**(8):e0202467

[90] Juma PA et al. Non-communicable disease prevention policy process in five African countries authors. BMC Public Health. 2018;**18**(Suppl 1):961

[91] Linegar DJ, van Walbeek C. The effect of excise tax increases on cigarette prices in South Africa. Tobacco Control. 2018;**27**(1):65-71

[92] van Walbeek C. The Impact of Tobacco Taxation on Consumption: The South African Experience. 2018

[93] WHO. WHO Commends South African Parliament Decision to Pass Tax Bill on Sugary Drinks. South Africa: WHO; 2017

[94] Hofman K, Lee R. Intersectoral Case Study: Successful Sodium Regulation in South Africa. Brazzaville, Republic of Congo: World Health Organization. Regional Office for Africa; 2013

[95] Juma K et al. From HIV prevention to non-communicable disease health promotion efforts in sub-Saharan Africa: A narrative review. AIDS. 2018;**32**(Suppl 1):S63-S73

[96] Ntwari DS. Kigali becomes an Exercise Hub Once Every Week. The East African. Nairobi; 2016

[97] Schwartz JI et al. Looking at non-communicable diseases in Uganda through a local lens: An analysis using locally derived data. Globalization and Health. 2014;**10**:77

[98] WHO. Report on the Status of Major Health Risk Factors for Noncommunicable Diseases: WHO African Region, 2015. Geneva: World Health Organization; 2016

[99] Kroll M, Phalkey RK, Kraas F. Challenges to the surveillance of non-communicable diseases – A review of selected approaches. BMC Public Health. 2015;**15**:1243

[100] Wandai M et al. Available data sources for monitoring non-communicable diseases and their risk factors in South Africa. South African Medical Journal. 2017;**107**(4):331-337

[101] Boateng D et al. Knowledge and awareness of and perception towards cardiovascular disease risk in sub-Saharan Africa: A systematic review. PLoS One. 2017;**12**(12):e0189264

[102] Raji YR, Abiona T, Gureje O. Awareness of hypertension and its impact on blood pressure control among elderly nigerians: Report from the Ibadan study of aging. The Pan African Medical Journal. 2017;**27**:190

[103] Bosu WK. The prevalence, awareness, and control of hypertension among workers in West Africa: A systematic review. Global Health Action. 2015;**8**:26227

[104] Porapakkham Y, Pattaraarchachai J, Aekplakorn W. Prevalence, awareness, treatment and control of hypertension and diabetes mellitus among the elderly: The 2004 National Health Examination Survey III, Thailand. Singapore Medical Journal. 2008;**49**(11):868-873

[105] Zhang X et al. Knowledge, awareness, behavior (KAB) and control of hypertension among urban elderly in

western China. International Journal of Cardiology. 2009;**137**(1):9-15

[106] Ojo TT et al. Exploring knowledge and attitudes toward non-communicable diseases among village health teams in eastern Uganda: A cross-sectional study. BMC Public Health. 2017;**17**(1):947

[107] Unwin N et al. The development of public policies to address non-communicable diseases in the Caribbean country of Barbados: The importance of problem framing and policy entrepreneurs. International Journal of Health Policy and Management. 2016;**6**(2):71-82

[108] Asiki G et al. Policy environment for prevention, control and management of cardiovascular diseases in primary health care in Kenya. BMC Health Services Research. 2018;**18**(1):344

[109] Allen LN. Financing national non-communicable disease responses. Global Health Action. 2017;**10**(1):1326687

[110] Mohamed SF et al. Facilitators and barriers in the formulation and implementation of tobacco control policies in Kenya: A qualitative study. BMC Public Health. 2018;**18**(1):960

[111] Beran D et al. The need to focus on primary health care for chronic diseases. The Lancet Diabetes & Endocrinology. 2016;**4**(9):731-732

[112] Siddharthan T et al. Noncommunicable diseases in east Africa: Assessing the gaps in care and identifying opportunities for improvement. Health Affairs (Project Hope). 2015;**34**(9):1506-1513

[113] Anyangwe SCE, Mtonga C. Inequities in the Global Health workforce: The greatest impediment to health in sub-Saharan Africa. International Journal of Environmental Research and Public Health. 2007;**4**(2):93-100

[114] Temu F et al. Integration of non-communicable diseases in health care: Tackling the double burden of disease in African settings. The Pan African Medical Journal. 2014;**18**:202

[115] Wang Q et al. Out-of-pocket expenditure on chronic non-communicable diseases in sub-Saharan Africa: The case of rural Malawi. PLoS One. 2015;**10**(1):e0116897

[116] Kankeu HT et al. The financial burden from non-communicable diseases in low- and middle-income countries: A literature review. Health Research Policy and Systems. 2013;**11**(1):31

[117] Allen L et al. Poverty and risk factors for non-communicable diseases in developing countries: A systematic review. The Lancet. 2016;**388**:S17

[118] Bukhman G, Mocumbi AO, Horton R. Reframing NCDs and injuries for the poorest billion: A lancet commission. The Lancet. 2015;**386**(10000):1221-1222

[119] Partners In Health. In: Bukhman G, Kidder A, editors. The PIH Guide to Chronic Care Integration for Endemic Non-Communicable Diseases. PIH, Kigali: Global Health Discourse & Tools; 2013

[120] Mwai D, Muriithi M. Economic effects of non-communicable diseases on household income in Kenya: A comparative analysis perspective. Public Health Research. 2016;**2016**:83-90

[121] Allen LN, Fox N, Ambrose A. Quantifying research output on poverty and non-communicable disease behavioural risk factors in low-income and lower middle-income countries: A bibliometric analysis. BMJ Open. 2017;7(11):1-7

Chapter 4

Health Promotion and Its Challenges to Public Health Delivery System in Africa

Edlyne Eze Anugwom

Abstract

The chapter examines the place and role of health promotion in the drive for sustainable and effective public health delivery in Africa. It conceptualizes health promotion from a multifaceted and multi-professional perspective hinged on the empowerment of communities and individuals to play active roles and adopt behaviour consistent with the goals of good health. The paper drawing on documentary data sees health promotion as critical to the achievement of health goals in the continent and equally reflects on the theories of health promotion, strategies for health promotion and challenges to health promotion in Africa. It argues that health promotion in the continent can be strengthened through such measures as appropriate legislations, robust funding, gender inclusiveness, stepping up research, regular needs assessment and evaluation, setting needs-driven priorities and building capacity of health promotion to target vulnerable and marginal members of the society, among others.

Keywords: health promotion, public health, challenges, Africa, health education, theories

1. Introduction: conceptualizing health promotion

According to Tannahill [1], health promotion is an umbrella term covering overlapping fields of health education, prevention and attempts to protect public health through social engineering, legislations, fiscal measures and institutional policies which entail the combination of the best in terms of both theory and practice from a wide range of expert groups (educationists, behavioral scientists, medical practitioners) and non-professionals including the communities involved. For him, health promotion stems largely from a new focus for health services that recognize some basic facts: many contemporary health problems are preventable or avoidable through lifestyle change; modern technology is a bundle of mixed blessings bringing both benefits and risks to health; medical technology is at the phase of diminishing returns (losing efficacy and connection to ordinary people); such non-medical factors as better nutrition, improved living conditions and public health measures have contributed to both health and longevity even more than medical measures; that doctors can cause as well as cure disease; and increasing public desire to attain better or improved quality of life and at the same time demystifying and demedicalising the attainment (achievement) of good health [1].

For the World Health Organization (WHO), health promotion is essentially about engendering a context in which the health and well-being of whole populations or groups are owned mainly by the people concerned, i.e., enabling citizens of local communities to achieve political control and determination of their health [2, 3]. Therefore, health promotion goes beyond mere healthcare but puts health on the policymaking agenda in all sectors and at all levels, directing policymakers to be cognisant or conscious of the health consequences of their decisions and accept responsibilities for health.

Health promotion can be seen as the whole process of enabling or empowering people to increase control over and improve their overall health. It focuses on creating awareness of health issues, engendering behaviour modification consistent with prevention and attitudes to ill health and motivating increased usage of available health facilities. In the pursuit of good health (physical, mental and social well-being), individuals and groups through health promotion are enabled to identify and realize aspirations, satisfy needs and change or cope with the environment in manners consistent with complete good health.

Health promotion is expected to contribute to programme impact by enabling prevention of disease, reduction of the risk factors or behaviors associated with given diseases, promoting and fostering lifestyles and conditions that are conducive to good health and enabling increasing use of available health facilities. Therefore, health promotion creates both the awareness and conscientisation that leads to disease prevention, control of health situations and usage of health services and facilities. It implies individual and collective control and participation in health focusing on behavioral change, socio-economic lifestyles and the physical environment.

Without doubt the WHO's Ottawa Charter definition of health promotion is very comprehensive and encompasses the core values and guiding objectives of health promotions [3]. It summarily sees health promotion as the process of enabling people to increase control over and improve their health. In line with the above definition, Macdonald and Davies [4] contend that it calls attention to the critical role of the concepts of process and control as the real essence of health promotion. For them, "the key concepts in this definition are 'process' and 'control', and therefore effectiveness and quality assurance in health promotion must focus on enablement and empowerment. If the activity under consideration is not enabling and empowering it is not health promotion" [4], p. 6.

As the burgeoning literature on health promotion over the years indicate it is a community-driven (inspired), multifaceted and multidisciplinary area of concern that also involves critical sociopolitical, economic and environmental elements and dynamics (see [4, 5–10]).

It is important to also understand that even though one can make a distinction between public health and health promotion, in reality both are interconnected and hardly practically separable. In other words, public health is built on health promotion and health promotion is imperative for public health delivery. As has been argued, public health "is synonymous with health promotion in that it aims to implement co-ordinated community action to produce a healthier society" [11], p. 315.

There is no gainsaying the fact that health promotion nowadays has an overwhelming sociopolitical component that is really definitive. In fact, as has been posited, "health promotion activities are by their nature inherently politically based and driven, thus making it impossible to divorce them from the political arena" [11], p. 314. Health promotion becomes a dynamic area of interface between public policy institutions (the state and its agencies), the public (community/people) and the professionals (ranging from the media professionals, public health advocates, social workers to medical practitioners).

The chapter depended on the desk review of extant literature and documents for its information. The main exclusionary criteria in this regard were materials not related to health promotion and materials published before 1984, which were considered extreme-dated. The inclusive criteria were determined by such concepts as public health, public health in Africa, health promotion, health education and awareness and theories and models in health promotion. Such prominent Internet information sites like the WHO, American Public Health Association (APHA), Health Resources and Services Administration (HRSA) and the Universitats Bibliothek Leipzig (UBL) Online Resources were utilized in gathering materials for the chapter.

2. Theories and models of health promotion

There is no gainsaying the fact that effective and result-oriented health promotion practice depends on sound theory [12]. In other words, theory becomes very informative of health promotion practice and activities. In recognition of the above, one would examine briefly the main theories that have implicated health promotion globally. It is important, however, to state here that the choice of a theory or model to guide health promotion should be determined largely by the specific nature of the health issue being addressed, the community or population in view and the sociopolitical context in question. This is because theories and models are simply used in practice in order to plan health programmes, explain and understand health behaviour as well as underpin the identification of appropriate intervention and implement such intervention in ways that are both effective and sustainable.

Despite a plethora of theories and models utilized in health promotion, I will only focus on five of the most popular and commonly used. These are ecological models of health promotion, the Health Belief Model (HBM), Stages of Change Model or the Trans-theoretical Model, Theory of Reasoned Action or Planned Behaviour and the Social Cognitive Theory.

2.1 The ecological models of health promotion

As the name implies, these models focus on the interaction of people with their physical and sociocultural environments. The approach thus recognizes that there are multiple levels of influence on health and health behaviour especially the health seeking behaviour and choices that people make. The ecological models are anchored on five overriding influences which determine and guide health behaviour and response to health issues [13–16]. These influences are intrapersonal or individual factors (these impact on individual behaviour, e.g., beliefs, knowledge, attitude, etc.); interpersonal factors (these are produced through living with and interacting with other people, e.g., family, friends and social groups/networks; these other people can function as both the source of solidarity and support as well as sources of barriers and constraints to health-promoting behaviour of the individual, e.g., dwelling among chronic smokers or having intense interaction with them may expose one to the dangers of either smoking or the influence of second-hand smoke); community factors (these make reference to social norms that are shared by groups or communities, and such norms whether formal or informal can influence health behaviour and health seeking behaviour of the individual and group members, e.g., relationship between institutions, groups and organizations); institutional factors (policies, rules, regulations and institutional structures that may constrain or even promote healthy behaviour in a given society, e.g., the workplace and voluntary organizations to which the individual belongs are prime examples); public policy factors (policies at different level of governance that regulate, structure or support

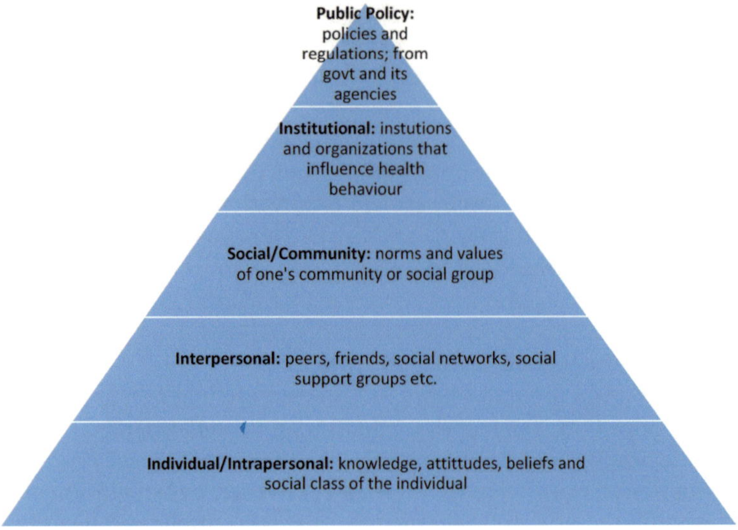

Figure 1.
Ecological models of health promotion (simplified).

actions and practices targeted at health outcomes like disease prevention policies and structures enabling early detection, control or response and management of health crisis in the society; these stem from the position of the government and are critical in achieving the goals of public health delivery) (**Figure 1**).

As the above pyramid, suggests the individual, interpersonal and community factors are at the base. These factors therefore exert more influence and pressure over the individual's health behaviour than the institutional and public policy factors as these are more important. In other words, the institutional and public policy factors are literally far from the individual and do not exert as much pressure on his behaviour as those factors that are very close to him both spatially and otherwise. In an age of increasing pessimism in government, people are much driven by interpersonal and community factors than what comes from a typical further off entity.

Given the above, it is obvious that the ecological approach is very pertinent in the understanding of the range of factors that influence people's health. Its main strength is that it can provide what is called a complete perspective on factors that affect health behaviour and response to health issues especially the role of social and cultural factors or normative patterns on health in the society. It is perhaps very well suited to health intervention and practice in developing societies with an overbearing influence of sociocultural factors on behaviour, attitudes and practice of the people.

2.2 The health belief model (HBM)

This is a theoretical model that has been found useful in guiding both health promotion and strategies for disease prevention. As the name suggests, it focuses on individual beliefs about specific health conditions which predict or direct individual health behaviour [17, 18]. The specific components of this belief that influence health behaviour include perceived susceptibility to the disease; perceived severity of the disease in question; perceived benefits of action (positive benefits of such action) as well as cues to action (awareness of factors that engender action); self-efficacy (belief that action would lead to success); and perceived barriers or obstacles to action (especially if such obstacles are seen as daunting or insurmountable or otherwise).

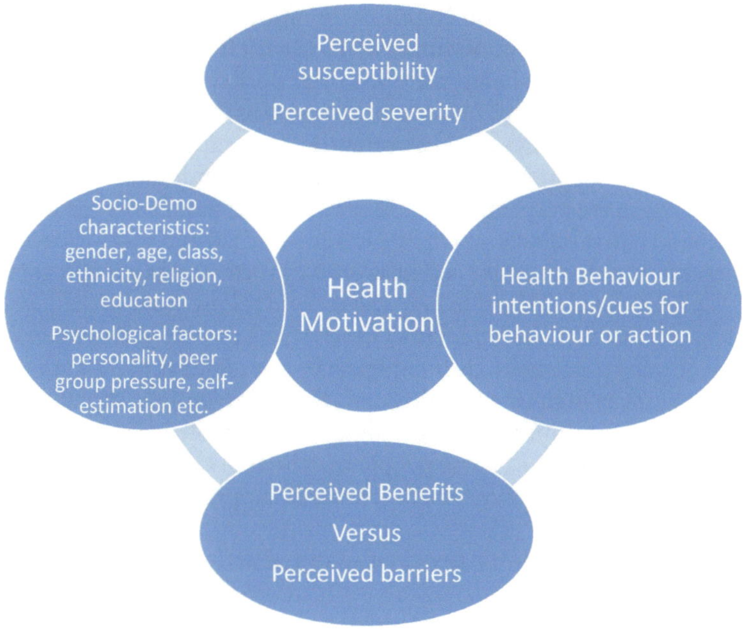

Figure 2.
Health belief model (HBM).

In the utilization of the HBM in health promotion, there are five main action-related segments that would help in identifying key decision-making points and thus facilitate the utilization of knowledge in guiding health intervention. These are: collection of information (through needs assessments; rapid rural appraisal, etc. in order to determine those at risk of the disease or affliction and specify which population or component of the population to be targeted in the intervention); conveying in unambiguous and clear terms the likely consequences of the health issue in question and its associated risk behaviors in order to facilitate a clear apprehension of its severity; communication (getting information to the target population on the recommended steps to take and the perceived or likely benefits of the recommended action); provision of needed assistance (help the people in both the identification of and reduction of barriers or constraints to action); and demonstration (actions and activities that enable skill development and support aimed at enhancing self-efficacy and increased chances of successful behaviour modification targeted at the health issue in question) (**Figure 2**).

In Africa, the HBM has been very useful in understanding people's response and behaviour to HIV/AIDS and other chronic diseases. Being a society very flushed with beliefs, the degree of responsiveness to a health situation is often the direct product of a set of beliefs held by the individual and/or by his immediate community.

2.3 Stages of change model (aka trans-theoretical model)

This model is focused on examining and explaining the individual's readiness to change his behaviour and sees such change as occurring or happening in successive stages. It therefore adopts a quasi-evolutionary framing of behaviour change in which behaviour change, sustenance and termination are encompassed in six stages. These stages are pre-contemplation (existence of no intention to take any action by the individual); contemplation (thinking about taking action and ruminating on plans to do this soon); preparation (signifies intention to take action and includes the possibility that some steps or preliminary steps to action have been taken already); action (discernible change in behaviour for a brief period of time); maintenance (sustenance of the action taken; behaviour change that is maintained in the long run or long-term behaviour change); and termination (the expressed and discernible desire never to return to prior negative behaviour by the individual concerned).

The above stages are very important in planning behaviour change or modification and recognize that behaviour change is both gradual and takes time. What is needed from the health promoter is that at each of these stages specific interventions or programmes are devised to help the individual progress to the next stage. Also, the recognition that the model may in reality be cyclical rather than lineal, i.e., individuals may progress to the next stage or even regress to previous or lower stages, is important in planning health promotion interventions utilizing this model. It also calls attention to understanding that there are individual differences in the adoption of change, i.e., some people may be swift in behaviour modification, while others may take longer time; but each needs support in order to pull through.

2.4 Theory of reasoned action (theory of planned action)

The main contention of this theory is that an individual's health behaviour is usually determined by his intention to exhibit or display a given behaviour. Therefore, the intention to exhibit a given behaviour (or behaviour intention) is predicated upon or predicted by two main factors, viz. personal attitude to the behaviour in question and subjective or personal norms (an individual's social and environmental context and the perception the individual has over that behaviour) related to that behaviour.

The basic assumption here is that both positive attitudes and positive subjective norms will generate greater perceived control of behaviour and increase the chances of intentions towards changes in behaviour. The theory generally provides information that can be used in predicting people's health behaviour and thus in planning and driving through health interventions. It anchors in recognizing the predictors of behaviour-oriented action and the need for supportive social and environmental contexts that facilitate and sustain desirable health behaviour.

2.5 The social cognitive theory (SCT)

This theory combines both the cognition of the individual and the social context of the individual in offering explanation and understanding of health behaviour and response. It seeks to describe the influence of the experience of the individual, his perception of the actions of other people near him and the factors in the person's immediate environment on health behaviour of the individual. It moves from this general perspective to provide opportunities for social support (defined as conducive to healthy behaviour) and reinforcements that generate behaviour change or modification. In this sense, the SCT depends on the idea of *reciprocal determinism* which denotes the continuing or uninterrupted interaction among the person's characteristics, his behaviour and the social context or environment in which the behaviour takes place.

However, the best way to appreciate the SCT is to examine the main components the theory isolates as related to behaviour change at the individual level. These are self-efficacy (belief in one's ability to control and execute behaviour within a given context); behaviour capability (thorough comprehension of behaviour and the ability to exhibit or perform it); expectations (outcomes or outputs of the behaviour change in question); expectancies (the assignation of value to the above outcome of behaviour

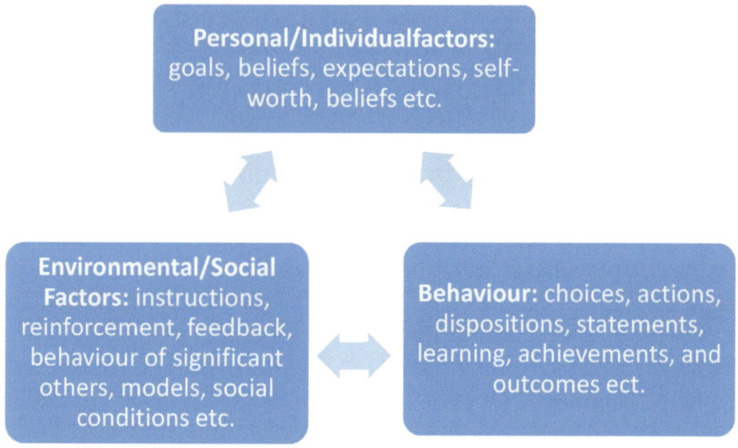

Figure 3.
Illustration of the social cognitive theory (SCT).

and which is important in sustaining the behaviour); self- control (the regulation and monitoring of behaviour of the individual); observational learning (the act of watching others performing the desired behaviour and the outcomes therein as well as modeling that behaviour in question); and reinforcements (incentives and rewards seen as eliciting, encouraging and sustaining behaviour change in the individual) [19].

The three components as the above diagram shows reinforce each other and in the process condition and determine behaviour of the individual even in the context of health as well as choices made therein (**Figure 3**). The SCT is very pertinent in contexts where desirable health outcomes can be achieved by behaviour modification or change. For instance, certain chronic diseases or health conditions can be tackled through healthy lifestyles and dieting that reduce risk factors and chances of individuals succumbing to such conditions. Therefore, the theory can help frame intervention programmes in this area that focus on changing people's behaviour and in the process achieve desirable health outcomes.

Theories and perspectives or models as already indicated are critical in providing explanations of a problem or issue (broadening our understanding and perspective as it were) and also very important in the effort to tackle a given problem or issue in the society especially by way of developing and implementing programmes and interventions. Perhaps, the above underscores why some scholars [20–22] would highlight the difference between the so-called theories of the problem and theories of action, meaning that while the former aids our apprehension of a given issue or social reality, the latter is important in terms of taking actions or evolving activities to tackle the issue in question.

3. Health promotion as sociopolitical engagement

Health promotion generally implicates a huge element of politics and power dynamics in the sense that only political will and cognition can build discernible changes in health. Lobbying and advocacy are critical tools of health promotion and function within the political arena. The sociopolitical contexts and influences are especially recognizable in the public health sector in the developing world where political will and doggedness are often necessary to drive through even the most salutary change or innovation in the health sector. Also, political forces are equally dominant in the provision of crucial health infrastructure and facilities as well as the reasonable funding demanded by any effective public health system. As Harrison opines health promotion "requires concerted, sophisticated and integrated political action to bring about change and requires professionals concerned with public health to engage with the politics of systems and organizations" [5], 165.

Therefore, health promotion seeks to empower and transform communities by getting them involved in activities that influence public health especially through agenda setting, lobbying and advocacy, consciousness raising and social education [11, 22]. All these are accomplished on terms that are either defined or strictly affected by the socio-economic realities of the people themselves. By its emphasis on the community, health promotion has a heavy sociological frame that prioritizes the values of society as well as mobilization and solidarity in the quest for good and sustainable health. It thus makes assumption that individual members of the society would give equal weight to their own health and the health of their neighbors. In other words, it is often anchored on the uncanny assumption that the health of the individual member of a given society is intertwined with the health of the community as a collective. This means the reference point of health promotion is that one's health is as good as the health of the members of the community or society as a whole, i.e., common health destiny. Therefore, such things as community empowerment, community competence and overwhelming sense of community are all apprehended as contributing to the health of the communities [23].

4. Approaches to health promotion

Traditionally there are five approaches utilized in health promotion. These are medical (the focus here is to make people free from medically defined diseases and afflictions; it is mainly anchored on prevention strategies and the role of the medical practitioner or expert in ensuring that the patients comply with recommendations); behavioural change (behaviour modification approach that recognizes that people's behaviour and lifestyles can be changed in order to enable them attain good health, i.e., facilitate adoption of healthy lifestyle); educational (provision of information and knowledge that enable understanding of health issues and build awareness for informed decision-making and choice among people); client-centred (in this situation health practitioners work with clients in order to identify what they know about a given disease and take appropriate action; emphasis on perceiving the client as equal and building the clients self-empowerment that enable them make good choices and control their health outcomes); and societal change (the focus here is on the society or community rather than the individual and seeks to change or modify both the physical and social environments in order to make them consistent with or conducive to good health).

The conventional health promotion methods (modes of operationalizing health promotion and achieving its goals) include health education (the conscious and systematic effort at providing education or knowledge to people on particular and general aspects of health; it is about enabling people through proper and right knowledge on what to do and how to do it; it is empowering and improving people's capacity to act with regard to their health issues and conditions), information, communication (the above three are often captured in the popular acronym IEC), social mobilization, mediation, community theater and advocacy and lobbying. However, while these methods are okay in differing contexts, a decision on the specific medium to use should be guided by both environment (community conditions) and the nature of the health issue involved. The use of more than one method in any given case is highly recommended especially in Africa where there are broad inequalities in access to social goods and the media. The increasing use of social media especially among young Africans calls attention to their deployment equally in core health promotion. Social media platforms like WhatsApp and blogs can be very potent in this regard.

5. Health promotion research in Africa

There is an undeniable need to give high priority to health promotion research in Africa. Such research should aim at enabling a realistic and focused achievement of the goals of health promotion. Broadly, health promotion aims inter alia at:

- The prevention of communicable and non-communicable diseases
- The reduction of risk factors associated with diseases
- The fostering of lifestyles and conditions in the general population that are consistent with overall well-being or good health
- The effective/maximal utilization of existing health services and stimulating demand for others where/when necessary

According to the WHO [24] Health Promotion Strategy for the African Region, the contributions of health promotion to the achievement of health objectives include increasing individual knowledge and skills especially through IEC; strengthening community action through the use of social mobilization; enabling the emergence of environments supportive and protective of health by making optimal use of mediation and negotiation; enabling the development of public policies, legislation and fiscal controls which enhance and support health and overall development using advocacy and lobbying; and making prevention and consumer needs the core focus of health services delivery. All these can be positively influenced by research and studies which evaluate the effectiveness of what has been done as well as explore new strategies suitable to the socio-environmental context in question.

However, while research is very critical to achieving the goals of health promotion, it should be concise and focus essentially on the priority health programmes which have been identified by the WHO for the continent. Some of such programmes include the Global Fund for Malaria, HIV/AIDS and Tuberculosis, Immunization, Mental Health, the Tobacco Free Initiative and Reproductive Health as well as the fight against recurrent scourge of Ebola, etc. Such research should focus on identifying effective health promotion approaches and communication media to embody and convey the outcomes to communities through community participation; the extent or effectiveness of these means and seeking to still improve overall programme effectiveness and sustainability. Therefore, health promotion research should focus on ascertaining goals/outcomes of health promotion (to guide policy), provide reliable conditions associated with these outcomes or goals, precisely define the changes intended and delineate reliable mechanisms and indicators of M and E of health promotion strategies in specific country/community contexts.

The importance of research is essentially derived from the fact that it calls attention to the need for verification and evidence-based activities in health promotion. These are without doubt the ways of knowing if real empowerment and enabling has been achieved in the process. Thus,

> *Health promotion is about enabling people to improve their health; and secondly, evidence relevant to health promotion should bear directly on factors that support or prevent enablement and empowerment (determinants of health) activities that support enablement and empowerment (health promotion) and assessing whether these activities have been successful (evaluation of health promotion). [25], p. 357*

The above clearly suggest that health promotion should be anchored on evidence or should rest on experience and reality regarding what works or what is possible and effective in any context. In this manner, "evidence-based health promotion involves explicit application of quality research evidence when making decisions" [26], p. 126. Research is even more foundational in health promotion since health promotion efforts need to be anchored on agreed definitions and values of health promotion. As Seedhouse contends the failure to be explicit about definitions and values generates conceptual confusion in research as well as sloppy practice [27].

The evaluation of health promotion which should be a core research activity may be based on the three main forms of evidence/knowledge associated with health promotion [28]: instrumental (controlling social and physical environments), interactive (understanding of diseases/health issues; lived experiences; solidarity) and critical (reflection and action; raising consciousness regarding causes and means of overcoming them). These three evidences are anchored on the given scientific/philosophical traditions, viz. instrumental (positivism, quantitative, experimental, scientific knowledge), interactive (constructivist, naturalistic, ethnographic/qualitative knowledge) and critical (materialist, structural and feminist theory).

There is also an overwhelming need for health promotion research to be aware of the difference between health promotion outcomes and health outcomes. Health outcomes crudely imply the consequences or benefits of healthcare delivery (e.g., reduction of mortality rate) related to a disease (which may be the case in spite of an increment in number of those affected by the disease). But health promotion outcomes signify the form of control and attitudinal re-orientation groups and individuals adopt in facing a given disease which may impact on the number of people affected by the disease and improve attitudes and behaviour towards those affected by the disease. Health promotion outcomes can be seen directly through community members' perception and interpretations of a given health issue which makes the achievement of control possible.

Health promotion research should utilize both quantitative and qualitative methods. In addition to complementing quantitative methods in health promotion research, qualitative research enables the researcher reach the heart of issues in engagement with community members. In Africa, where a good percentage of the population are still domiciled in the rural areas, qualitative approach offers the possibility of profound insights into the why and how of health behaviors which may not be possible or easily achieved with the quantitative or traditional biomedical approaches. As a result, "the increasing popularity of qualitative methods is as a result of perceived failure of traditional methods to provide insights into the determinants – both structural and personal – of whether people pursue or do not pursue health-promoting actions" [25], p. 359.

6. Challenges to health promotion in Africa

It is important to recognize that in spite of apparent good intentions, health promotion can actually generate negative or counterproductive effects when not well managed. Thus, "negative outcomes occur where professionally paternalistic and disempowering health policy decisions force health-related outcomes that are irrelevant to sustained community development and are not based on or resourced according to the social reality of the community" [11], p. 315. The above sentiments caution one against embarking on health promotion activities and initiatives that are not anchored on the health realities of the community concerned. Often, overzealous health professionals unintentionally betray the health priorities of communities by assuming knowledge of all there is to know about the health situations and needs of the people.

Perhaps a critical shortfall of some health promotion activities and processes is the adoption of what can be termed the pathogenic paradigm which over-relies on risk instead of emphasizing protective mechanisms. This essentially entails a focus on the failure of communities and individuals to avoid disease or their apparent susceptibility to diseases instead of seeking to unleash their potential and capacity to engender and sustain good health and development. It is an approach that relies too much on health practitioners and experts and hardly gives voice to the people and their own knowledge cum realities.

Generally health promotion in Africa suffers from some of the debilitating challenges which confront the practice of health promotion broadly in many countries in the continent. These challenges, among others, include:

- Poor definition and rudimentary elaboration of expected health outcomes
- Ambiguous elaboration of factors and conditions to be targeted in health promotions
- Ambiguity of health promotion policies and guidelines
- Lack of capacity (or inadequate capacity) to develop, implement and evaluate health promotion programmes
- A general context of inadequate investment in health promotion
- Underdeveloped sectoral collaboration
- Low political will and commitment to health promotion programmes as well as institutional corruption and resource mismanagement

The above challenges have implications for research in health promotions in the continent. There is no gainsaying the need for health promotion to be evidence based because essentially it is the only way to make it responsive to the health needs and interests of the people.

7. Resituating and reinforcing health promotion in Africa

Health promotion combines varied but complementary indicators like legislation, health finance including fiscal measures and taxation, gender inclusiveness, mapping of priorities and organizational change. In spite of their differences, these issues are in reality intertwined or systematically connected in the sense that, for the public health system to function well and optimally, there should be a synergy between these indicators. Briefly:

7.1 Legislation

This revolves around having the political will to make and drive through policies and laws that improve and sustain healthcare delivery. It also involves public health sector governance and leadership which aim at ensuring that only competent and qualified people lead the sector and that activities are governed by a democratic and free process which place emphasis on human rights, dignity and self-worth of all stakeholders.

7.2 Finance

Without doubt efficient health promotion and by implication the entire health delivery system cannot function without finance. In fact, the extent and impact of health promotion depend to a significant extent on the availability of funds. The problem of finance is especially critical in developing nations in Africa where political corruption and competing needs whittle down whatever gets to health from the yearly appropriation of government. However, there is a need to understand that a lot needs to be done in terms of the fiscal policies in these nations in order to achieve the desire for good health and improved life expectancy. In other words, the process of fiscal policymaking and budgetary allocation should prioritize health promotion and health delivery in these countries.

7.3 Organizational change

There is no gainsaying the fact that the health system as a whole is dynamic especially so in Africa where apart from battling known ailments new ones (or novel presentation of the old ailments) spring up now and then. The above entails that the health system calls for dynamic organizational setting that is robust enough to deal with changes while making improvements in the system. There is apparently no denying the fact that health promotion as a critical component of health delivery would benefit from organizational change. This is particularly so in the face of the reality that health promotion in most of the continent is still below the expectation. This is not to deny that health promotion has worked well in specific instances like the HIV/AID scourge and maternal health. However, such grab and slash system which focuses on only one of such delimited issues in the system cannot be seen as either robust or effective in the long run.

7.4 Gender inclusiveness

There is an obvious need to 'en-gender' health promotion as a very critical issue in Africa. This would entail ensuring that those involved in health promotion ensure that in all key phases of health promotion (planning, implementation and evaluation) women and men should be equal partners and collaborators. Gender, in this case, while calling attention to the needs of women, should also ensure that the men are not left behind even in approaching health issues traditionally seen as the concerns of women. Typical example here is in the area of family planning or reproductive health which demands the active collaboration or participation of both men and women to achieve desired results.

7.5 Mapping of priorities

For the WHO [24], the priority interventions in Africa in respect of health promotions include capacity building, development of plans, incorporation of health promotion components in non-health sectors and strengthening of priority programmes using health promotion interventions. These essentially mean pursuing health promotion through capacity building, action planning, advocacy and multisectoral orientation. They are also in tune with relating to the determinants of health promotion in the continent. These include socio-economic conditions and physical (environment), biological, and behavioral lifestyles which impact on health in Africa. Countries can be encouraged to map out their priorities taking into consideration such factors as disease and financial burdens, threats, intervention tools and agencies, acuity, management capabilities, persistent challenges, etc.

8. Conclusion and recommendations

Generally, there is a need for stepping up health promotion research in Africa in the areas of family and reproductive health targeting such issues as VVF, antenatal care, diabetes, cardiovascular issues, new disease forms/resurgence of old diseases (including Ebola), etc. especially in terms of communicating with those who are marginal to the formal sector of the society or who are less privileged by virtue of education, economic opportunities or physical/mental challenges, etc. in both urban and rural contexts. Health promotion can profit from an acute awareness of the fact that what works in one socio-geographical setting may not work in another since no two societies are exactly the same. This would entail designing programmes that even where the general principles or goals remain the same embody recognition of the socio-geographical peculiarities of the society/community concerned.

Given the usual paucity of funds in the continent, it makes sense that to minimize cost and save time, there should be incorporation of both needs assessment and evaluation into ongoing health promotion activities. This approach offers a smart way of pursuing health promotion goals without elaborate budget.

In spite of country differences and specific structural challenges, there is a need to build a culture of sharing and documenting outcomes and evidences of health promotion between different countries and organizations. This is a step towards achieving the desirable goal of multinational coordination especially for infectious diseases and epidemics. Equally, African nations need to invest more in capacity building for media and theater practitioners in both private and public sectors on health promotion. There is no gainsaying the media's crucial role in health information dissemination. Actually, health promotion is largely media driven and should be programmed as such.

In addition to media practitioners, there should be health programme or intervention specific to health promotion capacity building for different cadres of public sector workers. Such capacity building or training should be anchored on acute awareness of current research trends and best practices globally. There should also be increased attention to the need for specific health promotion for under-represented health issues and priority to non-communicable diseases should be targeted. It should also improve capacity on how to incorporate methods of targeting members of the society marginal or vulnerable within each country context.

Author details

Edlyne Eze Anugwom
Department of Sociology and Anthropology, University of Nigeria, Nsukka, Nigeria

*Address all correspondence to: akommiri@gmail.com

IntechOpen

References

[1] Tannahill A. Health promotion – Caring concern. Journal of Medical Ethics. 1984;**10**:196-198

[2] World Health Organization. Health Promotion: A Discussion Document on Concepts and Principles. Geneva: WHO; 1984

[3] World Health Organization. The Ottawa Charter for Health Promotion. Geneva: WHO; 1986

[4] Macdonald G, Davies J. Reflection and vision: Proving and improving the promotion of health. In: Macdonald G, Davies J, editors. Quality, Evidence and Effectiveness in Health Promotion: Striving for Certainties. London: Routledge; 1998. pp. 5-18

[5] Harrison D. Health promotion and politics. In: Bunton R, Macdonald G, editors. Health Promotion: Disciplines, Diversity and Developments. 2nd ed. London: Routledge; 2002. pp. 158-177

[6] Tones K. Why theorise? Ideology in health promotion. Health Education Journal. 1990;**49**(1):2-6

[7] Jones L. The politics of health promotion. In: Jones L, Sidell M, editors. The Challenge of Promoting Health: Exploration and Action. London: Macmillan; 1997. pp. 131-157

[8] MacDonald TH. Rethinking Health Promotion: A Global Approach. London: Routledge; 1998

[9] Victor C. Inequalities in health and health promotion. In: Pike S, Forster D, editors. Health Promotion for all. Edinburgh: Churchill Livingstone; 1995. pp. 157-170

[10] Webster C, French J. The circle of conflict: The history of the public health and health promotion movements. In: Adams L, Amos M, Munro J, editors. Promoting Health: Politics and Practice. London: Sage; 2002. pp. 5-12

[11] Whitehead D. Health promotion and health education: Advancing the concepts. Journal of Advanced Nursing. 2004;**47**(3):311-320

[12] Caplan R, Holland R. Rethinking health education theory. Health Education Journal. 1990;**49**(1):10-12

[13] McLeroy KR, Bibeau D, Steckler A, Glanz K. An ecological perspective on health promotion programmes. Health Education Quarterly. 1988;**15**:351-375

[14] Sallis JF, Owen N. Ecological Models. In: Glanz K, Rimer BK, Lewis FM, editors. Health Behaviour and Health Education: Theory, Research and Practice. 2nd ed. San Francisco: John Wiley; 1997. pp. 403-424

[15] Stokols D. Establishing and maintaining healthy environments: Towards a social ecology of health promotion. The American Psychologist. 1992;**47**(1):6-22

[16] Hancock T. Health, human development and the community ecosystem: Three ecological models. Health Promotion International. 1993; **8**(1):41-47

[17] Janz N, Champion VL, Strecher VJ. The health belief model. In: Glanz K, Rimer BK, Lewis FM, editors. Health Behaviour and Health Education: Theory, Research and Practice. 3rd ed. San Francisco: Jossey-Bass; 2002. pp. 45-66

[18] Strecher VJ, Rosenstock IM. The health belief model. In: Glanz K, Rimer BK, Lewis FM, editors. Health Behaviour and Health Education: Theory, Research and Practice. 2nd ed. San Francisco: John Wiley; 1997. pp. 41-59

[19] Bartholomew LK, Parcel GS, Kok G, Gottlieb NH. Intervention Mapping: Designing Theory and Evidence-Based Health Promotion Programs. Mayfield: Mountain View, CA; 2001

[20] Parker EA, Israel BA, Brakefield-Caldwell W, Keeler GJ, Lewis TC, Ramirez E, et al. Community action against asthma: Explaining the partnership process of a community – based participatory research project. Journal of General Internal Medicine. 2003;**18**(7):558-567

[21] Parker E. Application of health promotion theories and models for environmental health. Health Education and Behaviour. 2004;**31**(4):491-509. DOI: 10.1177/1090198104265601

[22] Whitehead D. Incorporating socio-political health promotion activities in clinical practice. Journal of Clinical Nursing. 2003;**12**:668-677

[23] Edmondson R. Social capital: A strategy for enhancing health? Social Science & Medicine. 2003;**57**:1723-1733

[24] World Health Organization. Health Promotion: A Strategy for the African Region. Geneva: WHO; 2001

[25] Raphael D. The question of evidence in health promotion. Health Promotion International. 2000;**15**(4):356-367

[26] Wiggers J, Sanson-Fisher R. Evidence-based health promotion. In: Scott D, Weston R, editors. Evaluating Health Promotion. Cheltenham, UK: Stanley Thornes; 1998. pp. 31-49

[27] Seedhouse D. Health Promotion: Philosophy, Prejudice and Practice. New York: John Wiley; 1997

[28] Park P. What is participatory research? A theoretical and methodological perspective. In: Park P, Brydon-Miller M, Hall B, Jackson T, editors. Voices of Change: Participatory Research in the United States and Canada. West Port CT: Bergin and Garvey; 1993. pp. 1-20

Chapter 5

Understanding the Science of Indigenous Health System: Key to Sustainable Collaborations

Mbulaheni S. Nemutandani, SJH Hendrick and FM Mulaudzi

Abstract

Most of the health systems in developing countries are dysfunctional and hardly responsive to the needs and demands of patients. Access to a plural healthcare system and reports of patients abandoning western medicine for indigenous medicine are signs of nonresponsive health system. The major contributing factors are the failures of the allopathic health system to recognize that indigenous medicine is a living and practised science, with its own philosophy, beliefs and practices developed over centuries. Indigenous communities and the patient's worldviews are intertwined with indigenous traditions, practices and beliefs. While the two health systems, allopathic and indigenous, coexist in Africa, they must collaborate in the management of patients. The two systems assign different etiological explanations and meanings to health, disease and illness based on worldviews, epistemologies and methodologies developed over time. Change of mindset, attitudes and practices through decolonization will lead to sustainable collaboration.

Keywords: indigenous health system, indigenous healers, living science, multiplicity of the epistemologies, colonization and destruction of indigenous practices, indigenous paradigms and euro-western paradigm, decolonization processes, change of mindset, attitude and practices, integration, sustainable collaborations

1. Overview

"Death is a spiritual illness to eradicate physical and biological life"

After reading this chapter, the reader should be able to appreciate the need to interrogate the predominant Euro-western mindset, attitudes and practices, which have existed as the results of centuries of colonization. There should be a new approach which enables the reader to explore the multiplicity of epistemologies and worldviews to include the voices of the indigenous communities and its science, which tend to be referred to as witchcraft, evil and inferior practices.

The reader is challenged to critically evaluate the power and extent of the influence of Euro-western history, its culture and philosophy on practices of medicine as science and monolithic approach to the search for answers to illness and diseases. The principles of the Euro-western approach are that if you do not know it, it does not exist and if you do not understand it, it's not science and therefore should be rejected. Their tendency is that of breaking it into pieces and flattening it to fit the mindset.

At the end of the chapter, the indigenous and Euro-western paradigms are compared in terms of what counts as scientific knowledge and ways of knowing, including the respective value systems applied in research. The reader is expected to continue to search for the path which will lead to full discovery of own truth.

As for the indigenous researchers, they should be able to remove the shackles which chained them to Euro-western practices and change their mindset of being loyal followers and consumers of western developed knowledge without considering the relevance thereof in the context of time, space and place. Where the content is alien to community beliefs and practices, it should be analyzed and interpreted through the worldview of the indigenous communities.

The institutions of higher learning, and especially those entrusted with the responsibility of approving, awarding and granting permission to conduct research, should consider whether they are promoting the discovery of unreported knowledge or whether they are promoting existing but unreported indigenous knowledge. Comments and questions from members of ethics committees, such as "Which methodology are you following?" and" Is there a similar approach reported in the literature?", suggest that those members do not understand that an indigenous approach to research and to access knowledge entails a ceremony which often involves communication with ancestors, facilitated by indigenous healers.

It must be indicated from the onset that an indigenous health system consists of multiple connections which indigenous communities experience with individuals around them, the environment, living and nonliving beings and objects in a state of physical, mental and spiritual consciousness. It is the frame of reference through which indigenous communities and their healers see the world and interpret events, including the diagnosis and management of illness and misfortunes in their environment.

It further exposes the reader to the existing ignorance and misunderstanding regarding the science behind indigenous health systems and the philosophy of Ubuntu applied in the management of patients in indigenous communities.

The authors strongly advocate that an environment of professional neutrality and open-mindedness should be the premise on which negotiations for collaboration between indigenous and Euro-western health systems are conducted.

2. Background

"When the body is smarter than the brain..."

Most of the Euro-western-based social and health sciences disciplines have inherited the logic that when they mediate and interact with indigenous communities, their disciplines constitute the gold standard [1]. This logic represents a colonial mindset of authority over and superiority to indigenous knowledge systems and is critical of any systems and science, which does not adopt or conform to their views of what constitutes science [2–4]. The sciences and philosophies of indigenous knowledge systems are labeled as witchcraft, pagan and barbaric. In the past this approach has resulted in representatives from indigenous communities to abandon their indigenous character, practices and own particular scientific reasoning and methodology [5, 6]. Where colonization to change indigenous practices failed after applying the conventional methods and means, it resorted to drastic and draconian actions such as banning it [7]. In order to survive the powers of colonialism, it appeared that those representing indigenous health systems and knowledge have adapted to "a new knowledge" and experienced their environment along the rules of a western system [8, 9].

Despite an increase in awareness of indigenous beliefs, forms of living and practices, the latter still get destroyed when they do not meet western standards. Destruction takes place through inquiries based on the relational realities and forms of knowing that are predominantly western, and anything not complying with this should be revised to fit the mold [9].

"Knowledge is acquired, without respect it's a self-imprisonment"

Ways of knowing follow a particular trajectory of searching for knowledge and is influenced by how one relates to the source of knowledge and the people who own and share that knowledge. Most of our understanding of science as determined by western standards is about compartmentalizing knowledge as it is being discovered and fragmentation thereof to fit the western model while ignoring the environment in which it is to be applied. It is common for practitioners of western-based science in the process of the so-called "new discoveries" of things that have existed in indigenous communities to disregard indigenous characters and names and rename them according to western concepts. Where there is poor understanding of the indigenous sciences, the *modus operandi* would be to destroy it to prevent it from competing with western standards. As Kaptchuk and Miller [10] explains it, western science seems not to understand that indigenous sciences do not characterize ways of knowing as higher and lower knowledge. The dominant Eurocentric model of thinking and relating to items and experiences is an attempt at homogenizing everything to become comprehensible [1, 11–14].

3. Indigenous health practitioners

There are different categories of indigenous health practitioners in Africa. Depending on the region, most of them are also known as a traditional healers, medicine doctors [15], etc. For our readers, an indigenous health practitioner is defined as someone who is recognized by the community in which she/he lives as a competent person to provide advice on the causation of disease, misfortunes and disabilities in their community and diagnose and provide treatment for both physical, spiritual and psychological conditions in individuals and the community as a whole [14]. The calling to become an indigenous health practitioner may manifest in different ways and at different ages or times in life. Some are "called" before they are born, while others are "called" during childhood or adulthood. Some are "called" through illness, while others are "called" by experiencing persistent unnatural occurrences in their lives such as dreams and visions of departed relatives and ancestors [1, 9, 15].

There are instances where the call is either not realized soon or sometimes the person ignored it [15]. If the "calling" is not obeyed, the person becomes ill or continues to suffer until he or she accepts the "calling" and enters into an apprenticeship with a more experienced indigenous health practitioner [12]. In South Africa, the process of training to become a health practitioner is called "u thwasa" [15]. The training period may range from a few weeks to months. During this period the intern/thwasana discovers his or her ancestors and means and methods in which they would communicate with and through him or her [9]. Visits by ancestors would often take place during the night, and prescriptions and directions would be provided on how and where to obtain treatment for the patients. Upon mastering the art of abiding and obedience to the ancestral spirits, a graduation function is organized [9].

While the knowledge about diseases is passed on from the training supervisor to the intern/thwasana during apprenticeship, the knowledge of medicines, preparation and application thereof is directly communicated to the thwasana by his/her ancestors only. Both the trainer and thwasana closely guard these secrets from the ancestors [9, 15].

Indigenous health practitioners are broadly categorized according to the techniques they employ and the methods of diagnosis [15]. The three main categories are discussed below.

3.1 Diviners

Diviners are a category of indigenous health practitioners who diagnose diseases and illness through divination. It's the unique and special process of interpreting the message of ancestors through possessed crafted objects such as bones, shells, wood, etc. This category of indigenous health practitioners also possesses the spirit to interpret misfortune and to perform family rituals to secure the protection and guidance of ancestors. They represent the memories of ancestors in human form and establish a crucial link between humans and the supernatural [2, 16, 17].

3.2 Herbalists

Unlike diviners, this category of practitioners are predominantly ordinary people who have acquired an extensive knowledge of herbal medicine and the application of plant components such as roots, barks, leaves, oils, minerals, etc. in treatment. It is a category in which skills are learned and acquired without the involvement of ancestors. They voluntarily decided to undergo training with an established herbalist and then practice independently. They diagnose and prescribe medicines to prevent and to alleviate illness and to provide protection against witchcraft and misfortune or evil, as well as to bring prosperity and happiness [16].

3.3 Traditional birth attendants

This category probably existed long before all other categories of health practitioners. Through the centuries their services had been utilized by all humanities albeit as a matter of necessity due to cultural beliefs or medical conditions which allopathic health practitioners were not able to explain and manage, such as birthmarks [15]. Their focus is on mother and child health, starting from conception right through till the child reaches the age of 5 years. The health of the nursing mother is managed together with that of the child. It is believed that the newborn will not survive unless prenatal conditions and infections that the mother may develop are left untreated. The traditional birth attendants are mostly elderly women of 60 years or older and use herbal medicines to treat their patients.

3.4 Spiritual healers/prophets/faith healers

The spiritual or faith healers and prophets have recently emerged as another category of indigenous health practitioners, and whether they should be recognized and accepted as indigenous health practitioners continues to be debated.

They use prophesy and faith in supernatural beings as the source of their power. A common practice among them is the use of prayer, candlelight and or water to heal their patients [18].

There is division within this category of indigenous health practitioners, and it is based largely on legitimacy and beliefs. Prophets/spiritual healers among themselves differ on the legitimacy of spiritual healers based on calling and supernatural sources of communication. One group of spiritual healers claim to have revelations and visions related to supernatural beings and a so-called heaven as their calling. This group also claim to communicate directly with God in the healing process and do not make use of roots and other raw plant materials to prepare traditional medicines. Instead, they use water and processed herbs to heal. However, the second group of spiritual healers claim to have visions of objects and people as their calling, similar to diviners.

4. Convergent and divergent views between allopathic health practitioners and indigenous health practitioners

Apart from a few areas of possible convergence between the two health systems, it is the divergent views which have obstructed the development of sustainable collaborations between allopathic and indigenous health practitioners. Some are highlighted in **Table 1** below.

The areas of convergence between the two systems are that both display sympathy towards their patients and care about the wellbeing of their patients. In addition, they accept accountability for their patients' health, work from a body of underlying empirical knowledge and both engage in elaborate processes of discernible empiricism in their efforts to diagnose and treat their patients [16]. There is, however, a view among allopathic health practitioners that indigenous medicine in terms of its body of knowledge and practices had remained stagnant during the course of human evolution [19]. The irony is that much of western knowledge, which is vowed to be scientifically based, originated from indigenous medicine by selecting certain practices from the latter, subjecting it to analyses and then

Indigenous health system	Characteristics	Allopathic health system
Diseases and illness are caused by supernatural forces (thuri[a]) and for a reason	Disease/illness	Disease and illness are the result of pathogens or physiological changes
God/supernatural powers in human/plant system; macro level	Source of healing/who heals patients	God/supernatural powers in the unit cell/energy: micro level
Plants, animal by-products Endogenous	Source of medications and treatment	Plants, animal by-products Endogenous
Ancestors/spirits/God Spirits do not forget Carried to next generation	Source of that knowledge Memory At death	Human, library/books and learning Rely on memory End of knowledge
Obedience to and compliance with wishes of ancestors	Improvements/growth	Training and development
Divinations Supernatural powers	Common diagnostic process/procedure	Investigations such as X-rays, FBC, examination, stethoscope, etc.
Biological and endogenous spiritual and exorcism	Treatment and intervention	Biological and endogenous
Ancestors/God	Ownership of knowledge	Individual
For spiritual/psychological cases	Ideal	For physical entities and body

[a]*Evil spells are thought to be in a form of a small nocturnal animal, capable of causing insanity.*

Table 1.
Simplistic comparison of the two health systems.

incorporating some of that into allopathic settings. Very little, if any, recognition is given to the science and philosophy of indigenous knowledge, let alone assigning intellectual ownership.

From the above table, it is evident that the two health systems display differences in their approach to knowledge and science. These differences could be explained using ontology as it evolved culturally and historically over time. The allopathic perspective is based on western science, while indigenous medicine is based on indigenous sciences. Allopathic health practitioners seem to find it difficult to accept the indigenous sciences into their "rational" scientific framework because it does not fit their model.

Another difference relates to the belief of what causes disease and illness. Allopathic medicine associates disease and illness with invading pathogens such as bacteria, parasites and viruses and or physiological changes. The indigenous system believes that disease and illness are caused by supernatural forces. Various explanations are offered for "why me and now" [20–22]. It can be as a result of the individual's own spiritual mishaps, provocation of ancestors by violating taboos, obligations or responsibilities or a mere "call" by ancestors to perform certain rituals. Witchcraft and evil spells are regarded as common causes [7].

Another aspect on which the two systems differ is on what is understood to be science. The point of departure would be on how knowledge or empiricism as a science is defined. Science as it is known from a western perspective in modern times is the accumulation of knowledge through experience/experimentation and observation, and it is stored in books or electronically [23]. In order to be educated, one has to read the books or access the information electronically. For this reason, allopathic medicine utilizes textbooks and other archived material to pass knowledge on. On the other hand, among indigenous health practitioners, knowledge is handed down, often verbally, from healer to apprentice, from one generation to the next [24, 25]. It provides the "paradigm" through which and by which they understand and interpret their environment. The entire constellation of beliefs, values, techniques, etc. is shared by the members of a given community as health practices [12, 18, 26].

The two systems have a different understanding and explanation of what constitutes a healthy individual and society and illness in the community. The allopathic health system subscribes to World Health Organization's (WHO) definition of health as "a state of complete physical, mental and social wellbeing and not merely the absence of disease or infirmity" [27]. This definition of health is limited to an individual within the society and does not comply with the indigenous standard of health. For the indigenous communities, health is not experienced at an individual level. It is defined in terms of the completeness of society as a whole, connectedness and harmonization between the living human kingdoms/beings and their ancestors, animal kingdoms and environment. It values health as a system, similar to the human system, with different components, and each component contributes to the functionality and completeness to purpose [28, 29].

There is growing evidence that the two main health systems—indigenous and allopathic—are operating side by side in Africa [9, 30]. Depending on the country and history of colonization, allopathic health practitioners tend to be well resourced and supported by the government, while neglecting and, in some situations, suppressing indigenous health systems and its practices. At times, the lack of communication and the adversarial relationships between the two systems impact negatively on the delivery of health services to communities [31, 32]. Patients are receiving conflicting advice from their health practitioners. Treatment overdose and drug interactions are very common, and this is not surprising as the two systems have divergent worldviews of the causes of diseases; why, when and how a person becomes ill; and finally the diagnostic tools, processes and approaches to management of patients [33]. Their understanding of what constitutes a diseased patient and or community and the healing process is largely influenced by their respective values and meaning of life and death. Why people get sick and why they should die or live longer will determine their acceptance of the outcome: death or recovery to health/healing. For example, if the death of a diseased individual is viewed as a means of joining the ancestors to provide guidance and advice to the living, the outcome of healing will not be considered as good and beneficial to the indigenous communities.

Indigenous health systems acknowledge that there are diseases and/or illness which infect or attack the human spirit without affecting the physical body [34]. The illness could be as a result of spiritual attacks by evil spirits or evil spells, demonic forces, ancestors' way of communicating with an individual, family and communities. While western science has not accepted this concept of disease, not everything that western science practices and observes meet their own standard of science. For example, western science believes that life in human beings constitutes the coexistence of the physical body, spirit or soul. The existence of the spirit as part of giving life to the body is not based on sciences, but on a belief system which is common to all [35–37].

Indigenous science believes that the spirit, which inhabits individuals, does not present with physical signs and symptoms which could be detected and diagnosed by modern technology as employed by allopathic health systems, e.g. a stethoscope, diagnostic radiography (X-rays), ultrasound, computed tomography (CT) scans, magnetic resonance imaging (MRI) scans and nuclear medicine scans. The opposite is also true. There are diseases, which infect/attack the physical body without affecting the spiritual aspect [35, 38–40]. Allopathic practitioners are well resourced to diagnose and manage both that of the body and spirit. At the centre of the two health systems is the phenomenon of dual consultation which is being exercised by patients based on their preferences of health provider, accessibility and affordability of the services and integration of the disease management model with their belief systems and practices. The perception created over the years under colonial rule by western authorities is perpetuated with the mindset suggesting that patients belong to the allopathic health system with no right of choosing and consulting health providers other than allopathic health practitioners [4]. Failure to recognize indigenous worldviews and beliefs had created a crisis for allopathic healthcare which persists to this day [41, 42].

This is particularly evident among HIV/AIDS and TB patients who are reported to be abandoning western treatment in favor of indigenous remedies and practices. In most cases allopathic health practitioners are made aware of this, often at an advanced stage of treatment, when patients who have been exercising their rights to choose disclose that they are also receiving treatment from indigenous health practitioners [43–45].

Without the recognition of patients' rights and the establishment of collaborations and referrals of patients between the two systems, the postcolonial health system will remain dysfunctional and ineffective to fully respond to the needs of the indigenous communities.

5. Integration of the two healthcare systems

The point of departure should be the interrogation and understanding of the existing health system which was operating in communities before colonization and globalization of their environment [46, 47]. The definition of indigenous in our context refers to the root, something natural or innate (to), a way of life, living, beliefs and practices which is an integral part of community culture. It is embedded in the culture and therefore tacit knowledge. It is communal, a shared form of knowledge achieved through experience. It is a linguistic phenomenon. This phenomenon serves cognitive interests of three types namely technical, moral and critical of own environment [48].

Due to globalization, indigenous communities have become increasingly exposed to foreign cultures and practices. There are no aspects of their social life, customary practices or traditional behavior which remained untouched. Communities are now living in countries without borders, and they seem to be short-changed by globalization and colonization. Foreign cultures and practices have intruded into indigenous inner self and being without respect and invaded their living space similar to a declaration of war against cultures that were different to that of the colonizers. The character and nature of globalization and colonization is to perpetuate the dominance of that which is being introduced to communities: western or foreign culture, language and health systems, including diseases against which indigenous communities had no innate immunity, constantly displacing indigenous knowledge systems of managing their patients.

For centuries, indigenous communities have maintained their dignity and trust in that which worked for their communities and which was gained through experience over many years. They rebelled against colonization and resisted to be mere bystanders and simply witness their indigenous norms and values to become extinct. With the rediscovery of self, communities are increasingly reclaiming their past and striving to retain their cultures and ways of knowing which were previously marginalized and dubbed unscientific and barbaric. This is no easy feat as they are split between claims of global science on the one hand and the equally compelling claims to recover the "African past" on the other hand.

Health systems are defined as all activities in the community which serve to promote, restore and maintain people's health. In a postcolonial and globalization context, both the indigenous and allopathic health systems are operating side by side. For the two systems to function optimally, it would require the leveling of the playing field through decolonization of mindsets, attitudes and practices. The desired outcome should be the gaining of knowledge, together with acknowledgment and recognition of the important role that indigenous health system plays in the delivery of primary healthcare services.

Globally, indigenous medicine has been declared a component of Primary Health Care (PHC) by the World Health Organization's Health Promotion: Strategy for the African Region. The strategy recommends that different countries should promote and incorporate their indigenous health practitioners into healthcare systems. The implementation of the recommendation has been met with resistance and criticism from allopathic practitioners [9]. A significant number of indigenous communities prefer indigenous medicine as their first choice. Indigenous medicine has always been acceptable, accessible, available, affordable and attainable to them. Several countries have adopted legislation promulgating traditional medicine initiatives. In response to the World Health Organization's Health Promotion: Strategy for the African Region, South Africa promulgated the Traditional Health Practitioners Act [49], to establish a regulatory body controlling the registration and education of THPs [49]. Despite this legislation, allopathic and traditional healthcare sectors remain in conflict and disjointed. Few allopathic health practitioners understand the philosophy, ontology and epistemology of indigenous medicine, let alone accept it as scientific with its own long-standing experiments and standards comparable to western medicine [4, 12]. Simply stated, most of the allopathic practitioners are not able to free themselves from the shackles and deeply embedded mindsets of colonization. Because there is no true understanding of indigenous healthcare systems and its sciences, allopathic health practitioners do not want indigenous medicine to be recognized as a health science [4, 12].

6. Misinterpretation and misrepresentation of indigenous healthcare system

The introduction of Euro-western culture, practices and religious beliefs, such as the Christian faith, dominated and disregarded the indigenous knowledge system. Indigenous still remained alive among communities even though it was not recognized by colonizers [4]. This had a significant impact on colonizing the minds of indigenous people. It enforced a change in indigenous culture, behavior, practice and belief. The continued alienation and exclusion of indigenous health practitioners in the management of patients is largely based on a monopolistic health system, which recognized allopathic health systems as the only practice of health systems emanating from the prevailing dominant practices by allopathic health practitioners and the lack of respect and recognition of traditional health systems [12]. In many of the formerly colonized countries, indigenous healthcare systems continue to be regarded as less important by Eurocentric healthcare providers and funders of healthcare services [12]. It is often perceived as a threat to western norms of standard of healthcare and at times associated with "witchcraft", actively discouraged and suppressed through powerful legislation [4].

Anecdotal actions, supported by published reports, reinforce the stereotype which appears to suggest that patients belong to allopathic health practitioners [4] and have no right to seek alternative opinions and treatment other than what western medicine prescribes. These actions go against the provisions of the Patient and Human Rights Charter in South Africa. In general, communities and patients are denied the power of self-determination, based on experience and informed by their understanding of health in their own particular context.

Most of the health training curriculums in universities and colleges do not expose students to the science of indigenous health systems, community belief systems and their particular worldviews. When confronted with patients demanding alternative health services from indigenous health practitioners, allopathic health practitioners have the perception that such demands for pluralism would lower their standard of heath service provision and result in inappropriate management of "their" patients by indigenous health practitioners through poor treatment, lack of compliance and a possible overdose of medication. These views of allopathic health practitioners have been commonly expressed to and reported by HIV/AIDS patients using traditional medicine concurrently with allopathic medicine.

Due to misinterpretation and misrepresentation, there is a lack of trust between the allopathic and indigenous healthcare sectors, which is exacerbated by a lack of understanding regarding the knowledge base of each sector. Allopathic healthcare providers simply expect indigenous health practitioners to use allopathic principles to treat ailments and promote health instead of indigenous practices. Throughout the era of colonization, and even during postcolonization in Africa, westernized healthcare training institutions have not incorporated traditional medicine and its philosophies in their curriculums. In instances where mention of indigenous health practices is made, it is usually done in a unilateral manner without incorporation of indigenous health practitioners as tutors and lecturers.

As a result, allopathic healthcare practitioners deny students the opportunity of exposure to the multitude of traditional health practices, among others the traditional preparation and packaging of medicines; reproductive health; indigenous preventative and promotive health practices; diagnostic measures; curative and rehabilitative practices; management of diseases and health promotion; lifestyle and dietary preferences; the status of women; music, ancestral drumming and dance and its influence on wellbeing; spirituality; types of traditional healers; traditional leadership; patient management; palliative care; and maternal and child health.

Although traditional health practices are considered to be primitive and backward, they continue to thrive due to its cultural importance among communities. In some communities, traditional healthcare practices are the only available healthcare services, given the prohibitive cost and inaccessibility of allopathic healthcare. It is estimated that to this day between 60 and 80% of patients in Africa consult indigenous health practitioners [41].

Despite years of colonization, the prohibition of indigenous health practices and its sciences, indigenous communities have not completely abandoned their ways of life, practices and beliefs [37]. For an outsider, this may be construed as being stubborn, backwards and ignorant of modern sciences and its achievements. For the local and indigenous communities, the allopathic health system has until now been unable to offer explanations for the onset of illness, the "Why me? Why now?" rationale which forms a crucial part of African indigenous understanding of health and healing [50]. In many instances the instructions by allopathic health practitioners to not use and mix allopathic medicine with traditional herbs confuse patients and do not achieve the desired effect [33]. Patients perceive it that they are expected to abandon their indigenous practices and roots and become part of the western culture.

If parity is to be reached, the two healthcare systems should embrace pluralism and respect the rights of choice for all communities. All parties should acknowledge that globalization created contemporary societies where there are different and coexisting competing health systems arising from different traditions, practices and bodies of knowledge. Although pluralism is now recognized as a global phenomenon, its application in colonized communities seems to remain a pipe dream. It will remain a challenge until such time as allopathic healthcare practitioners and students respectively provide and receive training based only on a western-orientated curriculum that excludes alternative methods of care acceptable to the indigenous communities. The worldviews that inform the current curriculum for allopathic healthcare practitioners are monolistic, hospital-centred and disease-oriented and exclude self-care or healing. Furthermore, the curriculum perpetuates health disparities and power imbalances that adversely affect patient outcomes [4, 12, 31].

6.1 Indigenous health systems as a living science

One of the common arguments by proponents of exclusivity health systems is that "our value system, science of medicine and standard of care will be compromised if we recognize and accept indigenous health practitioners to treat our patients" [4].

There are three fundamental problems associated with this approach, which require elaboration.

Firstly, it's the mindset and attitudes which seem to suggest that patients and communities are owned by health providers.

Secondly, the perception that allopathic medicine is the standard against which all health knowledge is measured.

Lastly, the notion that for "others" (indigenous health practitioners) to exist, function and be accepted by communities, it will require approval and support from allopathic health practitioners.

The plausible explanation for the above problems could be lack of knowledge and understanding of indigenous health systems and its sciences. In life, what we do not know or understand does not mean that it does not exist or does not make sense/work. It may possible mean that one does not understand and comprehend the whole picture and/or is not yet exposed to it.

Indigenous health systems constitute a life force of science practised by indigenous health practitioners before and after colonization; It has a history, origin, philosophy and epistemology [51–53]. Indigenous health system has its own level of excellence in providing an answer to-"why me, why now", resources, the dynamic that carries communities forward. Indigenous communities consider it as the knowledge inherent to its own identity, with its own science and technological advances beyond physical limitations. It is an institution in its own right, with consumers and pioneers [51, 52].

Long before colonial rule invaded indigenous communities, indigenous health practitioners were developed and advanced comparable to the allopathic health system. This is supported by a report by a Scottish medical anthropologist who witnessed the indigenous surgeons in Buganda performing a cesarean section (**Figure 1**).

The Scottish colonizers interacted with the indigenous communities and learnt from them while conducting studies through observation. It culminated in the publication of an article that appeared in the *Edinburgh Journal of Medicine* and in a dissertation titled "Ueber die Lage und Stellen bei der Geburt" which he submitted to the Marburg University in Germany in 1885 [53].

That article is now part of the *Annals of Obstetrics and Gynecology* history, describing in detail how cesarean section was performed. He gave an illustration of procedures and how they were carried out: anesthetics practices, aseptic measures, performance of the actual cesarean section, how the uterus was massaged and delivery progressed, the final postoperative measures and how the mother and baby responded were all included. From this it is evident that the procedures and the science practised by indigenous healthcare providers at that time compared to the best standard of performing a cesarean section that existed in Europe.

Research reports and dissertations published by medical anthropologists in 1885 confirmed that indigenous health practice is a field of health science practised by indigenous health practitioners with high ethical standard of care and value systems.

The question of what is defined as science, how it is practised and how the standard thereof is measured is worth exploring and explained in this context. It is not disputed that science is an art, a pathway and systematic process of finding solutions to societal problems. There are also different pathways of knowing and finding solutions to problems facing communities. Different communities had explored different mechanisms and at different times during the development of their healthcare systems, through experimentation and testing the efficacy of their different

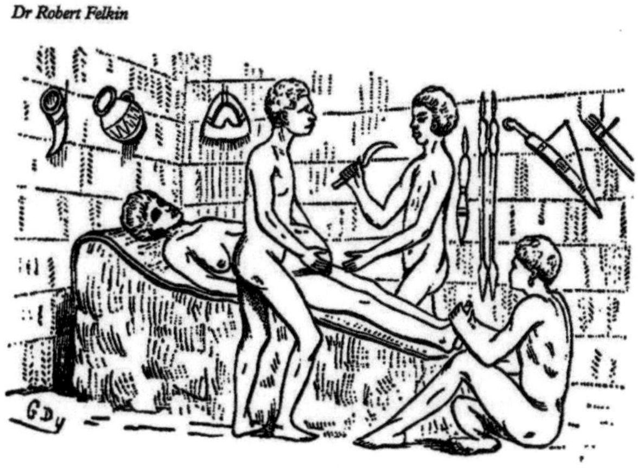

Figure 1.
Indigenous health practitioners of 18th century performing caesarean delivery.

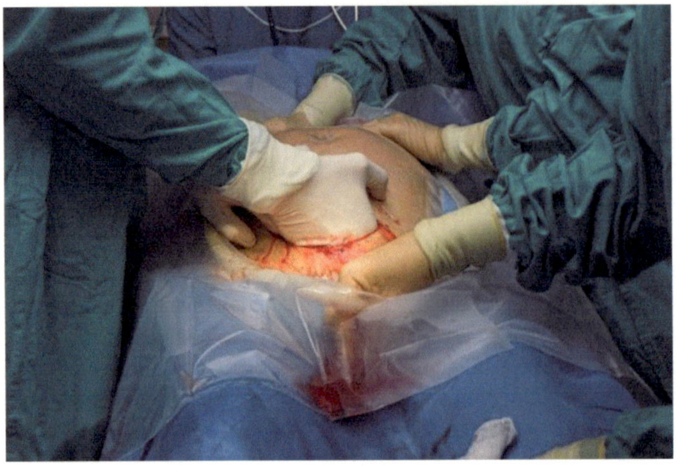

Figure 2.
Allopathic health practitioners of the twenty-first century performing caesarean delivery.

medicinal products, beliefs and practices. Some solutions are yet to be explored and discovered. Reports confirmed that indigenous health practitioners have perfected the art of sciences long before colonizers and missionaries introduced western medicine. Their processes of diagnosis and patient management are documented as being thorough, scientific and of comparable standard to other practices.

Despite what Felkin witnessed as being no different, in principle at least, from what modern doctors do, allopathic health practitioners of the twenty-first century do not recognize that indigenous health systems are a science and could play a significant role in existing health systems. There are several factors which contributed to poor working relationship between the two systems. Key among them is the effect and impact of colonization, globalization and commercialization of health and healthcare services as a commodity. Indigenous communities were encouraged to abandon their practices, beliefs and sciences. High levels of suspicion and mistrust supported the enforcement by law that prohibited the use of indigenous medicines.

There is no doubt that the impact of colonization extended beyond politics and the economic life of indigenous communities, for it disorientated and destabilized their psychosocial interactions with reality. There are perceptions that most scientific scholars raised and educated according to the western doctrine are unable to use their worldview to interrogate and interpret the world and environment, unless it meets the western worldview. They subscribe to western principles despite its limitations in African settings. While most of the colonized countries may have achieved political freedom from their erstwhile masters, the pervasive socioeconomic mindset persists and liberation from western scientific inclinations evades indigenous scholars.

Figure 2 Allopathic health practitioners of the twenty-first century applying similar principles, protocol and standards to that of indigenous health practitioners reported by medical anthropologist in 1885 during the delivery of a baby through Cesarean section (Google source).

7. Exploring the indigenous epistemologies and sustainable collaborations

The author argues for the need of a different approach to collaboration with indigenous communities who have experienced centuries of colonization and dehumanization of their traditional beliefs, health systems and practices. It is the author's view that postcolonial indigenous researchers should develop indigenous epistemologies and methodologies which dismantle, deconstruct and decolonize the Euro-western paradigms of thinking. It provides a platform for the rethinking of the indigenous health system, its philosophies and the sciences involved when a complete healthcare service was provided for centuries before colonization [54]. Although the two healthcare systems operate side by side at different levels of science, i.e. theory of disease causation and management of disease, a mutually agreed upon collaboration between the two systems could positively impact the establishment of a complete health system. A new trajectory and respect for the views that an individual or a community holds on health and diseases should be established, which will not only influence the interpretation of different health conditions and beliefs regarding causation of diseases but will also determine the type of providers who are consulted for the management, restoration of health and the wellbeing of communities. A sustainable collaboration would require exploring approaches that eliminate the "come join us" attitude and monopolistic health system of allopathic health practitioners who regard themselves as holding the gold standard against which all others are assessed.

8. Development of sustainable collaborations through decolonization processes

Studies show that the integration of allopathic and traditional medicine should include co-learning and mutual respect [19, 55, 56]. Traditional and allopathic healthcare practitioners already have common practices, for example, the physiotherapists' use of steam for inhalation therapy which is similar to ukugquma and using a warm towel compress which is similar to ukuthoba. Midwives recommending alternative positions during delivery is similar to methods used by traditional birth attendants throughout the ages.

Creating opportunities for collaboration and capacity development through training of allopathic healthcare practitioners in traditional healthcare practices is emancipatory, will stimulate awareness and creates a cultural sensitivity among allopathic healthcare practitioners [50, 57]. Collaboration will create an opportunity to enhance the transfer of skills and sharing of knowledge between the traditional and allopathic healthcare sectors [58, 59]. It should translate into curriculum transformation through co-teaching, co-supervision and transfer of knowledge on diagnostic measures applied by indigenous practitioners in preparation and packaging of traditional medicines. Through such a training process, trust will be fostered between the traditional and allopathic healthcare sectors, and co-operation will be facilitated, leading to sharing of critical information and ultimately empowerment of both types of healthcare practitioners [60].

Indigenous communities, through colonization, have been oppressed, stripped of human dignity and have died inside a long time ago. Existing collaborations have failed to recognize the importance of redressing the inequalities of the past and to acknowledge the importance of indigenous knowledge [4]. It is the belief that the experience gained when indigenous and allopathic health practitioners work alongside each other would result in lasting collaborations. The view has been expressed by indigenous scholars that decolonization of healthcare requires a change in mindset and the establishment of agendas that would allow for mutual exchange and recognition of indigenous knowledge [61]. The success of it relies on a change in attitude, recognizing the value of indigenous health systems, beliefs and the Ubuntu spirit in African communities.

The process of decolonization requires a participatory approach which requires commitment from all stakeholders [12, 62, 63]. It begins with demystifying traditional healthcare practices and community empowerment through honest and open discussion about the need for allopathic healthcare practitioners to learn from indigenous health practitioners. The main objective is changing the mindset and attitudes of the colonized indigenous and allopathic health practitioners through a participatory process. The demystifying stage involves the five phases of a decolonization process [4, 12, 62]: (1) rediscovery and recovery, (2) mourning, (3) dreaming, (4) commitment and (5) action (**Figure 3**).

8.1 Rediscovery and recovery process

This is the first phase in the process of decolonization. Allopathic healthcare practitioners are encouraged to rediscover and recover their historical cultural practices, languages and identities. They are to rediscover the many traditional practices including traditional methods of preparation and packaging of medicines; reproductive health, indigenous, preventative, promotive and diagnostic measures; curative and rehabilitative practices; management of diseases and health promotion; lifestyle and dietary preferences; the status of women; music, ancestral drumming and dance and its influence on wellbeing; spirituality; types of traditional healers, traditional leadership; patient management and palliative care; and maternal and child health.

Similarly, the colonized indigenous practitioners and communities should rediscover, interrogate and question the current status of their practices. Rediscovery and recovery give the oppressed and colonized people the ability to decontaminate their minds and thought process in which they can define their real world and problems associated with it. Indigenous practitioners should decide on their terms of references and rules for engagement among themselves and with others. In this case, allopathic healthcare practitioners go through the process of rediscovery and

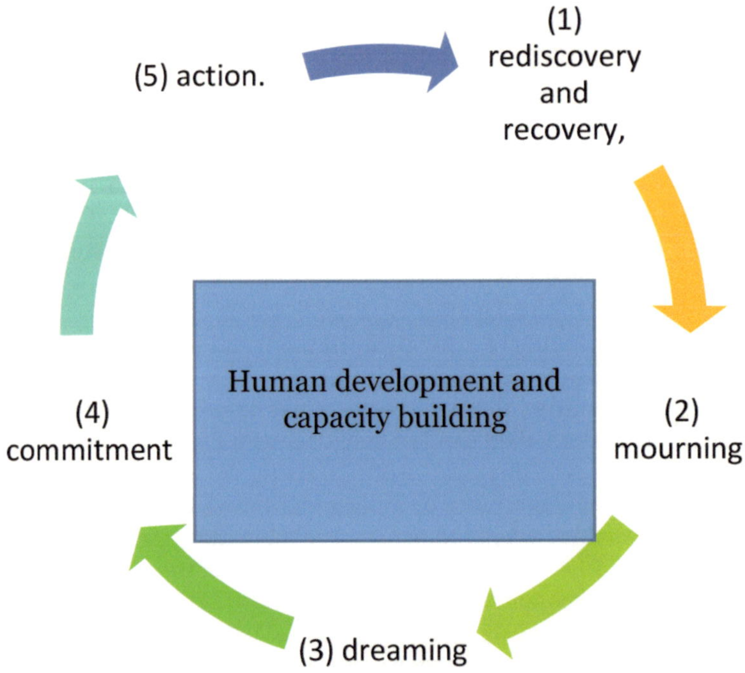

Figure 3.
Cyclical pattern of decolonization adopted from Nemutandani et al. [4].

recovery through learning about existing traditional healthcare practices, languages and identities. This process is the cornerstone for sustainable collaboration.

9. Mourning the disrespect of the indigenous medicine

This stage refers to the process of lamenting the injustices that have been done by colonization and how this has affected the self-esteem and image of the indigenous practitioners in the communities, including the impact it had on their practices and traditions. It has been argued to be an important part of healing and preparing for moving forward. The years of assault upon and damage done to the minds of indigenous people, their traditions, values and belief systems were reported on literature.

The scars from years of colonization and the indoctrination of African people to disown their own ways of living and of health practices are still evident years after achieving independence from colonizers. The perception that traditional beliefs and practices belong to the dark ages and uncivilized societies appears to have resulted in a refusal to accept indigenous heath practitioner.

Even the so-called educated and liberated middle-class African health professionals have not been prepared to free themselves of the limitations of colonization. "The main challenge is the existing negative perceptions you have about us. This is more prevalent among the educated and middle-class people... consult secretively, with skepticism, doubts and pride...." as quoted by an indigenous member in the study by Nemutandani and others [4].

9.1 Dreaming process

The third decolonization process involves dreaming in which the allopathic healthcare practitioners will allow the traditional healers to educate them about different possibilities of knowledge and skills that can still be helpful to offer alternative care. In the environment in which the dreaming should take place, two processes are required.

9.2 Commitment process

The allopathic healthcare practitioners should take on the positions of activism to advocate for incorporation of indigenous healthcare practices into the curriculum. They will therefore write monographs and textbooks to take the knowledge from tacit to explicit.

9.3 Action process

The last process in decolonization is the joint development of a plan of action by allowing indigenous health practitioners to build capacity among allopathic health practitioners. Dreams and commitments are translated into strategies for capacity building and skill transfer to ensure that their collaboration is sustainable.

The existing collaborations between the two health systems without understanding and acknowledging that the indigenous health system is a living science are not sustainable.

Finally, there are reports which found that allopathic and indigenous medicine are compatible in their sciences of treating and managing their patients. For example, allopathic health practitioners, using their existing biomedical knowledge of HIV-/AIDS-related illness, would set a course of treatment that emphasize antiretroviral medications and hospital treatment. On the other hand, indigenous health practitioners, invoking existing knowledge of sicknesses caused by spirits, set a course of treatment that emphasize herbal medicines, sacrifices and ritual ceremonies to appease ancestors. It can be argued that both approaches are typical of all medical systems in that they "frame problems in relation to the solutions they have to offer" and how they understand it to be according to their existing knowledge as defined by their health system—in textbook or through ancestors.

In conclusion, any health intervention which disregards the existing community health beliefs, traditions and cultural practices is likely to be resisted passively by communities if not openly by creating parallel systems acceptable to the communities.

Despite the existing bias against indigenous health practitioners and the negativities associated with those consulting them, collaboration between allopathic health practitioners and indigenous health practitioners in the management of patients is certainly possible.

Reflection: Why is it that indigenous health sciences are not incorporated in the curriculum of most health professional training institutions in Africa? Despite the strong beliefs and practical experiences of both academics and students being products of indigenous systems, few seem capable of associating with it. One could conclude that the prevailing educational system does not encourage either students or academics to think for themselves but rather follow the path traveled by their Euro-centric predecessors, despite well knowing that their environment is different. There seems to be a deeply embedded western paradigm of reasoning among members of human research committees who seem to be fixated on whether similar research had been done and whether tried and tested methods are being followed.

Reflection: For a long time, when we go out for research, if we are honest enough, what we are gathering or we went out for is a collection of existing information and raw data. It's only when we process it in our university (standards) that we call it knowledge. There are many of us who still go out and do research that way; it is the habit of the heart and mind and the habit of relating to people, society and healers as objects.

Author details

Mbulaheni S. Nemutandani[1]*, SJH Hendrick[2] and FM Mulaudzi[3]

1 Faculty of Health Sciences, School of Oral Health Sciences, University of the Witwatersrand, Johannesburg, South Africa

2 Faculty of Dentistry, University of Sefako Makgatho Health Sciences University, Garankuwa, South Africa

3 Department of Nursing, Faculty of Health Sciences, University of Pretoria, South Africa

*Address all correspondence to: simon.nemutandani@wits.ac.za

References

[1] Wreford J. Working with Spirit: Experiencing Izangoma. Healing in Contemporary South Africa. Oxford, UK: Berghahn Books; 2008

[2] Stoner BP. Understanding medical systems: Traditional, modern, and syncretic health care alternatives in medically pluralistic societies. Medical Anthropology Quarterly. 1986;**17**:44-48

[3] Bishop R. Freeing ourselves from neo-colonial domination in research: A Kaupapa Maori approach to creating knowledge. In: Denzin NK, Lincoln Y, editors. The Landscape of Qualitative Research. 3rd ed. Thousand Oaks, CA: Sage Publications; 2008

[4] Nemutandani SM, Hendricks SJ, Mulaudzi MF. Decolonising the mindsets, attitudes and practices of the allopathic and indigenous health practitioners in postcolonial society: An exploratory approach in the management of patients. The African Journal of Primary Health Care & Family Medicine. 2018;**10**(1):e1-e8

[5] Ashforth A. Madumo: A Man Bewitched. Chicago, IL, USA: University of Chicago Press; 2000

[6] Ashforth A. Witchcraft, Violence, and Democracy in South Africa. Vol. 10. Chicago, IL, USA: University of Chicago Press; 2018. pp. e1-e8. DOI: 10.4102/phcfm.v10i1.1518

[7] Government Printers. Witchcraft Suppression Act, No. 3 of 1957. Pretoria: Republic of South Africa; 1957

[8] WHO Kobe Centre. Formalisation of Traditional Health Services. Planning for Cost-Effective Traditional Health Services in the New Century, 2002. Available from: http://www.who.or.jp/tm/research/bkg/5_formalisation.html [Accessed: 02 June 2015]

[9] Kale R. Traditional healers in South Africa: A parallel health care system. British Medical Journal. 1999;**3**(10):1182-1185

[10] Kaptchuk TJ, Miller FG. Viewpoint: What is the best and most ethical model for the relationship between mainstream and alternative medicine: Opposition, integration, or pluralism? Academic Medicine. 2005;**80**(3):286-290

[11] Lett J. Science, religion, and anthropology. In: Anthropology of religion: A handbook. 1997. pp. 103-120

[12] Chilisa B. Indigenous Research Methodologies. United States: SAGE Publications Inc; 2012

[13] Kuper J. Sangoma's Power Challenges State. Mail & Guardian; 2015

[14] Mafukata MA. Mandevu. Journal of Arts and Humanities. 2015;**4**(1):14-26

[15] Bereda JE. Traditional healing as a health care delivery system in a transcultural society [MA disseration]. Pretoria: University of South Africa; 2002

[16] Puckree T, Mkhize M, Mgobhozi Z, Lin J. African traditional healers: What health care professionals need to know. International Journal of Rehabilitation Research. 2002;**25**:247-251

[17] Mehl-Madrona L. Coyote Medicine: Lessons from Native American Healing. New York, USA: Scriber; 1997

[18] Brownlee F. Some experiences of native superstition and witchcraft. African Affairs. 1940;**39**:54-60

[19] Farrand D. Is a combined western and traditional health service for black patients desirable? South African Medical Journal. 1984;**66**(17):779-780

[20] Van Dyk AC. "Why me and not my neighbour?" HIV/AIDS care and counselling in a traditional African context. Curationis. 2001;**24**(3):4-11

[21] Van Wyk NC, Bourne B, Gericke GJ, Mokoena JD, Mulaudzi FM, Van Wyk IWC. Integrative Healthcare: A Guide to Meet the Needs of Africa. Cape Town: Juta and Co Ltd. South Africa; 2009

[22] Van Wyk NC. Similarities in the meta-paradigm of nursing and traditional healing: An attempt to contribute to the integration of traditional medicine and western medicine in Africa. Health SA Gesondheid. 2005;**10**:14-22

[23] Clark VLP, Creswell JW. Understanding Research: A consumer's Guide. Pearson Higher Ed; 2014

[24] Conley RJ. Cherokee Medicine Man: The Life and Work of a Modern-Day Healer. Norman, OK, USA: University of Oklahoma Press; 2005

[25] Denzin NK, Lincoln YS, Smith LT. Handbook of Critical and Indigenous Methodologies. Thousand Oaks, CA: Sage Publications; 2008

[26] Keikelame MJ, Swartz L. A thing full of stories': Traditional healers' explanations of epilepsy and perspectives on collaboration with biomedical health care in Cape Town. Transcultural Psychiatry. 2015;**52**(5):659-680

[27] WHO. Definitions of Health/ Wellness, 1946. Available from: http:// www.pnf.org/Definitions of_Health_C. pdf [Accessed: 20 January 2013]

[28] WHO. Traditional Medicine Strategy 2002-2005. Geneva, Switzerland: World Health Organisation; 2002

[29] Struthers S, Eschiti VS, Patchell B. Traditional indigenous healing: Part I. Complementary Therapies in Nursing & Midwifery. 2004;**10**:141-149

[30] King R. Ancient Remedies, New Disease: Involving Traditional Healers in Increasing Access to AIDS Care and Prevention in East Africa. Geneva: Joint United Nations Programme on HIV/ AIDS (UNAIDS); 2002

[31] Peu MD, Troskie R, Hattingh SP. 2001. The attitude of community health nurses towards integration of traditional healers. Curationis. 2001;**24**(3):49-55

[32] Unge C, Ragnarsson A, Ekström AM, Indalo D, Belita A, Carter J. Ilako F, Södergård B. The influence of traditional medicine and religion on discontinuation of ART in an urban informal settlement in Nairobi, Kenya, AIDS Care 2011; 23(7): 851-858

[33] Schatz E, Gilbert L, McDonald C. 'If the doctors see that they don't know how to cure the disease, they say it's AIDS': How older women in rural South Africa make sense of the HIV/AIDS epidemic. African Journal of AIDS Research. 2013;**12**(2):95-104

[34] Kuokkanen R. Towards an "indigenous paradigm" from a Sami perspective. The Canadian Journal of Native Studies. 2000;**20**(2):411-436

[35] Loughlin M, Bluhm R, Fuller J, Buetow S, Upshur RE, Borgerson K, et al. Philosophy, medicine and health care—where we have come from and where we are going. Journal of Evaluation in Clinical Practice. 2014;**20**(6):902-907

[36] Lovell B. The integration of bio-medicine and culturally based alternative medicine: Implications for health care providers and patients. Global Health Promotion. 2009;**16**(4):65-68

[37] Madamombe I. Traditional healers boost primary health care: Reaching

patients missed by modern medicine. Africa Renewal. 2006;**19**:10-12

[38] Niehaus I. Witchcraft, Power and Politics: Exploring the Occult in the South African Lowveld. London, UK: Pluto Press; 2001

[39] Novins DK, Beals J, Moore LA, Spicer P, Manson SM. Use of biomedical services and traditional healing options among American Indians: Sociodemographic correlates, spirituality, and ethnic identity. Medical Care. 2004;**42**:670-679

[40] Makhubu N. SABS Urged to Standardize Traditional Cures. Available from: http://www.iol.co.za/news/special-features/the-zuma-era/sabs-urged-to-standardise-traditional-cures-1.1161993#.U-h5TvldV8E [Accessed: 08 July 2014]

[41] Freeman M, Motsei M. Planning health care in South Africa: Is there a role of traditional healers? Social Science & Medicine. 1992;**34**(11):1183-1190

[42] Madiba SE. Are biomedicine health practitioners ready to collaborate with Traditional health practitioners in HIV and AIDS Care in Tutume sub District of Botswana? African Journal of Traditional, Complementary, and Alternative Medicines. 2010;7(3):219-224

[43] Flint AG, Payne JR. Reconciling the irreconcilable? HIV/AIDS and the potential for middle ground between the traditional and biomedical healthcare sectors in South Africa. Forum for Development Studies. 2013;**40**:47-68

[44] Flint AG. Traditional healing, biomedicine and the treatment of HIV/AIDS: Contrasting south African and native American experiences. International Journal of Environmental Research and Public Health. 2015;**12**(4):4321-4339

[45] O'Brien S, Broom A. HIV in (and out of) the clinic: Biomedicine, traditional medicine and spiritual healing in Harare. SAHARA-J. 2014;**11**:94-104

[46] World Health Organization (WHO). Promoting the Role of Traditional Medicine in Health Systems: A Strategy for the African Region 2001-2010. Harare: World Health Organization; 2000

[47] WHO. The WHO Traditional Medicine Strategy: 2014-2023. Geneva.; 2013

[48] Bodeker G. Complementary medicine and evidence. Annals of the Academy of Medicine, Singapore. 2000;**29**:3-6

[49] Stuttaford M, Al Makhamreh S, Coomans F, Harrington J, Himonga C, Hundt GL. The Right to the Traditional Health Practitioners Act, Act 22 of 2007. Pretoria, Republic of South Africa: Government Printers; 2007

[50] Petersen I, Baillie K, Bhana A. Understanding the benefits and challenges of community engagement in the development of community mental health services for common mental disorders: Lessons from a case study in a rural south African subdistrict site. Transcultural Psychiatry. 2012;**49**:418-437

[51] Davies JN. The development of scientific medicine in the African kingdom of Bunyoro-Kitara. Medical History. 1959;**3**(1):47-57. DOI: 10.1017/s0025727300024248

[52] Felkin RW. Notes on labour in Central Africa. Edinburgh Medical Journal. 1884;**29**(10):922-930

[53] Meetings of Societies. Edinburgh Medical Journal. 1884;**29**(9):833-843

[54] Wilson S. Research Is Ceremony: Indigenous Research Methods. Manitoba, Canada: Fernwood; 2008

[55] Henneman HA, Lee JL, Cohen JI. Collaboration: A concept analysis. Journal of Advanced Nursing. 1995;**21**:103-109

[56] Campbell-Hall V, Petersen I, Bhana A, Mjadu S, Hosegood V, Flisher AJ. Collaboration between traditional practitioners and primary health care staff in South Africa: Developing a workable partnership for community mental health services. Transcultural Psychiatry. 2010;**47**(4):610-628

[57] Liverpool J, Alexander R, Johnson M, Ebba EK, Francis S, Liverpool C. Western medicine and traditional healers: Partners in the fight against HIV/AIDS. Journal of the National Medical Association. 2004;**96**(6):822-825

[58] Kayombo EJ, Uiso FC, Mbwambo ZH, Mahunnah RL, Moshi MJ, Mgonda YH. Experience of initiating collaboration of traditional healers in managing HIV and AIDS in Tanzania. Journal of Ethnobiology and Ethnomedicine. 2007;**3**:6-10

[59] Gqaleni N, Hlongwane T, Khondo C, Mbatha M, Mhlongo S. Biomedical and Traditional Healing Collaboration on HIV and AIDS in KwaZulu-Natal, South Africa. Vol. 2. Universitas Forum; 2011. Available from: http://www.universitasforum.org/index.php/ojs/article/view/62/240 [Accessed: 08 June 2014]

[60] Jernigan VB, Jacob T, Tribal Community Research Team, Styne D. The adaptation and implementation of a community-based participatory research curriculum to build tribal research capacity. American Journal of Public Health. 2015;**105**(Suppl 3): S424-S432

[61] Schrage M. Shared Minds: The New Technologies of Collaboration. USA: Random House; 1990

[62] Smith LT. Decolonizing Methodologies: Research and Indigenous Peoples. 2nd ed. United Kingdom: Zed Books Ltd; 2012

[63] Vogel V. American Indian Medicine. Norman, OK, USA: University of Oklahoma Press; 1970

Chapter 6

Public Health Effects of Wood Fuel in Africa: Bioenergy from Tree Commodities as a Sustainable Remedy

Serge Mandiefe Piabuo and Janice Tieguhong Puatwoe

Abstract

Globally, about 2.8 million people depend on solid wood fuel for energy, developing countries account for more than 90% of this population. About 70% of households in Sub-Saharan depend on wood fuel for energy. The combustion of solid wood fuel indoors and outdoors emits smoke with particles that have adverse effects on the health of users. This chapter investigates the health effects of wood fuel combustion on the users and evaluates the potential of bioenergy from tree commodities as a sustainable remedy. Through a literature review of literature on health effects of wood fuel, this chapter shows that acute respiratory infections, lung problems, cataract, cardiovascular diseases and bronchitis are common public health issues that wood fuel users suffer from. Bioenergy provides a clean and healthier alternative energy for rural households; tree commodities provide a more sustainable option for millions of Africans who depend on tree commodities for their livelihoods. Estimates show that between 4.26E+06 and 1.14E+07 MW of bioelectricity can be generated from tree commodities, while 6.26E+08 to 1.71E+09 litres of bioethanol and 4.27E+08 to 1.14E+09 litres of biodiesel can potentially be generated from tree commodities. Significant government support, financial investment, public-private partnerships and community sensitisation are required for tree commodities to sustainable provide clean and healthy bioenergy to rural Africa.

Keywords: solid wood fuel, respiratory infections, bioenergy, tree commodities

1. Introduction

Renewable energy remains the most dominant energy source in Africa with wood sources accounting for a large share of biomass energy. Although wood energy accounts for only 10% of global primary energy, about 2.8 million people depend on wood fuel for cooking and heating [1, 2]. The extraction and use of wood for energy is prominent in developing countries with more than 70% of households in Sub-Saharan Africa depending on wood energy. Access to modern energy remains a major problem in developing countries; however, poorer countries suffer more from energy access problems [3]. Poor access to modern energy rates in less developed countries (LDCs) and Sub-Saharan (SSA) countries remain high at 91 and 83%, respectively. In SSA, the access to electricity and modern energy remains a major constraint with 560 and 625 peopled deprived, respectively. Poor access to modern energy equally varies between urban and rural areas in Africa; in SSA, 66% of the population use solid fuels for heating and cooking, 13% use charcoal while kerosene, electricity and LPG follow with 7, 6, and 5%, respectively [4].

The global use of wood fuel for cooking and heating has devastating negative health effects with 2 million deaths annually from pneumonia, cancer and chronic lung diseases due to exposure to pollution from biomass combustion. Women and children are most affected by these diseases with about 44% of these deaths being children and 60% of adult death being women [3]. More than 50% of deaths from pneumonia, cancer and chronic lung diseases in LDCs and SSA is due to combustion of solid fuels, while only 38% for developing countries in general [3]. Household air pollution (HAP) is a major driver of global health emergencies with about 4.3 million premature deaths; non-communicable diseases (NCDs) account for 3.8 million deaths (WHO, 2016). HAP accounts for more than 33% deaths related to chronic obstructive pulmonary in both low- and middle-income countries, 17% of deaths related to cancer, 15% of ischaemic heart disease and 25% stroke-related deaths (WHO, 2016). This chapter seeks to review the different diseases caused by incomplete combustion of biomass for energy and how bioenergy from tree commodities can be a sustainable remedy.

2. Solid fuelwood combustion and health effects in rural Africa

Several scientific publications have reported significant health effects of wood fuel combustion for cooking especially through open fire in rural areas [5, 6]. Childhood respiratory infections such as pneumonia and otitis media have been highly associated with fuel wood combustion [5]. Among women, there is a high association between fuelwood combustion and high risk of chronic bronchitis and chronic obstructive pulmonary disease, especially asthma and cataract. Indoor combustion of fuelwood has been called the 'kitchen killer' because about 1.6 million deaths have been registered as a result, accounting for 2.7% of global disease burden (WHO, 2007).

The combustion process generates smoke; this smoke contains a complex mixture of numerous particles and substances composed of varied organic and inorganic compounds [7, 8]. These compounds are toxic and dangerous to the health system of human beings; they contain carbon monoxide (CO), nitrogen and sulphur oxide (NO_2, CO_2), aldehydes, particulate matter PM (PM10), volatile organic compounds, chlorinated dioxins, free radicals and polycyclic aromatic hydrocarbons [8]. The health effects on children less than 5 years and women are not homogenous. Respiratory infections such as pneumonia are common in young children less than 5 years, while chronic obstructive pulmonary disease (CORP) and lung cancer are common in women. Other health effects such as adverse pregnancy and eye diseases are equally common [9, 10].

To better appreciate the health effects of fuelwood combustion, a review of literature for over 17 papers was done. The objective was to capture the most prevalent health outcomes as a result of indoor and outdoor fuelwood combustion. The table below (**Table 1**) shows the results of the reviewed papers in a summary form [11].

The exposure to smoke due to cooking fuel accelerates respiratory-related illnesses such as dry cough and nose irritation; further analysis equally underscores high association with headache, dry cough and hypertension [25]. The review above shows significant health effects related to respiratory-related diseases, of the 17

Author(s)	Study carried out	Country/region	Methodology	Major findings	Discovered health outcomes
Bruce et al. [12]	Indoor biofuel air pollution and respiratory health: the role of confounding factors among women in highland Guatemala	Guatemala	Cross-sectional analysis	The prevalence of reported cough and phlegm was significantly high among women using open fire	Cough and phlegm
Vinod et al.	Biomass cooking fuels and prevalence of tuberculosis in India	India	Logistic regression	Substantial prevalence of active tuberculosis in person living in households using biomass cooking fuels (wood or dung)	Tuberculosis
Neelam et al. [13]	Indoor air pollution from biomass combustion and its adverse health effects in central India: an exposure response study	India	Qualitative analysis with the use of peak expiratory rate flow	Exposure to biomass smoke causes health related problems	Eye irritation, headache, bronchitis, cataract and respiratory problems
Rajiv [14]	Disease burden of fuelwood combustion pollutants in rural households of the Himalayas	India	Qualitative analysis	The use of fuelwood has an impact on health	Acute lower respiratory infection, chronic obstructive pulmonary disease and lung cancer
Zschauer [15]	Households' energy supply and the use of fuelwood	Kenya (case of Taita Hills)	A qualitative analysis	The use of fuelwood has a negative impact on health	Eye problem, respiratory problems (coughing irritation of the lungs and sniffles), tuberculosis
Silwal and McKay [16]	The impact of cooking with firewood on respiratory health	Indonesia	A unique Indonesian household survey	Individuals living in households that cook with firewood have lower lung capacity than those that cook with cleaner fuels; impact being larger on women and children	Lower lung capacity
Agrawal and Yamamoto [17]	Effect of indoor air pollution from biomass and solid fuel combustion on symptoms of preeclampsia/eclampsia in Indian women	India	Logistic regression	Women living in households using biomass and solid fuels have two times higher likelihood of reporting preeclampsia/ eclampsia symptoms than those living in households using cleaner fuels	Preeclampsia/eclampsia
Sharma et al. [18]	Types of cooking stove and risk of acute lower respiratory infection among under five children: a cross sectional study in Rasuwa, Nepal	Nepal	Cross-sectional survey	The presence of acute lower respiratory infection among users of biomass fuels	Lower respiratory infections
Zoë et al.	Residential heating with wood and coal: health impacts and policy options in Europe and North America	Europe and North America	Qualitative analysis	Evidence links emissions from wood and coal heating to serious health effects	Respiratory and cardiovascular mortality and morbidity

Author(s)	Study carried out	Country/region	Methodology	Major findings	Discovered health outcomes
Tao et al. [19]	Residential solid fuel combustion and impacts on air quality and human health	Mainland China	A qualitative analysis	Evidence showed that household air pollution in china causes a range of health outcomes	Respiratory diseases; asthma, lung cancer, cardiovascular diseases; heart diseases, stroke and immune system impairment
Zidago & Wang [20]	Charcoal and fuelwood consumption and its impacts on environment	Cote d'Ivoire (Case Study of Yopougon Area)	A qualitative analysis through the households was used	The production and consumption of charcoal have a negative impact on the health of its producers and consumers	Burns, chronic cough
Das et al. [21]	Biomass cooking fuels (firewood, Charcoal) and health outcomes for women in Malawi	Malawi	Cross-sectional sample analysis	The use of firewood and charcoal for cooking is associated with five categories of health outcomes.	cardiopulmonary, respiratory, neurologic, eye health and burns
Kadafa et al. [22]	The health impact of fuelwood Utilisation on users	Nigeria (case study of Yelwa Village)	A qualitative analysis	It was discovered that fuelwood has health implications on its users	Eye problem, respiratory problem and heart diseases
Mbanya and Sridhar [23]	PM10 emissions from cooking fuels in Nigerian households and their impact on women and children	Ibadan, Nigeria	Qualitative analysis	Majority of the respondents complained of health-related issues during and after cooking with cough, breathing problems, skin and eyes irritation being the most common	Cough, breathing problems, skin and eyes irritation
Badamassi et al. [24]	The effects of particulate matter (PM2.5) from household combustion on life expectancy in SSA	43 SSA countries	GMM and panel cointegration model	Household particulate matter (PM2.5) is significantly and negatively associated with higher life expectancy in the long run especially with females	Lower life expectancy
Mohapatra et al. [25]	Health impact on women using solid cooking fuels in rural area of Cuttack District, Odisha	Cuttack District, Odisha	Cross-sectional study with the use of Chi-square test	Exposure to smoke from cooking fuel is significantly associated with the prevalence symptoms of headache, dry cough and hypertension	Headache, dry cough and hypertension

Table 1.
Review of health effects of fuelwood combustion on users.

studies, 13 underscore respiratory tract infections as major outcome of fuelwood combustion. The most common forms of the respiratory tract infections are dry cough, breathing problems, neurologic problems, cardiopulmonary, cardiovascular diseases, asthma and lung cancer [20, 23, 25].

Lower life expectancy has equally been reported by Badamassi et al. [24]; they underscore that combustion of particulate matter (PM2.5) has adverse effect on life expectancy in the long run, with a greater negative effect on female life expectancy. Their study equally shows higher life expectancy for exposed households in urban areas and countries with higher GDP per capita; this can be explained by the fact that these groups can have better access to health care. Cardiovascular diseases have equally been reported to be associated with fuelwood combustion [19]. Other diseases such as asthma, stroke and immune system impairment have equally been attributed to indoor and outdoor pollution as a result of fuelwood combustion [19].

3. Bioenergy as a sustainable and health energy source

The precedent section underscores that about 700 million (82%) of Africans are at high risk of household air pollution due to the use of solid-fuel for cooking with an average 581,000 deaths annually [26]. Globally, the demand for solid-fuel for cooking has reduced considerably, average 50–40%; however, Africa stagnates at 80% over the decades. Escalating fuel cost, population growth and supply interruptions have accounted for reduced demand in modern fuel demand. Even when households use modern fuel for cooking, they often combine with solid-fuel cooking stoves [27, 28]. The production of energy from biological waste using modern production techniques has been promoted as a way out of this public health crisis. Significant efforts have been made through different cross-country projects aimed at producing clean and modern bioenergy such as liquid and gel biofuels. Efforts to promote more clean energy sources such as ethanol stoves and clean cooking stoves have not met required objectives due to poor market penetration and high subsidisation cost [26]. However, in West Africa, ethanol businesses have registered steady growth with over 200,000 stoves reported in different countries over 3 years.

Biogas projects in East Africa played an important role in changing mindsets and providing a cleaner alternative for households. In Kenya, three biogas operating units have been constructed by the Taita Taveta Wildlife Forum (TTWF) as part of a pilot project aimed at improving access to clean energy. This is promoted because biogas produces clean energy, with less indoor and outdoor pollution, thus reduced chances of respiratory tract infections and heart infections. The biogas production process equally generates nitrogen and liquids rich in nutrients that can serve as fertilizers.

The use of bioenergy as an alternative to solid-fuels is encouraged because through the different conversion techniques, energy is generated which enhances good combustion with limited emission of air pollutants. This form of energy is good both for indoor and outdoor use at urban and rural areas. The promotion of this form of energy is equally backed by the constant availability of biomass for bioenergy conversion, with by-products that are equally good for crop cultivation.

4. Bioenergy from tree commodities as a sustainable remedy

Tree commodities commonly referred to as 'money trees' are trees grown principally for cash by many African countries. These trees are often the principal source of income for most farmers in Sub-Saharan Africa. In Africa, cocoa, coffee, oil palm, industrial round wood, cashew, almonds and walnuts are the principal tree commodities. These tree commodities are a source of income to millions of Africans and accounts for tons of agricultural biomass produced annually. Agricultural biomass after extraction of the fruit of these products is often left to rot in the farms while farmers suffer from energy shortages. Residue from tree commodities such as husk of cocoa and coffee, empty fruit bunch of oil palm, forest thinning from timber exploitation and shell of almonds are potential sustainable feedstock for bioenergy generation.

With the appropriate technology and adoption by community members, tree commodities can serve as a pathway for sustainable bioenergy generation without changing land use and without extra efforts from the farmer to find feedstock. The potential of using bioenergy for reducing health effects of traditional biomass for combustion is backed by the fact that tree commodities are often found in rural areas, with serious energy deficiencies, high prevalence of respiratory tract infections as a result of solid wood fuel combustion.

The potential of using bioenergy from tree commodities as a clean energy source is evaporated in this chapter by looking at two aspects: (1) by evaluating the potential in terms of quantity of bioenergy that can be generated by tree commodities and (2) operational framework for bioenergy from tree commodities to effectively serve rural population as a renewable and healthy energy source.

4.1 Evaluating the potential quantity of bioenergy from tree commodities in Africa

To evaluate the potential of bioenergy from tree commodities, seven tree commodities were chosen for analysis based on the number of farmers or population affected by the different tree commodities. The chosen tree commodities are coffee (*Coffea arabica* and *Coffea canephora*), cocoa (*Theobroma cacao*), oil palm (Arecaceae), walnuts (*Juglans*), cashew (*Anacardium occidentale*), almonds (*Prunus dulcis*) and industrial round wood. When evaluating bionenergy potential from tree commodities, provisions are taken for the use of residue for other uses, such as soil nutrient. The extraction equally considers other aspects such as weather, soil types, crop yields, harvesting technique and wind patterns [29, 30]. Researchers have evaluated different soil systems and uses of residue from biomass and conclude that 44–64% of biomass residue can sustainably be used for biomass generation [29–31]. Using a more conservative approach, this chapter uses a 20% extraction rate to estimate bioenergy production from tree commodities. Data from the FAO (2018) database serve as a basis for estimation in this chapter. Sustainable extraction rates were gotten from literature review from a variety of sources; residue to product ratio and moisture content was extracted from OECD/IEA [32]. Moisture content for coffee and cocoa was obtained from NREL [33], oil palm from Husain et al. [34], walnuts from Uzan and Yaman [35], cashew from Mohod et al. [36], industrial round wood from FAO [37] and almonds from [38]. **Table 2** below shows the results of bioenergy potential from tree commodities for bioelectricity, biochemical ethanol and diesel.

Bioenergy generation from tree commodities in Africa can potentially generate between 4.26E+06 and 1.14E+07 MW of bioelectricity from the seven-tree commodities while 6.26E+08 and 1.71E+09 L of bioethanol can potentially be generated from tree commodities. Tree commodities equally can equally serve as an important potential source for diesel, estimates from tree commodities show that 4.27E+08–1.14E+09 L can be generated from tree commodities.

Tree commodity	Average	Type of residue	Residue to product ratio	Moisture content	Lower heating value	Residue (wet tons)	Residue (Bone dry tons)	Residue. 30% Sustainable Extraction (bone dry tons)	Energy potential (bone dry x MK/kg) GJ	bioelectricity		Biochemical ethanol		Thermochemical syngas to Ficher Tropsch diesel	
										15% efficiency MW h (low)	40% efficiency MW h (high)	(low) litres	(high) litres	Low (litres)	High (litres)
Coffee	1,149,511	Husk	2.10	0.15	12.56	2.41E+06	2.05E+06	6.16E+05	7.73E+06	3.25E+05	8.66E+05	6.77E+07	1.85E+08	4.62E+07	1.23E+08
cocoa	3,398,572	Pods, Husk	1.00	0.15	15.48	3.40E+06	2.89E+06	8.67E+05	1.34E+07	5.63E+05	1.50E+06	9.53E+07	2.60E+08	6.50E+07	1.73E+08
oil palm	19,402,457	empty fruit bunch (EFB)	0.25	0.60	15.51	4.85E+06	1.94E+06	5.82E+05	9.03E+06	3.79E+05	1.01E+06	6.40E+07	1.75E+08	4.37E+07	1.16E+08
Walnuts, with shell	37,471	shell	2.00	0.15	16.70	7.49E+04	6.37E+04	1.91E+04	3.19E+05	1.34E+04	3.57E+04	2.10E+06	5.73E+06	1.43E+06	3.82E+06
Cashew	1,713,285	Shell	2	0.15	23.98	3.43E+06	2.91E+06	8.74E+05	2.10E+07	8.80E+05	2.35E+06	9.61E+07	2.62E+08	6.55E+07	1.75E+08
Industrial round wood	28,764,846	forest thinning	0.5	0.4	18.3	1.44E+07	8.63E+06	2.59E+06	4.74E+07	1.99E+06	5.31E+06	2.85E+08	7.77E+08	1.94E+08	5.18E+08
Almonds, with Shell	281,549	shell	2	0.15	18.86	5.63E+05	4.79E+05	1.44E+05	2.71E+06	1.14E+05	3.03E+05	1.58E+07	4.31E+07	1.08E+07	2.87E+07
Total									**1.02E+08**	**4.26E+06**	**1.14E+07**	**6.26E+08**	**1.71E+09**	**4.27E+08**	**1.14E+09**

Table 2.
Tree commodities as a source of bioenergy, bioelectricity, biochemical ethanol and diesel.

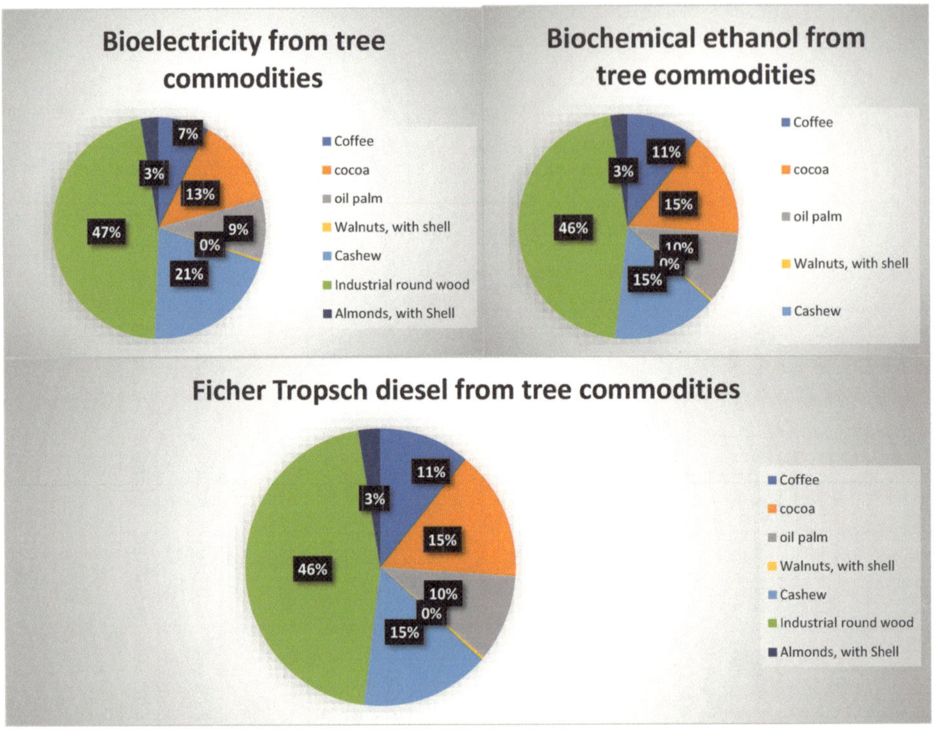

Figure 1.
Percentage of bioenergy generated from different tree commodities.

The figure above (**Figure 1**) shows that bioenergy generation from industrial round wood is the highest averaging 46% for the bioelectricity (47%), bioethanol (46%) and Fischer-Tropsch diesel (46%). Cashew shell can equally contribute significantly bioenergy production accounting for 15% of diesel and bioethanol and 21% of electricity. Cocoa comes third as the highest contributor, accounting for 13% of bioelectricity and 15% of bioethanol and diesel. Coffee follows representing 7% of bioelectricity production and 11% of bioethanol and diesel. Oil palm equally contributes significantly to this potential, with 9% of total potential of bioelectricity and 10% of bioethanol and diesel potential production. These percentages underscore the significant potential contribution of tree commodities in generation clean, modern bioenergy than can potentially reduce public health diseases associated with the combustion of solid-fuel biomass. However, for this to be a reality, a lot of policy and operational tools must be put in place and readily available at local level.

4.2 Operational framework for bioenergy from tree commodities to effectively serve rural population as a renewable and healthy energy source

For modern bioenergy to serve as a potential clean energy source for rural African communities and millions of Africans at risk of respiratory tract infections and cardio-vascular diseases, several important pre-requisites are required.

i. **Government support**: For modern bioenergy to be a mainstay in rural Africa and reduce incidences of deaths through solid-fuel combustion, government authorities must support the development of modern bioenergy infrastructure. This requires significant shift in policy and investment from the government and different multi-lateral partners. The understanding of policy makers of the health advantages of developing modern bioenergy systems coupled with sustainable management practices is key to pushing a policy reform agenda for modern bioenergy generation in Africa.

ii. **Significant financial investment:** Developing modern bioenergy generation systems for tree commodities requires significant financial investment. Multi-lateral development agencies aimed at reducing carbon emissions and promoting healthy living of populations can shift their funding streams to bioenergy generation. For this to happen, they must understand that modern bioenergy does not only reduce carbon emission, deforestation but can equally save the lives of millions of people potentially at high risk of respiratory tract infections as a result of solid-fuel combustion. This financing should go along way in investing not only in infrastructure for bioenergy development but equally in community adapted distribution mechanisms that will enhance adoption of new form of energy. These new energy sources should be cheaper and more efficient for adoption to be faster.

4.3 Sensitization and training on modern bioenergy generation from tree commodities

The acceptance and adoption of new bioenergy as an improved energy source required that users understand the key advantages. Thus, sensitisation at different levels with a clear distinction of advantages over traditional solid-fuel combustion should be made. Adoption can equally be facilitated by developing simple modern bioenergy generation systems that are adapted to rural context with minimal investment. This will enhance adoption especially when the cost of generation is relatively low and accrued advantages and multi-scaled.

i. **Public-private partnerships and cooperation**: The developments of sustainable modern bioenergy systems stakeholder buy-in a different levels and scales. Thus, a public-private partnership scheme is very important. The private sector with similar objectives can collaborate with government agencies in developing the bioenergy agenda as financial partners, technical support agents, or for policy advocacy. International cooperation is equally important for broad-based decision-making with local impacts coupled with strategic deployment frameworks adapted to different contexts. Understanding different stakeholders from different countries is paramount to advancing bioenergy generation.

Author details

Serge Mandiefe Piabuo[1*] and Janice Tieguhong Puatwoe[2]

1 World Agroforestry Centre (ICRAF), Yaounde, Cameroon

2 Technical Training Research Centre for Development (TTRECED), Yaounde, Cameroon

*Address all correspondence to: p.mandiefe@cgiar.org

References

[1] IEA. Annual Report 2006, IEA Bioenergy. IEA BIOENERGY: EXCO; 2007:01. 2006. Available from: http://www.globalbioenergy.org/uploads/media/0707_IEA_-_Bioenergy_annual_report.pdf

[2] World Bank. World Development Indicators 2016 (English). World Development Indicators. Washington, D.C: World Bank Group; 2016. Available from: http://documents.worldbank.org/curated/en/805371467990952829/World-development-indicators-2016

[3] WHO. WHO Natural Ventilation for Infection Control in Health-care Settings. 2009. Available from: https://www.who.int/water_sanitation_health/publications/natural_ventilation/en/ed^eds: World Health

[4] WHO. World Health Statistics. 2010. ISBN: 978 92 4 156398 7. Available from: https://www.who.int/gho/publications/world_health_statistics/EN_WHS10_Full.pdf?ua=1

[5] World Health Organization. The health effects of indoor air pollution exposure in developing countries/by Nigel Bruce, Rogelio Perez-Padilla, and Rachel Albalak. 2002. World Health Organization. Available from: https://apps.who.int/iris/handle/10665/67496

[6] UNDP and WHO. The Energy Access Situation in Developing Countries: A Review Focusing on the Least Developed Countries and Sub-Saharan Africa. © Copyright UNDP and World Health Organization. 2009. Available from: https://www.undp.org/content/dam/undp/library/Environment%20and%20Energy/Sustainable%20Energy/energy-access-situation-in-developing-countries.pdf

[7] Zelikoff JT, Schermerhorn KR, Fang K, Cohen MD, Schlesinger RB. A role for associated transition metals in the immunotoxicity of inhaled ambient particulate matter (pm). Environmental Health Perspectives. 2002;**110**(Suppl 5): 871-875. DOI: 10.1289/ehp.02110s5871

[8] Naeher LP, Brauer M, Lipsett M, Zelikoff JT, Simpson CD, Koenig JQ, et al. Woodsmoke health effects: A review. Inhalation Toxicology. 2007;**19**: 67-106

[9] Bruce N, Perez-Padilla R, Albalak R. Indoor air pollution in developing countries: a major environmental and public health challenge. Bulletin of the World Health Organization. 2000;**78**: 108-1092. PMID: 1101945

[10] Ezzati M, Lopez AD, Rodgers A, Murray CJL. Comparative Quantification of Health Risks: Global and Regional Burden of Disease Attributable to Selected Major Risk Factors. Geneva: World Health Organization; 2004

[11] Tao S et al. Quantifying the rural residential energy transition in China from 1992 to 2012 through a representative National Survey. Nature Energy. 2018;**3**:567-573

[12] Bruce N, Neufeld L, Boy E, West C. Indoor biofuel air pollution and respiratory health: The role of confounding factors among women in highland Guatemala. International Journal of Epidermiology. 1998;**27**(3): 454-458

[13] Neelam DS, Narlawar UW, Phatak MS. Indoor air pollution from biomass combustion and its adverse health effects in Central India: An exposure-response study. Indian Journal of Community Medicine. 2012;**38**(3):162-167. DOI: 10.4103/0970-0218.116353

[14] Rajiv R. Disease burden of fuelwood combustion pollutants in rural

households of the Himalayas. India. Indian Council of Forestry Research & Education. Indian Journal of Public Health. 2012;**9**(1):71-79. DOI: 10.2427/5631

[15] Zschauer K. Households' Energy Supply and the Use of Fuelwood in the Taita Hills. Kenya: University of Helsinki; 2012

[16] Silwal, McKay. The Impact of Cooking with Firewood on Respiratory Health: Evidence from Indonesia. Working Paper Series No. 72. 2014. Available from: https://www.sussex.ac.uk/webteam/gateway/file.php?name=wps-72-2014.pdf&site=24

[17] Agrawal S, Yamamoto S. Effect of indoor air pollution from biomass and solid fuel combustion on symptoms of preeclampsia/eclampsia in Indian women. 2015. Available from: www.ncbi.nlm.nih.gov.

[18] Sharma S, Bhandari N, Bhandari R, Wagle K, Adhikari M. Types of cooking stove and risk of acute lower respiratory infection among under-five children: A cross sectional study in Rasuwa, a Himalayan district of Nepal. Health Prospect Journal of Public Health. 2015; **14**(1):1-7. DOI: 10.3126/hprospect.v14i1.1236

[19] Tao S, Cao J, Kan H, Li B, Shen G, Shen H, et al. Residential solid fuel combustion and impacts on air quality and human health in mainland China. Global Alliance for Clean Cook stoves. 2016

[20] Zidago AP, Wang Z. Charcoal and Fuelwood consumption and its impacts on environment in cote d'Ivoire (case study of Yopougon area). Environment and Natural Resources Research. 2016;**6**(4):2016. DOI: 10.5539/enrr.v6n4p26

[21] Das I, Jagger P, Yeatts K. Biomass cooking fuels and health outcomes for women in Malawi. EcoHealth. 2017; **14**:7-19

[22] Kadafa A, Medugu N, Stephen DK, Medan J. The health impact of fuel wood utilization on users in Yelwa Village, Nasarawa state, Nigeria. International Journal of Sciences: Basic and Applied Research. 2017;**24**(6):174-191

[23] Mbanya V, Sridhar M. PM10 emissions from cooking fuels in Nigerian households and their impact on women and children. Health. 2017;**9**: 1721-1733. DOI: 10.4236/health.2017.913126

[24] Badamassi A, Xu D, Mahaman Y, Boubacar H. The effects of PM2.5 from household combustion on life expectancy in sub-Saharan Africa. International Journal of Environmental Research and Public Health. 2018; **15**(4):748

[25] Mohapatra I, Das SC, Samantaray S. Health impact on women using solid cooking fuels in rural area of Cuttack district, Odisha. Journal of Family Medicine and Primary Care. 2018; 7:11-15

[26] World Bank. World Bank Annual Report 2014—Open Knowledge Repository. 2014. Available from: https://openknowledge.worldbank.org/bitstream/handle/10986/20093/WB%20Annual%20Report%202014_EN.pdf?sequence=13 [Accessed: 15 December 2019]

[27] Hiemstra-Van der Horst G, Hovorka AJ. Reassessing the "energy ladder": Household energy use in Maun, Botswana. Energy Policy. 2008;**36**:3333-3344. DOI: 10.1016/j.enpol.2008.05.006

[28] Masera OR, Saatkamp BD, Kammen DM. From linear fuel switching to multiple cooking strategies: A critique and alternative to the energy ladder model. World Development. 2000;**28**:

2083-2103. DOI: 10.1016/S0305-750X(00)00076-0

[29] Helwig T, Jannasch R, Samson R, DeMaio A, Caumartin D. Agricultural Biomass Residue Inventories and Conversion Systems for Energy Production in Eastern Canada. Ste. Anne-de-Bellevue, QC, Canada: Resource Efficient Agricultural Production (REAP); 2002

[30] Lal R. Crop residues as soil amendments and feedstock for bioethanol production. Waste Management. 2008;**28**:747-758

[31] Scarlat N, Martinov M, Dallemand J-F. Assessment of the availability of agricultural crop residues in the European Union: Potential and limitations for bioenergy use. Waste Management. 2010;**30**:1889-1897

[32] OECD/IEA. Sustainable Production of Second-Generation Biofuels, Potential and Perspective in Major Economies and Developing Countries. Information Paper. Paris, France: OECD, IEA; 2010

[33] National Renewable Energy Laboratory. Sustainability Report. 2008. Available from: https://www.nrel.gov/docs/gen/fy09/45638.pdf [Accessed: 18 December 2019]

[34] Husain Z, Zainal ZA, Abdullah MZ. Analysis of biomass-residue-based cogeneration system in palm oil mills. Biomass & Bioenergy. 2003;**24**:117-124. Available from: https://www.nrel.gov/docs/gen/fy09/45638.pdf [Accessed: 16 December 2019]

[35] Uzun BB, Yaman E. Thermogravimetric pyrolysis of walnut shell an assessment of kinetic modeling. In: International Conference on Industrial Waste and Waste Water Treatment Valorization, held in Athens, Greece. 21st–23rd May 2015

[36] Mohod A, Jain S, Powar A. Cashew nut shell waste: Availability in small-scale cashew processing industries and its fuel properties for gasification. ISRN Renewable Energy. 2011;**2011**:1-4. DOI: 10.5402/2011/346191

[37] FAO. Fuelwood Supplies in the Developing Countries, by de Montalembert MR. Clement J. Rome; 1983

[38] Parikh J, Channiwala SA, Ghosal GK. A correlation for calculating HHV from proximate analysis of solid fuels. Fuel. 2005;**84**:487-494

Chapter 7

Cultural Practices and Health Consequences: Health or Habits, the Choice Is Ours

Radiance Ogundipe

Abstract

Human beings are social animals with an innate desire to conform to socially accepted norms and values. Over periods of time, some of these norms become standards that all members of the community are expected to adhere to. Deviance from these standards is seen as absurd, wrong, or frankly abnormal. However, many of these cultural mores have no scientific basis and, some of them actually promote behaviors with negative health consequences. This chapter examines the cultural practices of some communities in Africa and their health consequences and, explores ways to address the challenges.

Keywords: communities, cultural practices, communal behaviour, health, behavioral change, motivation

1. Introduction

Human beings are social animals with an innate desire to conform to socially accepted norms and values. Over periods of time, some of these norms become standards that all members of the community are expected to adhere to. Deviance from these standards is seen as absurd, wrong, or frankly abnormal. However, many of these cultural mores have no scientific basis and, some of them actually promote behaviors with negative health consequences. While the health consequences of many of these practices may not be of public health significance, some have major short and long term impact on the health of individuals in the community. The more difficult ones to appreciate are those practices that do not immediately appear to have deleterious health consequences but, may have direct and indirect long term impact on the health of individuals, families and the community.

It must be appreciated that not all cultural practices are deleterious to health. Some are actually beneficial. For example, many communities in rural Africa forbid intimacy between a newly delivered mother and her partner for some months. This practice encourages child spacing and allows the mother to adequately breastfeed the new baby [1].

Cultural practices are varied across different contexts. They have usually been viewed as the normal way of life and may be actively encouraged in the communities.

This chapter is a review of literature on some cultural practices with overt health consequences. It seeks to highlight some of these practices in Africa as prototype and explore ways they can be addressed at public health level.

2. Search strategy

The searches were conducted on Google Scholar and PubMed using the following mesh terms: cultural practices; culture; health impact; and health consequences:

1. health consequences and cultural practices/"health consequences," "cultural practices";

2. "health risks," "cultural practices," and "culture";

3. how cultural practices affect health; and

4. "health implications" and "cultural practice."

A review of the abstracts of many of the articles got from the search did not provide the information desired for this chapter. However, a few articles provided the information extracted and was systematically reviewed.

3. Female Genital Mutilation (FGM)

This is a cultural practice that has attracted worldwide concern due to its profound deleterious consequences on the health, reproductive ability and psychological wellbeing of women [2]. It is a cultural practice common in parts of Africa, Asia and Middle East. Part of, or the entire external female genital is cut off as a cultural practice believed to reduce libido and enhance the chastity of women. More than 200 million girls and women mostly from the above mentioned areas have experienced FGM. The procedure is usually done by traditional attendants using unsterile devices on girls from the ages of infancy to about 15 years of age. Apart from the risk of infections from the unhygienic way the procedure is carried out and the unsterile equipment used, there can be severe bleeding, injuries to the urinary tract as well as subsequent increased risk of complicated childbirth and death of the newborn [1]. The paradox of the practice is that rather than promote sexual chastity as believed by the practitioners, FGM actually causes painful sexual intercourse and difficulties achieving sexual satisfaction. It has absolutely no health benefit for the women and it has been associated with depression, anxiety, post-traumatic stress disorder and low self-esteem [1].

4. The Wodaabe's wife stealing night dance

This is a cultural practice found among the Wodaabe tribe, a sub-group of the Fulani ethnic communities of the northern parts of Nigeria, northeastern Cameroon, the western region of Central African Republic and southwestern Chad [3]. The tribe holds a cultural dancing festival at night. While dancing, a man is allowed to steal and carry home any woman he likes whether the woman is married or not. The health implication of this cultural practice is obvious. Sexually transmitted infections including HIV as well as unwanted pregnancies may result, with attendant consequences.

5. The Chawe cultural corpse washing ritual

Among the Chawe community, a Bantu tribe mostly found in Malawi, when a member of the tribe dies, the throat of the corpse is sliced open and water is run through then squeezed out until it comes out looking clear [3]. This water from the corpse is collected and used to prepare a meal for the entire community.

The health implication of this cultural practice is the spread of infectious diseases, which may have led to the death of the deceased tribal member in the first instance. Gastrointestinal diseases like gastroenteritis, food poisoning, hepatitis, enteric fever or cholera among others, may result from this cultural practice.

6. The Banyankole tribe's potency test

In many tribes of Africa, older females play advisory roles as matrons to newly wedded couples [3]. They usually advise on how the woman especially, should relate to her husband so that they can avoid marital frictions. Some of these advice include how the woman is expected to behave in bed with her husband so that he does not stray out for sexual satisfaction. However, the Banyankole tribe of Uganda take this innocuous and possibly helpful cultural practice to another dimension. The older female who plays the role of the matron to the couple is required to test the sexual potency of the intending husband by having sexual intercourse with him. In addition, she has to test the "purity" of the intending wife by examining for her hymen before they are allowed to marry.

Here again, this cultural practice may promote sexually transmitted infections, female genital tract infection as well as lower the self-esteem of the vulnerable young couple, who may be ridiculed if declared to have fall short by the more experienced matron.

7. Bull jumping ritual in Ethiopia

Young boys in some communities in Ethiopia are required to prove their manliness by stripping naked, running and jumping on the back of a bull [3]. This is followed by running on the backs of a line of several bulls held by their horns and tails by the adults. This cultural practice is called Hamar. Female friends of the young boy are then required to prove their loyalty to him by smearing their bodies with ochre mixed with fat and dancing while being given several lashes on their bare backs.

This cultural practice may result in trauma, fractures or even loss of life. Infections like tetanus may result from contamination of the injuries and abrasions caused by the lashes.

8. Sharo beating ritual of Benin

Among the Fulani tribe of Benin, an intending husband may be required to endure severe beating to prove his worthiness of the wife [3]. If the husband is unable to endure the flogging, the marriage is called off.

Many intending husbands have died from the flogging ritual and consequently, it is no longer a compulsory requirement for marriage. Apart from a fatal consequence, the Sharo beating cultural practice portends physical and psychological trauma to the intending husband.

9. The wife exchanging culture of northern Namibia

The nomadic tribes of Ovahimba and Ovazimba communities of Kunene and Omusati regions in northern Namibia, express their appreciation of their friend or visitor by giving the friend or visitor their wife to have sexual intercourse with for the night [4]. This cultural practice is called okujepisa omukazendu. This practice is deeply rooted in the communities, they believe that it deepens their friendship and prevents promiscuity.

In a country with one of the highest prevalence of HIV infection, a cultural practice like this may be contributing to the spread of the disease. It will be interesting to find out if the wives given as sexual gifts to friends and visitors have a say in the decision and, if they appreciate the cultural practice.

The cultural practices described above are examples of the obvious ones with possibly deleterious health consequences. Some others are not as obvious but nevertheless may have significant adverse heath impact. An example is the cultural upbringing of male children to assume dominant and aggressive roles in relationship with the more docile brought up female partner. This cultural practice is common in many parts of Africa and has been associated with tolerance in the communities for violence by husbands on their wives and, intimate partner violence [5–7].

10. How do we address cultural practices with adverse health consequences?

Female genital mutilation (FGM) was declared a public health concern due to the widespread practice of the culture and, the huge number of girls and women whose physical, psychological, and reproductive health have been adversely affected [2]. The international collaborative response to the practice involved the World Health Organization (WHO), the United Nations Children's Fund (UNICEF) and the United Nations Population Fund (UNFPA). The modality for the concerted efforts to stamp out FGM includes [1]:

- wider international involvement to stop FGM;
- international monitoring bodies and resolutions that condemn the practice; and
- revised legal frameworks and growing political support to end FGM (this includes a law against FGM in 26 countries in Africa and the Middle East, as well as in 33 other countries with migrant populations from FGM practicing countries).

Though the sustained and collaborative efforts resulted in reduced prevalence of the cultural practice, research revealed that if the communities that practice FGM themselves decide to abandon the cultural practice, FGM will be quickly eradicated [2].

So, how then do we get communities to be aware of the health consequences of aspects of their culture that have adverse consequences on health? I propose a multi-dimensional, sustained and motivational approach; similar to the motivational interviewing used medically to influence changes in individual behaviors that have undesirable health consequence [8].

This approach requires identification of influential individuals and stakeholders in the community and developing a relationship of respect and mutual trust in these identified people. Then, without being overtly critical of their cultural practice, they can be made aware of the health impact of the practice using subtle methods such as drama, movies and carefully prepared literature [7]. When the influential individuals and stakeholders are motivated to appreciate the harmful effects of the cultural practice, they may then be involved in peer influence of others in their communities. This will require careful and meticulous documentation of the health consequences of the cultural practice. The process of presenting the documented health consequences have to be very well planned, gradual and packaged in neutral non-offensive ways.

11. Conclusion

It should be expected that motivating a change in a cultural practice that has been held and believed in by a community for decades or centuries would require tact, patience and sustained, multidimensional, collaborative effort. It may be several years before any appreciable change is achieved but nevertheless, it is expedient to start the change process.

Conflict of interest

The author declares no conflict of interest.

Author details

Radiance Ogundipe
Department of Family Medicine, Faculty of Medicine, University of Botswana, Botswana

*Address all correspondence to: docradiance@gmail.com

References

[1] Ojua TA, Ishor DG, Ndom PJ. African cultural practices and health implications for Nigeria rural development. International Review of Management and Business Research. 2013;**2**(1):1-7. ISSN: 2306-9007. www.irmbrjournal.com

[2] World Health Organization. Female Genital Mutilation. 2018. Available from: https://www.who.int/news-room/fact-sheets/detail/female-genital-mutilation

[3] Murori K. Takudzwa Hillary Chiwanza Cultural Practice of Exchanging Wives. 2016. Available from: https://www.africanexponent.com/post/7260-5-unusual-african-cultural-practices

[4] Murori K. Kajuju Murori African Exponent. 2019. Available from: https://www.africanexponent.com/profile/Murori

[5] Btoush R, Campbell JC. Ethical conduct in intimate partner violence research: Challenges and strategies. Nursing Outlook. 2009;**57**(4):210-216

[6] Machisa M, Dorp R. Botswana Gender Violence Indicators Study. UNDP. 2012. Available from: http://www.bw.undp.org/content/botswana/en/home/library/democratic_governance/gender-based-violence-indicators-study-botswana.html [Accessed: 01 January 2016]

[7] Ogundipe RM, Woollett N, Ogunbanjo G, Olashore AA, Tshitenge S. Intimate partner violence: The need for an alternative primary preventive approach in Botswana. African Journal of Primary Health Care & Family Medicine. 2018;**10**(1):1699. DOI: 10.4102/phcfm.v10i1.1699

[8] Stover CS, Meadows AL, Kaufman J. Interventions for intimate partner violence: Review and implications for evidence-based practice. Professional Psychology: Research and Practice. 2009;**40**(3): 223-233. DOI: 10.1037/a0012718

Chapter 8

Mitigating the Hazard of Lightning Injury and Death across Africa

Mary Ann Cooper, Ronald L. Holle and Richard Tushemereirwe

Abstract

Lightning injuries, deaths, and the economic consequences of lightning damage to property and infrastructure continue to be a significant public health challenge and economic development issue in many tropical and subtropical areas of the world, especially sub-Saharan Africa. This chapter will discuss the scope of the hazard, known risk factors including common cultural beliefs that inhibit public education, existing data sources, medical effects and long-term disability, lightning formation and detection, injury mechanisms, existing lightning safety programs and their challenges, and the work being done to decrease injuries, death, and property damage from lightning in Africa by the African Centres for Lightning and Electromagnetics Network (ACLENet).

Keywords: ACLENet, lightning, lightning strike, lightning fatalities, lightning injury, lightning safety, lightning occurrence, disaster risk reduction, lightning detection, mechanisms of injury, lightning myths

1. Introduction

This chapter will summarize the hazards of lightning injury, death, and property damage in Africa. Lightning kills and injures not only people but their livestock, still a frequent measure of a family's worth. It threatens economically challenged countries with damage to infrastructure including utilities, mining, aviation, and many other industries, as well as causes losses from downtime, food spoilage, lost work, lost data, and other problems from damaged electronics [1].

2. Methodology

The number of lightning safety researchers is small and well known to each other. A significant portion of the literature since 1990, particularly for Africa, has been written, mentored, or summarized in papers by the first two authors of this chapter. Most of the literature on lightning safety and injury prevention is published in engineering and physics journals and may not be available to medical or public health experts through the usual search engines. An extensive bibliography on safety and demographics of lightning casualty papers, maintained by Mr. Holle, serves as the basis for this chapter [2].

3. History and limitations of lightning injury studies

Unlike many infectious diseases and other causes of injury, lightning injury is not reportable to any government agencies or databases worldwide. A number of other data sources and collection techniques have been used with varying degrees of completeness [3, 4].

For example, the general public in the United States might expect that everyone injured by lightning would seek immediate medical care so that hospital diagnoses or admission information would be a good source for the number of lightning injuries and deaths. However, a sizeable number of survivors do not seek care until a few days after the injury when symptoms do not resolve [5]. Those cases do not make it into any databank. Additionally, not all patients seen in emergency departments require admission, and emergency physicians may use symptom-based complaints such as pain, weakness, or mental status changes rather than "lightning injury." Even coroner's reports may not list "lightning injury" [5, 6].

Prior to the internet, U.S. death and injury statistics were collected as news reports provided by contracted clipping services for Storm Data, a monthly publication of the National Centers for Environmental Information [7]. **Figure 1** shows the death rate per million population collected for more than a century in the United States. During the clipping service era, studies showed that between 30 and 70% of deaths were unreported and injuries much more so [8–11]. Data on property damage, while included in Storm Data, are even less well documented than injuries, particularly because insurance companies are loath to share their claims information [12–15].

Of those injured by lightning, 90% survive, although many have permanent disabilities [6, 16]. The derivative 10:1 injury/death ratio has long been used for projecting total injuries in developed countries.

With the development of the internet, online news reports, and online searches have made up-to-the-minute collection of deaths in the U.S. routine with deaths caused by lightning well documented in the United States and studied in many developed countries [17–20].

Even with the internet as a source, there have been few studies in developing countries, and press coverage is marginal [21, 22] (**Figure 2**). As communication

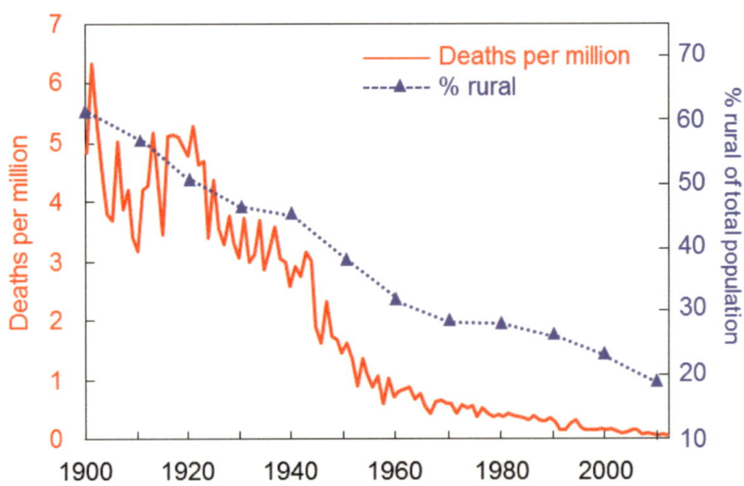

Figure 1.
Solid red line: U.S. lightning deaths per million people from 1900 to 2013 [20]. Dashed blue line: Percent rural population. (©Ronald L. Holle).

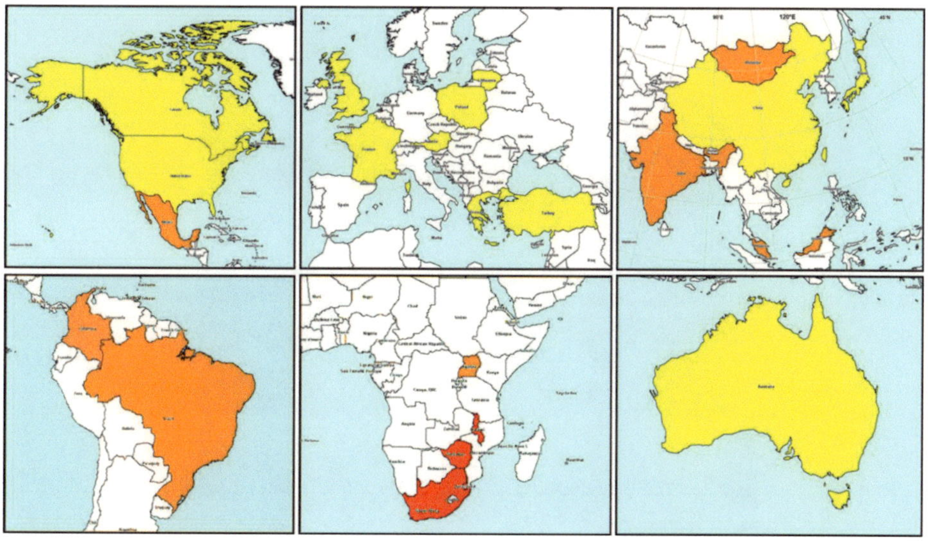

Figure 2.
Lightning fatality rate per million people per year by continent. Red shading indicates rate > 5.0 fatalities per million per year, orange indicates 0.6–5.0, and yellow indicates 0.5 or less. White indicates no national summaries have been published for datasets ending in 1979 or later (updated from [22]). (©Ronald L. Holle).

technology improves and cell phone penetrance grows, it is expected that more incidents will be reported in African media sources. However, for the foreseeable future, single deaths, nonfatal injuries, smaller incidents, and those in distant or hard-to-reach areas are less likely to be reported than those involving multiple people, animals, and children in school [1]. The first source to collect injury data in Africa, the nonprofit African Centres for Lightning and Electromagnetics Network (ACLENet), has been posting news reports across Africa for several years [23].

Different papers have estimated total annual global deaths as 6–24,000 [24–27]. Applying the 10:1 injury/death ratio projects up to 240,000 annual injuries. However, survival and disability rates have not been studied in developing countries, and numbers may be considerably higher for both deaths and injuries.

Lightning researchers have proposed mathematical models and other strategies for estimating lightning injuries and deaths using lightning stroke density data (number of lightning strokes per km^2 per year), population density, socioeconomic measures, and other factors [5, 26–28], but these need refining and validation before they can be used as predictive tools for developing countries. Although lightning may cause fewer deaths worldwide than some other public health threats, the consequences of lightning strike to individuals, families, communities, schools, and economic progress in countries that are already economically challenged should not be underestimated [21, 29–38].

4. Demographics of lightning injury

Lightning was the second largest storm killer in the United States for over a century, exceeded only by floods [5]. Since data collection began in the United States, lightning deaths have roughly paralleled the percentage of the population living in rural areas ([20], **Figure 1**). Although this has been a consistent finding in countries as they become "developed" [24], urbanization is not the only factor governing lightning injury. In Africa, as people move to cities to find work, huge shantytowns often arise on the periphery of cities (**Figure 3**). These dwellings do not meet the

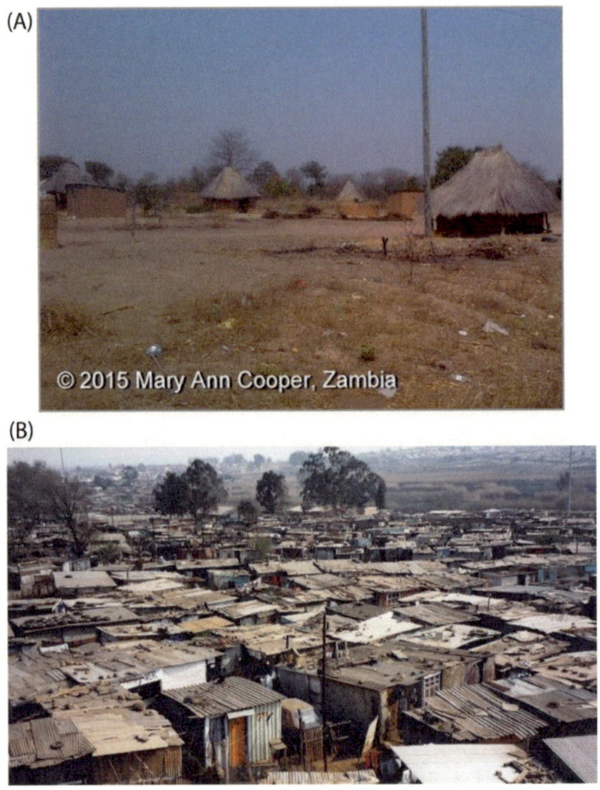

Figure 3.
Typical African dwellings and work areas, particularly in rural areas [1]. (A) Mudbrick with generations-old thatch roofs or sheet metal held down by rocks. In some areas, chicken wire may be cast over the thatch to prevent monkeys and baboons from disrupting the roof. In others, car tires may be placed on the roof because it is thought that their "rubber" will protect the building from lightning. (B) Soweto shantytown. Soweto is a million-plus populated southwest township near Johannesburg, South Africa, and the birthplace of Nelson Mandela. (courtesy Derek Elsom).

definition of "lightning-safe": a substantial, fully enclosed building with plumbing, wiring, and metal structural components running through the walls. Not only do buildings with these features tend to be less likely to collapse in a storm, but the metal and pipes act as a modified "Faraday cage" channeling lightning through the walls and around the inhabitants [5]. Lightning safety advocates avoid using the world "shelter" as almost all "shelters" are not lightning-safe (bus shelters, golf shelters, rain shelters, picnic shelters, etc.) [5].

Another "lightning-safe" area to choose in a thunderstorm is nearly any fully enclosed metal vehicle such as a school bus, automobile, truck, and most mechanized farming equipment. Open carts, including boda bodas, golf carts, and others are not lightning-safe [20, 21].

To illustrate the difference substantial, lightning-safe construction makes, **Figure 4** compares the relative frequency of locations of U.S. deaths from lightning from the 1890s, before indoor plumbing and wiring was common, with the most recent decade for which data was available [39]. In the 1890s, over half of the U.S. population lived in rural areas where few buildings had indoor plumbing, electrical wiring, or what would nowadays be considered reasonably lightning-safe construction. **Figure 4** shows that the largest percentage of deaths in the 1890s occurred indoors because when lightning hit them, they were likely to collapse on the inhabitants and any surviving inhabitant was likely to have lightning injuries.

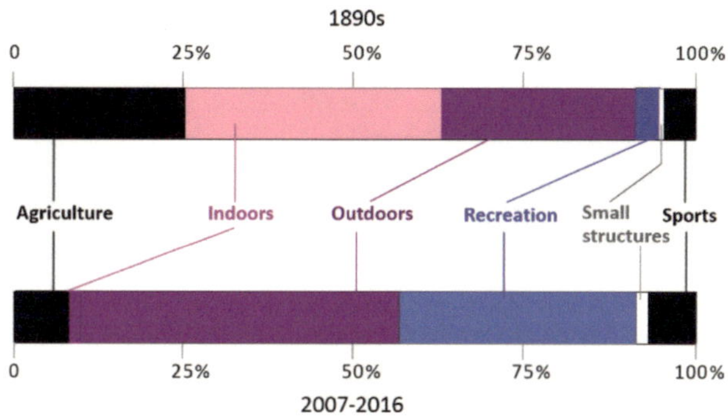

Figure 4.
Comparison of the percentage of locations where U.S. lightning fatalities occurred in the 1890s versus the 2007–2016 decade (updated from [39]). (©Ronald L. Holle).

As housing construction became more substantial and more likely to be lightning-safe, the share of indoor lightning deaths decreased to nearly zero and has certainly been less than one per year for the past two decades in the United States. Similarly, as farming in the United States became mechanized, fewer people were "exposed" to lightning. Nowadays, the vast majority of people killed by lightning in the Unites States and other developed countries are pursuing recreational and other outdoor nonwork activities such as organized sports, gardening, fishing, boating, or running and are almost always within a few feet of safety [1].

Figure 4 shows the second most common location of U.S. deaths in the 1890s was for labor-intensive outdoor activities with farming coming a close third. **Figure 4** is useful because the U.S. 1800's data gives a reasonable approximation of where to expect lightning deaths to occur in developing countries including sub-Saharan Africa where over 90% of buildings are not lightning-safe.

The fatality rate from lightning in the United States is now more than two orders of magnitude lower than a century ago ([1, 20, 40], **Figure 1**). Over the last decade, lightning deaths in the United States have averaged 27 per year or less than 1 in 12,000,000 population [39]. The fatality rate per capita has become very low in developed countries during the last century due to widespread availability of "lightning-safe" structures and metal-topped, fully enclosed vehicles, extensive public education by broadcast meteorologists and in-print and electronic media, mechanized agriculture, weather apps, good forecasting that incorporates lightning warnings, and other factors, including the fact that there is simply less lightning in most developed countries, which tend to be in temperate climates, compared to tropical and subtropical areas of the world [1, 5, 40].

Table 1 shows many differences in known demographics of lightning injuries between developed and developing countries. In developed countries, it is well known that the injury to death ratio is about 9:1, so that 90% survive [6, 16, 41]. The injury/death ratio in Africa and developing countries is unknown but is expected to be lower since fewer lightning-safe locations are available, resulting in a higher proportion of deaths. More people die per lightning event in the developing world than in the United States and other developed countries, particularly in agricultural and school events [42, 43]. Injuries, in general, are less well documented as some victims may not seek medical care immediately and most countries do not require reporting of these medical visits nor of lightning-related diagnoses [5, 6].

Whereas the male-to-female fatality rate in developed countries is consistently about 3:1 [2], many developing countries have a large portion of their population involved in labor-intensive agriculture during the daytime when thunderstorms are

Measure	Developing countries	Developed countries
Deaths/million	Unknown	Well documented (0.01–0.5/million)
Number of deaths per event	Multiple deaths	Single deaths
Injury/death ratio	Unknown, expected to be lower due to lack of "lightning-safe" areas	10:1
Male/female deaths	Tends to be more equal	3:1
Age range	Equal risk for everyone	Males age 15–30

Table 1.
Demographics of lightning injury (©MACooper).

most common. No lightning-safe locations are typically available to these people, and deaths and injuries are often nearly equally distributed between males and females [5, 41, 44–46]. A recent study of labor-intensive agriculture in India and Bangladesh shows that 47% of the fatalities and injuries were females as they worked during the daytime hours when thunderstorms are most frequent [39, 46]. In addition, dwellings occupied outside of working hours often are not lightning-safe due to their construction of mud brick with thatch or sheet metal roofing (**Figure 3**).

While lightning deaths in developed countries rarely involve more than one person, and injuries to groups are few, deaths in developing countries often involve more than one person, sometimes with more than ten deaths per event [35]. Sometimes this is because people, particularly students, are packed together in classrooms and churches or walking with several others [1]. This leads some experts to hypothesize that ground current, responsible for at least 50% of deaths in developed countries, may play an even larger role in these situations [20, 47].

Multiple studies done by Holle [2] have shown that the majority of those killed die during the afternoon hours when thunderstorms are more likely to occur. In more developed countries, the dominant profile of lightning casualties is the young male. Risk-taking in recreation, workplaces, and organized sports tends to be dominated by males between about 15 and 30 years old. In lesser developed countries, the distribution by ages is much more dispersed. The lack of lightning-safe dwellings, schools and workplaces means that all ages and both genders are equally vulnerable at all times [27, 34, 42, 46].

5. Risk factors for lightning injury

The factors that increase the risk of lightning injury are well known ([1], **Table 2**). Like infectious diseases, lightning injuries are related to exposure. Exposure is related to the amount of lightning that occurs in a given area over time (**Table 2**, dark orange), common socioeconomic factors (mid-orange), and cultural beliefs (light orange and **Tables 2** and **3**) about lightning that affect behavior.

The frequency of lightning in a given area is measured as strokes/km^2/year (stroke density), which can vary substantially depending on season, topography, and other factors but, in total, is reasonably unchanging from year to year [38]. Most lightning occurs in cloud (IC) than cloud-to-ground (CG), but *all* lightning is dangerous because any stroke can change direction and start toward the ground where people are located. Worldwide lightning data over decades has shown no change that can be attributed to climate change, despite speculations to the contrary [48].

Lightning stroke density is higher in tropical and subtropical areas of the world, precisely where people are less likely to have substantial, developed housing and

Factors that increase risk	Factors that decrease risk
High lightning stroke density	Low lightning stroke density
Large rural population	Mostly urban population
Increasing population	Stable or decreasing populations
Labor-intensive, outdoor work such as farming, fishing, and animal husbandry	Mechanized farming and stricter laws governing work conditions
Inadequate building construction. No lightning protection mandated for public and frequently inhabited buildings; lack of technical knowledge about lightning protection; use of lightning protection materials that are not compliant with international lightning protection codes	High-quality building construction involving wiring, plumbing, and metal components in the walls and roof combine to act as a 'Faraday cage' to safely divert lightning energy around inhabitants. Code-compliant lightning protection mandated for public buildings and those frequently inhabited by large numbers of people
Lack of lightning-safe areas for easy evacuation; lack of proven actions that individuals can take to decrease risk	Easy availability of lightning-safe buildings and fully enclosed metal vehicles within easy reach. Widespread personal knowledge of lightning injury avoidance behavior
No or little lightning detection data or nonavailability to the public	High-quality lightning detection data incorporated into weather forecasts
Lack of reliable and timely weather forecasts or forecasts that are only available to specific sectors of the economy, primarily aviation	Weather forecasting systems with high-quality forecasts and weather apps available to the public on a free and real-time basis
Delayed or nonexistent access to high-quality medical care	Easy access to high-quality medical care
Low literacy rate; multiple languages	High literacy rate
Little or no valid public education on lightning safety; strongly held beliefs that injuries are inevitable, regardless of personal behavior, and that lightning is called down by witches and other cultural beliefs	An active media; news reports of injuries; enthusiastic public education with wide access to lightning safety information; knowledge of how lightning is formed and where it is statistically more likely to hit

Table 2.
Risk factors for lightning injury and death. Modified from Cooper and Tushemereirwe [1] ©MACooper.

where work is more often outdoors [48]. The Democratic Republic of the Congo and Lake Maracaibo in Venezuela are hotspots for the highest stroke density in the world [48]. **Figure 5** shows stroke density map of Africa.

Despite studies showing stable negative population growth in most developed countries, the population of Africa continues to increase, putting more people at risk.

The vast majority of factors determining risk of lightning injury are socioeconomic and, therefore, could be modified given adequate resources, education, and infrastructure improvement. During the day, people are at higher risk of lightning injury when they are involved in labor-intensive outdoor work such as animal husbandry and farming, when they do not have access to "lightning-safe" buildings for habitation and work, and when they are exposed as they walk to the market, work near their homes or on fishing boats, or attend school and church either outdoors or in non-lightning-safe buildings [1, 35–37]. At night, as people sleep in lightning-unsafe dwellings, entire families are at risk. It is difficult for people who have not worked extensively in Africa to understand life there, but the fact is that nearly everyone in sub-Saharan Africa is at risk 24/7/365 regardless of the activities they are pursuing [10, 16–26, 29–37, 42, 49–51].

A small sample of common beliefs about lightning in Africa
Lightning is punishment from a god for wrongdoing.
Thunder is a warning that the god who controls lightning is walking on the earth.
Muti (folk medicine in Africa) can ward off lightning damage to a house.
Wearing red attracts lightning.
Mirrors should be covered during thunderstorms because they can attract or reflect lightning to kill someone nearby.
Individuals can call lightning down to harm others; witches can be hired to call down lightning on an enemy.
It is necessary to hire a sangoma to assure good weather for your wedding or other important event. If the weather is bad, it is because someone who wishes you harm hired a stronger sangoma.
A person who has been injured by lightning requires purification by traditional healers before it is safe to touch them (delaying resuscitation and first aid efforts) or before the person can be prepared for burial.

Table 3.
Common cultural beliefs about lightning. (©MACooper).

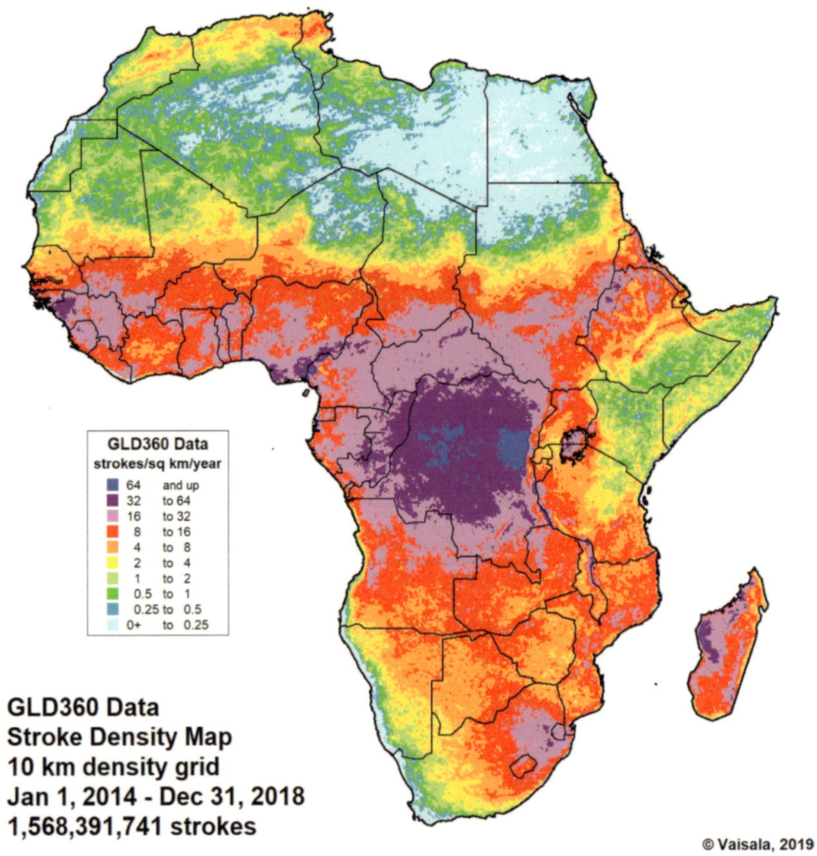

Figure 5.
Lightning stroke density per square km per year from the global lightning dataset GLD360 network from 2014 through 2018. The density map depicts 1,568,391,741 strokes. Scale is at lower left; grid size is 10 by 10 km [48].

Most developing countries do not have or may not enforce building codes that require lightning protection (LP) for public buildings such as schools, churches, hospitals, and other frequently inhabited buildings. Proper LP is delineated in internationally recognized codes [52, 53]. The design and installation of LP is a very specialized field and beyond discussion in this chapter [47]. In practice, it is seldom part of the curricula for engineers or architects and is nearly always "learned on the job" although more countries are instituting LP training and certification. Because of this complexity, it is nearly impossible for the average local official, school principal, or administrator to judge between code-compliant plans and those offered by fast-talking charlatans or by well-meaning but untrained LP purveyors. Further discussion of the unvalidated claims of those using early streamer emitters (ESE) and other fraudulent practices is beyond this text, although an overview can be accessed at [47]. Unfortunately, the infiltration of purveyors of ESE and other unproven philosophies of lightning protection has resulted in multiple countries adopting lightning protection codes that are not compliant with the international IEC standards, notably France, Spain, Turkey, and many others. All wishing to have LP installed should inquire what code will be used before accepting a contract or design [47, 52, 53].

A factor that makes lightning injuries strikingly different in the developing world is the combination of keraunoparalysis (KP) (kerauno—lightning) and building construction using dry thatch [5, 54–57]. Lightning injury often causes a temporary paralysis that lasts for at least several minutes to hours. This is particularly a problem for families working or sleeping inside their mudbrick home roofed with tinder-dry, generations-old thatch. KP can prevent even the most fit young person from escaping a home as the burning thatch starts to fall ([5, 54, 55], **Figure 6**). These are the injuries that result in the media writing "burned beyond recognition" or "charred," terms that are never seen in the United States or other developed countries [21, 55].

Governmentally, many developing countries have little or no access to lightning detection data sources. Most meteorological authorities, while mandated to serve a country's airports to assure international flights, commerce, and tourism, have limited resources and no mandated obligation to warn citizens of droughts, floods, lightning, or other weather hazards [40, 47, 58, 59]. There are no weather apps in most of these countries, and those that exist may access poor data sources or incorporate time lags of 20–30 minutes, making their displays useless for lightning safety and injury prevention. Near-real-time warnings (delayed by less than 30 seconds) are available on a subscription basis from several vendors but are largely unaffordable or unknown to industry, government meteorological authorities, and the public in Africa [40, 47]. ACLENet is piloting this type of warning system at a few schools in Uganda.

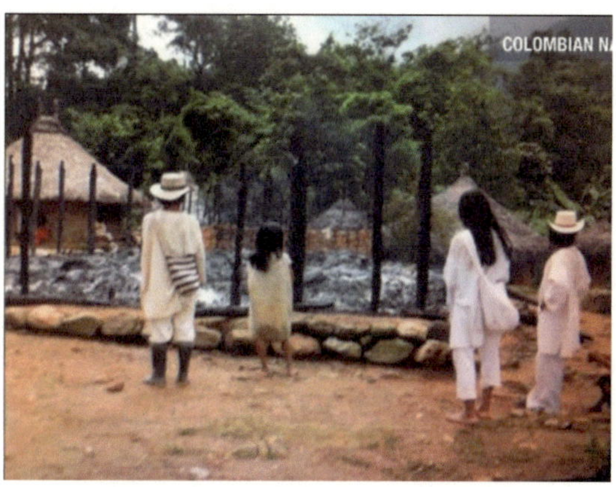

Figure 6.
Eleven tribal leaders were killed when the thatch building where they were meeting caught fire from a lightning strike. (used with tribal permission).

Many of the most lightning injury-prone countries have inadequate or hard-to-reach medical care and other supports such as trained personnel, ambulance services, first aid providers, and other first responders [47]. Besides the high exposure and risk of lightning strike, victims also have less chance of survival during the acute phase or access to specialized services such as cognitive therapy and chronic pain management for those who survive [5, 16, 55].

All of the socioeconomic factors listed in **Table 2** could be addressed and improved, but the cost and time to do so would be enormous and prohibitive for most African countries which may already be economically challenged. Public education, however, does not need to cost nearly as much as revising buildings and medical infrastructure [18, 60, 61], and it is probably the easiest and fastest way to make a difference [18, 60–62]. ACLENet has worked with other agencies in Uganda to begin public education through television broadcasts and newspaper inserts which teachers often hang as classroom posters and use for lesson plans [63].

The third major set of contributors to risk are the long-held cultural beliefs about lightning (**Table 2** light orange), a small sample of which are listed in **Table 3**. These beliefs have been taught for generations and are nearly impossible to counter except by persistent public education or by community elders who have been trained [64–66]. In some countries, if a family member has been injured by lightning, communities may shun the family, believing the family to be cursed and forcing them to leave their communities, property, and friends to start over [30]. In the Democratic Republic of the Congo, a head teacher and two teachers at a private school were imprisoned after being accused of "calling down lightning" to kill students at the public school in order to induce parents to enroll their children in their private school [65]. Widows or other women with no family to protect them may be stoned as witches if someone in their village is killed by lightning [64]. Other common myths can be found in the monthly ACLENet newsletters [65].

6. Mechanisms of lightning injury

Medically, lightning injury could be investigated from a number of different approaches including cellular physiology or electrical field effects, flashover versus internal flow of energy, and others [5, 47]. However, considering the five common electrical mechanisms of injury is the most useful for prevention and lightning safety education [5, 67]. To complicate further, these can be combined, and blunt or concussive trauma/barotrauma may be overlaid on any of the five [5, 67, 68]. **Figure 7** shows the relative distribution of these mechanisms in developed countries. The distribution is not known in developing countries, but it is suspected that ground current plays an even larger role.

Ground current (also called earth potential rise and step voltage): The mechanism that kills the most people is ground current, where lightning strikes the surface of the earth and spreads to nearby people. It can affect a large number of people either inside or outside an unprotected building. Children crowded together in unprotected school buildings are at particular risk [42].

Side flash/splash: This occurs when trees, poles, towers, and many other objects that are not necessarily tall are struck and a portion of the lightning jumps to a nearby person.

Upward streamer (leader): As a thundercloud moves above the earth, opposite charges are induced on the surface of the earth and in objects on the ground under the cloud whether they are a tree, a home, a person, or a blade of grass. Upward streamers, not usually visible from these objects, will reach up and attempt to

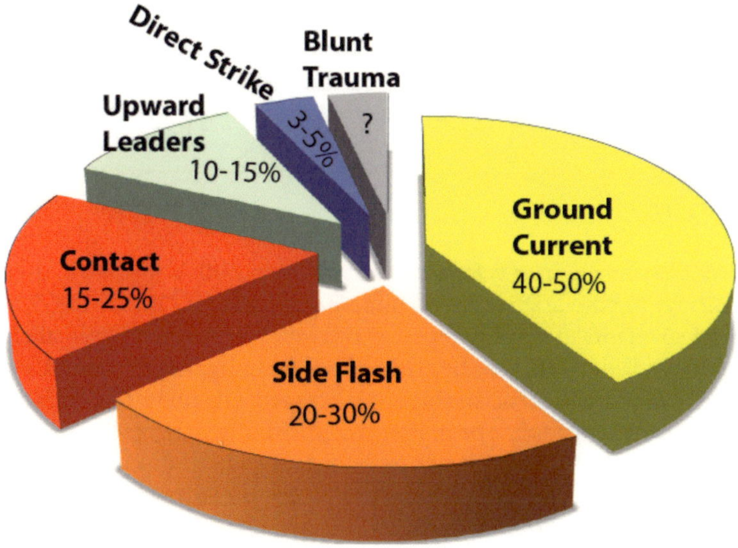

Figure 7.
This chart shows the frequencies of the primary lightning fatality mechanisms [67]. (©MACooper/RLHolle).

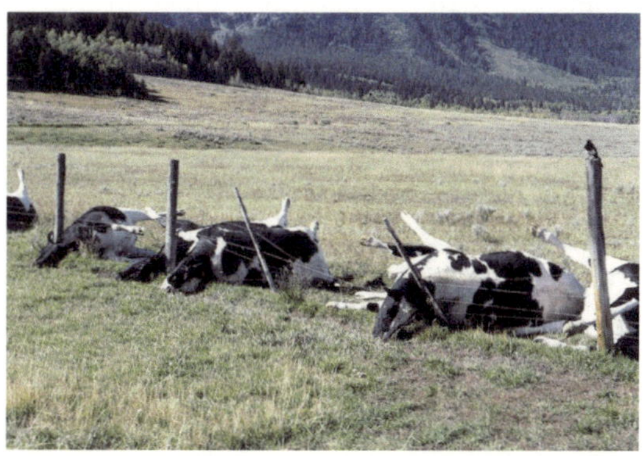

Figure 8.
Cows killed by lightning as they gathered by an ungrounded wire fence. This is a common occurrence and can be from contact injury as lightning energy is conducted from a distance or from ground current. Sideflash from the fence is less likely. (©MACooper).

connect with the downward-moving lightning channel. The upward leader is strong enough to cause injury even if the lightning channel is not completed [69–72].

Contact: This occurs when the person is in contact with conducting paths such as plumbing, corded telephones or appliances, headsets, or wiring, either outdoors or inside structures. Contact injury may also occur as animals gather next to long metal wire fences (**Figure 8**).

Direct strike: Contrary to public belief, direct strike is the least common mechanism causing only perhaps 3–5% of deaths [5, 40, 67, 73]. A direct injury occurs when the lightning stroke attaches directly to the victim and is most likely to occur in the open. While it is intuitive that a direct strike might be the most likely to cause fatalities, this has not been shown in any studies.

Blunt trauma (concussive/explosive trauma, barotrauma): Blunt trauma has long been suggested as a mechanism of lightning injury [5]. As lightning passes through the air, rapid heating and expansion of the air occurs so that those nearby may experience a concussive force as if they were near an explosion. Blumenthal investigated barotrauma in his dissertation and likened it to being near a 5 kg of TNT blast [68]. Barotrauma is independent of the other electrical mechanisms of injury but may potentially overlay any of them [5, 40, 68]. People may also be thrown by opisthotonic contractions and experience musculoskeletal injuries as would be expected [5, 66].

7. Lightning injury

As noted in Section 3, in developed countries, nearly 90% of those injured by lightning survive but are often left with disabling sequelae [5, 10, 11, 16, 55, 67]. The percentage of survivors in developing countries may be considerably smaller where people are exposed 24/7/365, may be affected by keraunoparalysis in unsafe structures that catch on fire, and cannot access high-quality medical and rehabilitative care.

A large range of injuries has been reported including damage to the ears, eyes, skin, heart, and brain. For a more complete and referenced discussion, see Cooper et al. in Auerbach [5]. The proximate cause of death is cardiac arrest and anoxic brain injury at the time of the strike, even if a partially successful resuscitation delays the legal pronouncement for a few days [5, 11, 74]. Later, deaths may be due to suicide as survivors become despondent when they cannot find help for their brain injury and other sequelae, may not be able to return to work and lose their homes, or lose the support of their friends and family due to personality changes and other stressors [75, 76]. Others may self-medicate with alcohol, drugs, or herbs for their post-injury chronic pain and frustration [76].

People tend to take their experience with common household electricity and scale it up, predicting that lightning must cause horrible burns [5, 66]. They may even have heard of the destructive injuries caused by high-voltage injuries. However, in developed countries, lightning burns tend to be superficial and insignificant compared to the neurologic injuries that are suffered. Less than ½ of lightning survivors surveyed by the Lightning Strike and Electric Shock Survivors, International (LSESSI) support group several years ago had damage of any kind to their skin [16, 74–76]. Given the majority of injuries are not direct strikes or direct injuries but from mechanisms where the strength of the strike has been mitigated by dissipation across longer distances or other factors (ground current, contact injury, upward streamer), this is a reasonable finding. However, the lack of burns will often result in physician skepticism and legal disputes with worker insurance denial [5, 57, 75, 76].

Long term, lightning survivors may suffer temporary or permanent neurological sequelae including chronic pain syndromes and cognitive damage similar to those reported in the now widely recognized post-concussive syndrome with attention deficit, memory problems, learning difficulty, frontal lobe damage causing irritability and personality changes, and loss of multitasking and executive function, all resulting in inability to return to their previous level of employment [5, 16, 75, 76]. Blunt injury from being thrown may also cause musculoskeletal pain [5, 68]. As with other brain injured people, frustration, impatience, instant rage, and other personality changes may drive away family members, further compromising the survivor's recovery [5, 16, 75, 76].

Disability may significantly affect a family's socioeconomic status if the survivor is unable to return to work or needs chronic care [5, 16, 40, 49, 57, 75, 76]. A further setback to the victim's family, particularly in developing countries such as those in Africa, is a common belief that a family affected by lightning injury is "cursed" or was punished for bad behavior such as beating their wives or children. The community may shun the entire family so that they have little choice but to leave their community, home, and employment to start over in a new community where their tragedy is unknown [5, 30, 40].

Currently there is no way to reverse or decrease the damage cascade that is set in motion when the injury first occurs. The Lightning Strike and Electric Shock Survivors, International is a support group that has helped hundreds of survivors and their families to find help and knowledge about their injuries [16, 47, 75, 76]. Treatment is standard for pain syndromes, anoxic brain injury, eighth nerve tinnitus and balance problems, and cognitive disability. Unfortunately, this type of care is expensive and seldom available in developing countries. In the developed world, some survivors may return to work, but it may be in a different field or with lesser responsibility and income.

As in most injuries and illnesses, prevention is far better than caring for those injured by lightning. In developed countries, lightning injury prevention through public education is simple and cost-effective [17, 18, 60, 62, 77]. However decreasing lightning injuries in developing countries is a much more complex task than in countries where lightning-safe structures and vehicles are common and almost universally close at hand.

8. African Centres for lightning and electromagnetics network, Inc.

The African Centres for Lightning and Electromagnetics Network (https://ACLENet.org) is a pan-African network of national centers dedicated to reducing deaths, injuries, and property damage from lightning across Africa [1]. It was formed with multiple goals in mind (**Table 4**). Among its many activities, ACLENet is attempting to establish an injury and damage database by collecting news reports for each of the countries in Africa and working with citizen reporters to document injuries and deaths as well as property damage [23].

The majority of lightning deaths can be avoided if there are "lightning-safe" areas to evacuate to, if good weather forecasts and warning systems are available to the public, and if individuals have been educated in actions they can take to avoid injury [1, 17, 18]. Almost none of these are available to the vast majority of sub-Saharan Africans, particularly in rural areas, leaving entire families at risk 24/7/365 whether they are working in their fields, walking to the market, cooking near their homes, worshipping, or in school [1]. Children in school tend to be at particular risk because typical classes have about 50 children packed into classrooms that are not protected and are not lightning-safe [1, 42].

In June 2011, 18 children were killed by one lightning strike with another 38 children injured and transported to the hospital from Runyanya Primary School in Kiryandongo, Uganda [78]. Prior to this incident, the head teacher related that

ACLENet's multifaceted goals
To assess the impact of lightning on each nation's citizens and economy
To educate teachers, parents, pupils, and the public on lightning safety and injury prevention
To work with governments to assure that code-compliant lightning protection systems are designed for new schools and other important buildings
To work with universities to train Africa's own lightning experts for the future
To improve engineering training and professional qualifications in lightning protection
To advise on code-compliant lightning protection of utilities and other economically important industries
To improve the availability of accurate and timely lightning data, weather forecasting, and warnings

Table 4.
Modified from Cooper et al. [1] (©MACooper).

the school had 600 pupils attending. After the incident, parents were afraid to send their children, and children were afraid to attend school where they had seen their friends die. The enrollment fell to under 400. Children cannot learn if they are anxious about being killed every time dark clouds roll across the sky. After lightning protection was installed at the school by ACLENet, the head teacher related that enrollment climbed to over 1100 [79].

Perhaps more alarming than deaths is the fact that lightning is survivable but can leave survivors with permanent disabilities that make adults unable to return to work to support themselves and their families and children less able to learn in school to become contributing, productive citizens [5, 16, 55, 75, 76]. As with any significant disability, the family suffers at least as much as the survivor does, and the economic impact to the family can be great.

In addition to deaths and disabling injuries to people, lightning often destroys livestock, the main source of income and wealth for many families in developing countries (**Figure 9**) [40]. Sometimes these incidents are reported by the media, but there is little reliable data on total livestock deaths or on damage to infrastructure such as utilities, mining, agriculture, and other industries. Additionally, the hundreds of languages in Africa confound good data gathering.

The effects of lightning damage to property has not only direct effects on the structure but also indirect economic effects including food spoilage from lack of refrigeration after electrical failure, electrical parts and repairs unaffordable or not available for days, hospitals without power, and expensive, nearly irreplaceable electronics damaged along with their databases and records [1, 40, 80]. It is estimated that aggregate economic losses to unprotected installations, both due to damage and downtime, will grow exponentially as a result of the explosive growth in usage of electronics, the extension of national power grids into rural areas, and mushrooming communication towers across Africa [35, 81–83]. Lightning damage to infrastructure occurs in countries that can ill afford more economic threats due to already struggling with issues such as drought, HIV, underemployment, or civil strife.

In developed countries, lightning damage is almost always covered by insurance. However, in Africa, studies indicate lack of penetration of insurance across the African continent. Conservative estimates put the extent of insurance coverage at as little as 3.5% of the potential African market [84]. For public health threats like lightning, lack of insurance can be devastating. In Africa, emergency response and medical care to victims without health insurance is limited or nonexistent. Businesses without insurance coverage may be forced to close.

Two stories illustrate the outcome lack of insurance coverage for lightning events can cause:

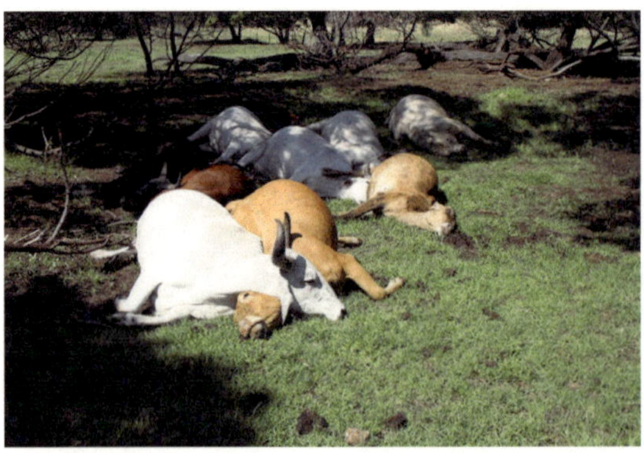

Figure 9.
Cattle killed by lightning in South Africa. (photo courtesy Ian Jandrell).

1. Reported on October 17, 2019, 11 head of cattle belonging to 1 farmer were killed by lightning at Mboza in northeastern KwaZulu-Natal, leaving the farmer unable to provide for his family as cattle farming was his only means of subsistence [85].

2. When a community radio station in northern Uganda was hit by lightning destroying a major part of their infrastructure and equipment, lack of insurance forced it to close down [86].

The African Centres for Lighting and Electromagnetics Network (ACLENet - https://ACLENet.org) is a nonprofit organization dedicated to decreasing deaths, injuries, and property damage from lightning across Africa. It seeks to change the toll of lightning across Africa (**Table 4**) by addressing lightning from many aspects:

1. Establishing a database of news reports of injuries and property damage and encouraging individuals and the media to report them so that the impact of lightning on each nation's citizens and economy can be assessed [23].

2. Educating the public on how lightning occurs, mechanisms of injury, and what individuals can do to protect themselves and their families [63, 87]. Due to extensive public education with involvement of the media, U.S. lightning deaths have decreased from over 100/year to less than 30/year for the past decade [17, 18, 62]. Fortunately, all the National Oceanographic and Atmospheric Administration (NOAA) lightning safety materials, curricula for schools, games, animations, posters, and public service announcements are free to download and use from the website [41]. Further, the authors of most of these materials are willing to work with African lightning safety advocates to "Africanize" the settings, languages, and idioms (personal communications).

3. Protecting schools with code-compliant designs ([52], **Figure 10**). If children and teachers feel secure from lightning injury, they are more likely to attend school and continue their studies despite thunderstorms. One of the schools

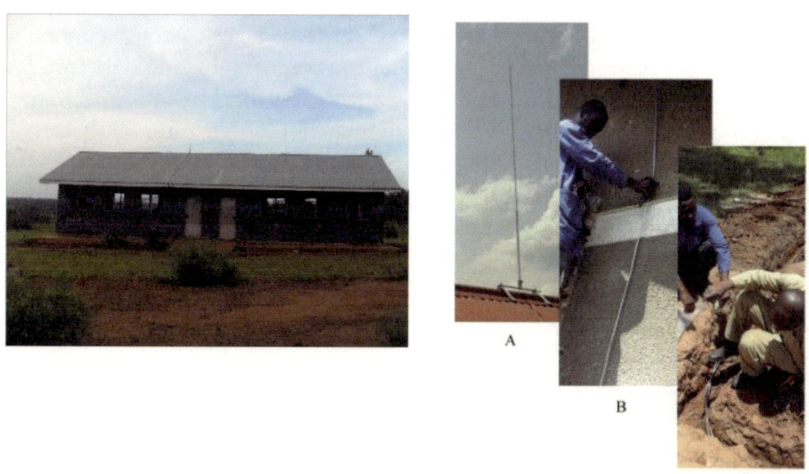

Figure 10.
Installation of lightning protection system at a typical classroom building at Runyanya school, Uganda. Details: (A) air terminal; (B) down conductor; and (C) ground terminal or "earthing ring." (©ACLENet).

protected by ACLENet has written detailing that the surrounding community now feels safe to use the school as a meeting place since it was protected [88]. Effective lightning safety education and behavior change for communities begins with children in so many ways!

4. Decreasing the cost of LP by using local materials to avoid expensive imports and developing "templates" for schools and other common buildings that can be used across Africa.

5. Fostering graduate education to train Africa's own experts. The University of Zambia is accepting the first class in lightning science and electrical engineering, a program developed under the mentorship of one of ACLENet's founders, Chandima Gomes, to start January 2020.

6. Working with governments to assure implementation of internationally recognized lightning protection codes consistent with IEC 62305-1,2,3,4 [52].

7. Working with utilities, mining, aviation, and other industries to provide lightning protection for infrastructure as well as lightning safety education for their staff.

8. Advocating improved training and professional qualifications for LP designers, engineers, and installers.

9. Conclusions

Lightning is a significant cause of weather-related death and injury across Africa [1, 5, 40]. While it is a largely preventable death in developed countries where "lightning-safe" areas are usually readily available and within a few feet of those threatened [1, 17, 18, 60, 77], the majority of sub-Saharan Africans are at risk 24/7/365 due to living in dwellings that are not lightning-safe. Further risk factors include engaging in largely outdoor, labor-intensive work such as farming and shepherding [39]. Worshippers often meeting outdoors and children walking to or attending school, roadside shopkeepers, those walking to the market, working in mines, or other outdoor activities are also all at risk [1, 42]. Poor or nonexistent lightning detection systems, little or no incorporation of lightning data into forecasting, no warnings to the public and those at risk, cultural beliefs, and many other factors keep injuries, deaths, and property damage from lightning a substantial threat to entire families, schools, villages, and populations [1].

ACLENet was founded to address many aspects of lightning safety, public education, and injury prevention and to work with governments and other agencies with similar goals [89].

Author details

Mary Ann Cooper[1]*, Ronald L. Holle[2] and Richard Tushemereirwe[3]

1 ACLENet (African Centres for Lightning and Electromagnetics Network), River Forest, IL, USA

2 ACLENet (African Centres for Lightning and Electromagnetics Network), Oro Valley, AZ, USA

3 ACLENet (African Centres for Lightning and Electromagnetics Network), Kampala, Uganda

*Address all correspondence to: macooper@uic.edu

References

[1] Cooper MA, Holle RL, Tushemereirwe R, Andrews CJ, African Centres for Lightning and Electromagnetics Network (ACLENet). Progress report. Preprints. In: 34th International Conference on Lightning Protection; 2-7 September 2018; Rzeszow. Poland: ICLP; 2018. 7pp

[2] Holle RL. Bibliography on Safety and Demographics of Lightning Casualties [Internet]. Ongoing. Available from: https://aclenet.org/news-publications/publications/lightning-safety.html [Accessed: 25 Ocotber 2019]

[3] Navarrete-Aldana N, Cooper MA, Holle RL. Lightning fatalities in Colombia from 2000 to 2009. Natural Hazards. 2019;**74**:1349-1362

[4] Richey S, Holle RL, Cooper MA. A comparison of three data collection methods for reporting of lightning fatalities in Florida from 1995 to 2004. In: International Conference on Lightning and Static Electricity, August 28-31, 2007; Paris, France; 2007. Paper: Ic07/PPR KM01

[5] Cooper MA, Andrews CJ, Holle RL, Blumenthal R, Navarrete NA. Lightning-related injuries and safety. In: Auerbach P, editor. Wilderness Medicine. 7th ed. Philadelphia, Pennsylvania: Elsevier; 2017. pp. 71-117

[6] Cherington M, Walker J, Boyson M, Glancy R, Hedegaard H, Clark S. Closing the gap on the actual numbers of lightning casualties and deaths. Preprints. In: 11th Conference on Applied Climatology; 10-15 January 1999. Dallas, Texas, USA: American Meteorological Society; 1999. pp. 379-380

[7] Storm Data and Unusual Weather Phenomena. Monthly Publication of National Centers for Environmental Information, National Oceanographic and Atmospheric Administration. [Internet]. Ongoing. Available from: https://data.nodc.noaa.gov/cgi-bin/iso?id=gov.noaa.ncdc:C01036 [Accessed: 25 October 2019]

[8] Cherington M, Holle RL, Heitkamp TA. Deaths, injuries, and property damage due to lightning in Colorado from 1950 to 1991 based on storm data. NOAA Technical Memorandum ERL NSSL-103. Norman, OK; 1994. 45pp

[9] Lushine JB. Underreporting of lightning deaths in Florida. Preprints. In: International Lightning Detection Conference; November 6-8, 1996; Tucson, Arizona. Tucson: Global Atmospherics, Inc.; 1996. 5pp

[10] Andrews CJ, Darveniza M. Telephone mediated lightning injury: An Australian survey. Journal of Trauma. 1989;**29**:665

[11] Cooper MA. Lightning injuries: Prognostic signs for death. Annals of Emergency Medicine. 1980;**9**(3):134-138

[12] Roberts SK, Elsom DM. Analysis of storm insurance claims in the United Kingdom, 1997-2001. In: Abstracts, European Conference on Severe Storms 2002, August 26-30, 2002; Prague, Czech Republic; 2002. pp. 109-110

[13] Holle RL, López RE, Ortiz R, Watson AI, Smith DL, Decker DM, et al. Cloud-to-ground lightning related to deaths, injuries, and property damage in central Florida. In: Proceedings, International Aerospace and Ground Conference on Lightning and Static Electricity, 1992; Atlantic City, NJ; 1992. pp. 66-1-66-11

[14] Holle RL, López RE, Arnold LJ, Endres J. Insured lightning-caused property damage in three western

states. Journal of Applied Meteorology. 1996;**35**:1344-1351

[15] Holle RL, López RE, Curran EB. Deaths, injuries, and property damages from lightning by state in the United States. Preprints. In: International Lightning Detection Conference, November 16-18, 1998. Tucson, AZ: Global Atmospherics, Inc.; 1998. 12pp

[16] Cooper MA. Disability, not death, is the main problem with lightning injury. National Weather Digest. 2001;**25**:43-47

[17] Jensenius J. A detailed analysis of lightning deaths in the United States from 2006 through 2015. Preprints. In: 6th International Lightning Meteorology Conference; 18-21 April 2016; San Diego, California: Vaisala; 2016. 8pp

[18] Jensenius J. NOAA's lightning safety awareness efforts—What we've accomplished in 15 years. Preprints. In: 6th International Lightning Meteorology Conference; 18-21 April 2016; San Diego, California: Vaisala; 2016. 5pp

[19] Elsom DM. Factors contributing to a long-term decrease in national lightning fatality rates: Case study of the United Kingdom with wider implications. International Journal of Disaster Risk Reduction. 2018;**31**:341-353

[20] López RE, Holle RL. Changes in the number of lightning deaths in the United States during the twentieth century. Journal of Climate. 1998;**11**:2070-2077

[21] Cooper MA. Whether the medical aspects of lightning injury are different in developing countries. Preprints. In: 33rd International Conference on Lightning Protection; 2-7 September 2012; Vienna. Austria: ICLP; 2012. 6pp

[22] Holle RL. A summary of recent national-scale lightning fatality studies. Weather, Climate, and Society. 2016;**8**:35-42

[23] Injury Reports—By Country and Year. [Internet]. Ongoing. Available from: https://aclenet.org/news-publications/country-news/ [Accessed: 25 October 2019]

[24] Holle RL, López RE. A comparison of current lightning death rates in the U.S. with other locations and times. Preprints. In: International Conference on Lightning and Static Electricity; 16-18 September 2003; Blackpool. England: Royal Aeronautical Society; 2003. 7pp

[25] Gomes R, Ab Kadir MZA. A theoretical approach to estimate the annual lightning hazards on human beings. Atmospheric Research. 2011;**101**:719-725. DOI: 10.1016/j.atmosres.2011.04.020

[26] Cardoso I, Pinto Jr O, Pinto IRCA, Holle RL. A new approach to estimate the annual number of global lightning fatalities. In: Preprints of the 14th International Conference on Atmospheric Electricity; 8-11 August 2011; Rio de Janeiro. Brazil: ICAE; 2011. 4pp

[27] Syakura R, Ab Kadir MZA, Gomes C, Elistina AB, Cooper MA. Comparative study on lightning fatality rate in Malaysia between 2008 and 2017. In: 34th International Conference on Lightning Protection; 2-7 September 2018; Rzeszow, Poland; 2018. 5pp

[28] Roeder WP, Cummins BH, Ashley WS, Holle RL, Cummins KL. Mapping lightning fatality risk. Preprints. In: 5th International Lightning Meteorology Conference; March 20-21, 2014. Tucson, Arizona: Vaisala; 2014. 13pp

[29] Nibigira E, Gomes C. Lightning environment in Burundi. In: 32nd International Conference on Lightning Protection. Shanghai, China: ICLP; 2014. 4pp

[30] Mulder MB, Msalu L, Caro T, Salerno J. Remarkable rates of lightning strike mortality in Malawi. PLoS One. 2012;7:1. DOI: 10.1371/journal.pone.0029281.2012

[31] Dlamini WM. Lightning fatalities in Swaziland: 2000-2007. Natural Hazards. 2009;**50**:179-191

[32] Mary AK, Gomes C, Gomes A, Ahmad WFW. Lightning accidents in Uganda. In: 32nd International Conference on Lightning Protection. Shanghai, China: ICLP; 2014. 10pp

[33] Blumenthal R. Lightning fatalities on the South African Highveld: A retrospective descriptive study for the period 1997-2000. The American Journal of Forensic Medicine and Pathology. 2005;**26**:66-69

[34] Kalindekafe L, Katonda V, Nthara TK, Chinsenga C, Gomani P, Mkandawire M, et al. Lightning fatalities in Malawi: A retrospective study from 2010 to 2017. In: 34th International Conference on Lightning Protection; 2-7 September 2018. Rzeszow, Poland: ICLP; 2018

[35] Holle RL, Cooper MA. Lightning fatalities in Africa from 2010-2017. In: 34th International Conference on Lightning Protection; 2-7 September 2018. Rzeszow, Poland: ICLP; 2018

[36] Lubasi FC, Gomes C, Ab Kadir MZA, Cooper MA. Lightning related injuries and property damage in Zambia. In: 31st International Conference on Lightning Protection; 2-7 September 2012; Vienna, Austria; 2012

[37] Mary AK, Gomes C. Lightning safety of under-privileged communities around Lake Victoria. Geomatics, Natural Hazards and Risk. 2014;**6**:1-17. DOI: 10.1080/19475705.2014.922506

[38] Pasha E. Injuries caused by Lightning in Africa. Nature. 1888;**37**:582-583

[39] Holle RL, López RE, Navarro BC. Deaths, injuries, and damages from lightning in the United States in the 1890s in comparison with the 1990s. Journal of Applied Meteorology. 2005;**44**:1563-1573

[40] Holle RL, Cooper MA. Lightning occurrence and social vulnerability. In: Atmospheric Hazards – Case Studies in Modeling, Communication, and Society Impacts. Rijeka, Croatia: InTech; 2016. DOI: 10.5772/63001. 18pp

[41] Lightning Safety Tips and Resources [Internet]. Ongoing. Available from: https://www.weather.gov/safety/lightning-victims [Accessed: 25 October 2019]

[42] Holle RL, Cooper MA. Lightning-caused deaths and injuries at schools. Preprints. In: 33rd International Conference on Lightning Protection; 25-30 September 2016. Estoril, Portugal: ICLP; 2018. 5pp

[43] http://global-growing.org/en/content/fact-1-majority-sub-saharan-africans-live-rural-areas-europeans-predominantly-cities [Accessed: 06 July 2019]

[44] Holle RL, Cooper MA. Overview of lightning injuries around the World. In: The 11th Asia-Pacific International Conference on Lightning; 12-14 June 2019. Hong Kong, China: APL; 2019. 5pp

[45] Dewan A, Hossain MF, Rahman MM, Yamane Y, Holle RL. Recent lightning-related fatalities and injuries in Bangladesh. Weather, Climate, and Society. 2017;**9**:575-589

[46] Holle RL, Islam AKMS. Lightning fatalities in Bangladesh in May 2016. Postprints. In: 8th Conference on the Meteorological Applications of Lightning Data. Seattle, Washington, USA: American Meteorological Society; 2017. 4pp

[47] Cooper MA, Holle RL. Reducing Lightning Injuries Worldwide. New York: Springer; 2019. DOI: 10.1007/978-3-319-77563-0

[48] Holle RL, Said RK, Brooks WA. Monthly GLD360 lightning percentages by continent. In: 7th International Lightning Meteorology Conference, 2018. Fort Lauderdale, FL, USA: Vaisala; 2018. 4pp

[49] Cooper MA, Holle RL. Casualties from lightning involving motorcycles. In: International Conference on Lightning and Static Electricity; 28-31 August 2007. Paris, France: ICOLSE; 2007. 6pp

[50] Holle RL. Lightning-caused casualties in and near dwellings and other buildings. Preprints. In: International Lightning Meteorology Conference; 21-22 April 2010. Orlando, Florida: Vaisala; 2010. 19pp

[51] Holle RL. Lightning-caused deaths and injuries in the vicinity of trees. Preprints. In: International Conference on Lightning Protection; 2-7 September 2012; Vienna, Austria; 2012. 8pp

[52] IEC-62305 Code. Available from: https://webstore.iec.ch/home [Accessed: 25 October 2019]

[53] NFPA Code. Available from: https://catalog.nfpa.org/NFPA-780-Standard-for-the-Installation-of-Lightning-Protection-Systems-P1367.aspx [Accessed: 25 October 2019]

[54] Villamil DE, Navarrete NA, Cooper MA. Keraunoparalysis—An explanation for the more severe lightning injuries reported in developing countries. In: International Symposium on Lightning Protection (XV SIPDA); 30th September–4th October 2019. São Paulo, Brazil: SIPDA; 2019. 5pp

[55] Cherington M. Spectrum of neurologic complications of lightning injuries. NeuroRehabilitation. 2005;**20**(1):3-8

[56] Jandrell IR, Blumenthal R, Anderson RB, Trengove E. Recent lightning research in South Africa with a special focus on keraunopathology. In: Proceedings of the 16th International Symposium on High Voltage Engineering, 2009; Johannesburg, South Africa; 2009

[57] Andrews CJ, Reisner AD, Cooper MA. Post electrical or lightning injury syndrome: A proposal for an American Psychiatric Association's diagnostic and statistical manual formulation with implications for treatment. Neural Regeneration Research. 2017;**12**:1405-1412

[58] Nag A, Murphy MA, Schulz W, Cummins KL. Lightning locating systems: Insights on characteristics and validation techniques. Earth and Space Science. 2015;**2**:65-93. DOI: 10.1002/2014EA000051

[59] Cummins KL, Murphy MJ. An overview of lightning locating systems: History, techniques, and data uses, with an in-depth look at the U.S. NLDN. IEEE Transactions on Electromagnetic Compatibility. 2009;**51**(3):499-518

[60] Roeder WP. Teaching lightning safety—A five level method. In: International Conference on Lightning and Static Electricity; 28-31 August 2007; Paris, France; 2007. 7pp

[61] Cooper MA, Tushemereirwe R, Holle RL, Villamil DE. African Centres for Lightning and Electromagnetics Network (ACLENet)—Application to South America? In: International Symposium on Lightning Protection (XV SIPDA); 30th September–4th October 2019. São Paulo, Brazil: SIPDA; 2019. 6pp

[62] Cooper MA. A brief history of lightning safety efforts in the United

States. Preprints. In: 4th International Lightning Meteorology Conference; April 4-5, 2012. Broomfield, Colorado: Vaisala; 2012. 5pp

[63] Newspaper Inserts [Internet]. 2019. Available from: https://aclenet.org/news-publications/publications/newspaper-inserts.html [Accessed: 25 October 2019]

[64] Trengove E. Lightning myths and beliefs in south africa: Their effect on personal safety [Dissertation]. Johannesburg: South Africa University of the Witwatersrand; 2013

[65] ACLENet Newsletter. Myths that Can Kill You—Issue 2019-4 [Internet]. 2019. Available from: https://us14.campaign-archive.com/?u=7831fb96742ec9ee9e7fe8c29&id=68674907cb [Accessed: 25 October 2019]

[66] Cooper MA. Myths, miracles, and mirages. Seminars in Neurology. 1995;**15**(4):358-361

[67] Cooper MA, Holle RL, Andrew CJ. Distributions of lightning injury mechanisms. Preprints. In: International Lightning Detection Conference; 21-23 April 2008. Tucson, Arizona, USA: Vaisala; 2008. 4pp

[68] Blumenthal R, West NJ. Investigating the risk of lightning's pressure blast wave. South African Journal of Science. 2015;**111**(3/4):2014-0187. 5pp

[69] Anderson RB. Does a fifth mechanism exist to explain lightning injuries? IEEE Engineering in Medicine and Biology. 2001;January/February:105-113

[70] Anderson RB, Jandrell IR, Nematswerani HE. The upward streamer mechanism versus step potential as a cause of injuries from close lightning discharges. The Transactions of the South Africa Institute of Electrical Engineers. 2002;**93**:33-43

[71] Cooper MA. A fifth mechanism of lightning injury. Society for Academic Emergency Medicine. 2002;**9**:172-174

[72] Holle RL, Zhang D. So You Think You Know Lightning: A Collection of Electrifying Fast Facts. Vaisala. 2017. 64pp. Available from: https://www.vaisala.com/en/lp/so-you-think-you-know-lightning

[73] Cooper MA, Holle RL. Mechanisms of lightning injury should affect lightning safety messages. Newsletter, National Weather Association. 2011;June:2-3

[74] Cooper MA. Emergent Care of lightning and electrical injuries. Seminars in Neurology. 1995;**15**:3

[75] Cooper MA, Marshburn S, Marshburn J. Lightning strike and electric shock survivors, international. National Weather Digest. 2001;**25**(1,2):48-50

[76] Cooper MA, Marshburn S. Lightning strike and electric shock survivors, international. NeuroRehabilitation. 2005;**20**(1):43-47

[77] Roeder WP, Holle RL, Cooper MA, Hodanish S. Lessons learned in communicating lightning safety effectively. Preprints. In: 4th International Lightning Meteorology Conference; 4-5 April 2012. Broomfield, Colorado, USA: Vaisala; 2012. 20pp

[78] Lightning Strike Kills 18 Children in Uganda, The Telegraph [Internet]. 2011. Available from: https://www.telegraph.co.uk/news/weather/8606238/Lightning-strike-kills-18-children-in-Uganda.html [Accessed: 06 July 2019]

[79] Testimonial. ACLENet Homepage [Internet]. 2019. Available from: https://ACLENet.org [Accessed: 25 October 2019]

[80] Uganda Resolution to Establish the African Centres for Lightning Information and Research (ACLIR), 7 February 2013; Kampala. Uganda [Internet]. 2013. Available from: https://aclenet.org/news-publications/publications/declarations.html [Accessed: 06 July 2019]

[81] Akello RJ. Lightning protection in the Republic of Kenya. In: 4th IEEE AFRICON; 24-27 September 1996. AFRICON; 1996. pp. 687-692

[82] Gijben M. The lightning climatology of South Africa. South African Journal of Science. 2012;**108**:3-4

[83] Gijben M. Investigating the plausibility of a model-based lightning risk indicator for South Africa. In: XV International Conference on Atmospheric Electricity; June 2014. Norman, Oklahoma, USA: ICAE; 2014. pp. 15-20

[84] Tapping Into Africa's Insurance Market [Internet]. 2019. Available from: https://www.ntusbfcas.com/african-business-insights/content/tapping-into-africa-s-insurance-market-growth-opportunities-risks [Accessed: 06 July 2019]

[85] 11 Cattle Killed by Lightning in KZN, The Public News Hub, 17-Oct-2019 [Internet]. 2019. Available from: https://www.publicnewshub.com/11-cattle-killed-by-lightning-in-kzn/ [Accessed: 26 October 2019]

[86] Lightning Strikes Radio Palwak in Pader District, Uganda Radio Network [Internet]. 2012. Available from: https://ugandaradionetwork.com/story/lightning-strikes-radio-palwak-in-pader-distric [Accessed: 26 October 2019]

[87] Lightning, TV Broadcast [Internet]. 2019. Available from: Part 1 https://www.youtube.com/watch?v=D2oFHt5IRDQ&list=PLypI5FX3f0AYy1bLyeDV7sXaIRp_RVBBp&index=5; Part 2 https://www.youtube.com/watch?v=B6zhzCkpWr8&list=PLypI5FX3f0AYy1bLyeDV7sXaIRp_RVBBp&index=4 [Accessed: 26 October 2019]

[88] Thank You Letter, Nkurungiro School [Internet]. 2019. Available from: https://aclenet.org/programs/lightning-protection-of-schools/thank-you-letters-from-schools-aclenet-has-protected.html [Accessed: 26 October 2019]

[89] Cooper MA, Tushemereirwe R. The Formation of ACLENet: NAM S&T Centre's Involvement in Preventing Lightning Injuries and Deaths. NAM S&T Commemorative Compendium; 2019

Chapter 9

Leprosy: Prevention and Control

Vaseem Anjum

Abstract

Hansen's disease is one of the most ancient diseases that is still prevalent in the world. The causative agent, Mycobacterium leprae (*M. leprae*) has a long incubation period, clinical features after infection are identified late and these acid fast bacilli cannot be cultured – making leprosy a difficult disease to eradicate. Therefore the prevention and control of disease becomes more important. The shift of treatment from dapsone monotherapy to multidrug therapy regimen has given a new hope. The multidrug therapy coupled with the newer vaccines promise better results to prevent further transmission. Globally and locally the efforts to decrease the burden of leprosy by using different strategies has resulted in elimination of leprosy. But there is still a long way to go to make world free of this dreaded disease.

Keywords: leprosy, prevention, vaccine, disability, multidrug therapy, rehabilitation

1. Introduction

Mycobacterium leprae (*M. leprae*) is an acid fast bacilli that is the causative agent of leprosy disease which mainly effects the skin and peripheral nerves. In olden times leprosy was common in temperate climates (e.g. Europe), today it is mainly confined to tropical and subtropical regions. Mode of transmission in leprosy is mainly through inhalation of droplets containing the bacteria. But skin contact is also claimed by many leprologists. The disabilities and deformities associated with leprosy due to neuropathy leads to long-term consequences, including. This in turn is associated with stigma.

The immunity of the host plays an important role in disease progress and control. Thus, fortunately 95% of patients exposed to *M. leprae* will not develop this disease. The variation in incubation period ranges from 2 to 20 years, or even longer.

Leprosy has been successfully eliminated as a public health problem in 2000 globally and at the national level in 113 countries out of 122 by 2005 [1]. Elimination of leprosy is defined by World Health Organization as a point prevalence below 1 per 10,000 population [2]. However, the number of new patients diagnosed with leprosy is still significant, at more than 200,000 in 2016 globally. The new case detection rate of the disease (NCDR) is only slowly declining (**Figure 1**) [3].

The long incubation period, silent symptoms, long duration MDT and unavailability of effective vaccine makes this disease difficult to identify, treat and eradicate. To add to the misery the stigma associated with the disease is another challenge. In such circumstances, prevention and control of disease gains utmost importance.

IntechOpen

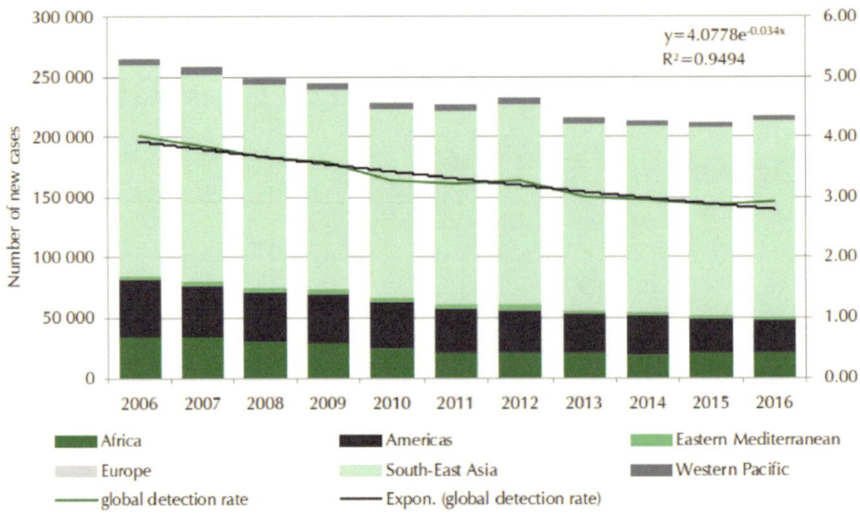

Figure 1.
Trend in case detection and case detection rate, by WHO region, 2006–2016 [3].

2. Burden of disease

In 2017, 192,713 patients were on treatment globally which makes the prevalence rate of 0.25 per 10,000 population [4]. Total of 210,671 new cases were reported in same year from 150 countries making NCDR of 2.77 per 100,000 population. **Figure 2** below shows the trends over the past decade (2008–2017) in new case detection of leprosy cases globally in the reporting countries of World Health Organization (WHO) [4].

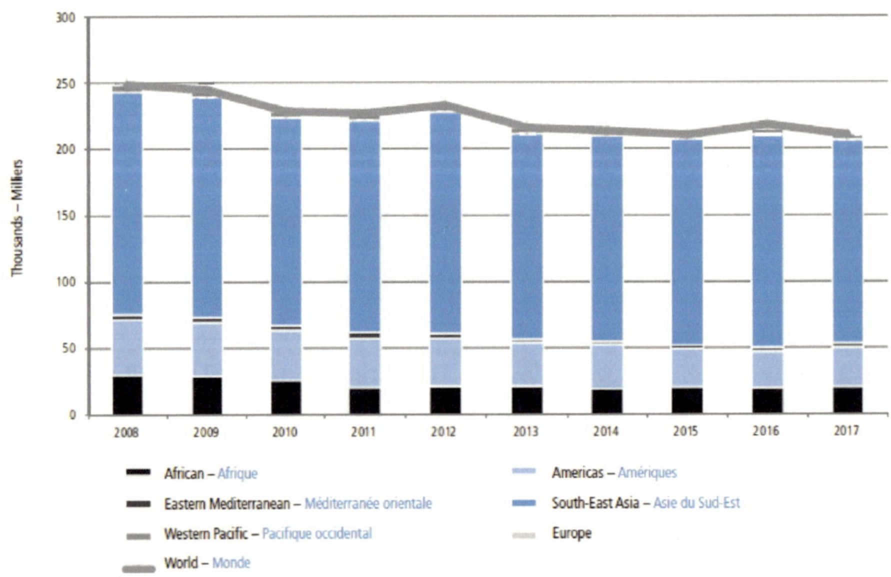

Figure 2.
Country-wise trends of detection of new leprosy cases from 2008 to 2017 [4].

3. Control of leprosy

The three main goals of control of leprosy are

a. To detect the pathology early and treat the patient completely.

b. To prevent the transmission to the others.

c. To prevent the disabilities and other complications.

Thus the following modalities are adopted to control leprosy:

1. Medical measures

2. Social support

3. Program management

4. Evaluation

4. Medical measures

4.1 Estimation of the burden of leprosy

The control of leprosy starts with the estimation of size and magnitude of the problem. Most common epidemiological survey method of collection of data is "Quick random sample survey." Information about the prevalence of leprosy, age and sex-wise distribution, various forms of leprosy and the health facilities available should be gathered. Roughly the total prevalence of leprosy in an area would be about 4 times that of the cases found among school children [5, 6]. These estimates are essential to plan, implement and to evaluate the results of the control program.

4.2 Early Case Detection

The objective is to detect all the cases as early as possible and to register them. Active case finding is important as the disease is symptomless in the early stages. Cases can be detected by the Contact surveys, Group surveys and Mass surveys. Contact surveys consists of examination of all household contacts with a lepromatous case, particularly children, in areas with prevalence less than 1 per 1000. Contact surveillance of households is recommended for a minimum period of 10 years after case is declared bacteriologically negative, and for 5 years in households with a non-lepromatous case from the time of diagnosis of the index case. Group surveys are done in areas where prevalence of leprosy is more than 1 in 1000 population. This consists of screening certain groups such as school children, slum dwellers, military recruits, industrial workers, etc. through "Skin camps." Lastly, mass surveys consists of examination of each and every individual by house-to-house visits in hyperendemic areas (prevalence – 10 or more per 1000 population). These are generally carried out by repeated annual examinations of school children which yield better results at relatively low cost [5, 6]. The data of each case is entered in the standardized proforma developed by WHO.

4.3 Chemotherapy

Since an effective vaccine is unavailable for leprosy the secondary prevention (early treatment) becomes more important. Until 1981, Dapsone (Diamino Diphenyl Sulphone—DDS) was used to treat leprosy which resulted in the development of resistance and relapse, making leprosy control difficult.

Multidrug Therapy: In 1982, WHO recommended Multidrug Therapy (MDT) for all leprosy patients. Introduction of MDT has opened a new avenue in the control of leprosy in the world. Aim of MDT is to convert the infectious case into noninfectious as soon as possible, so as to reduce the reservoir of infection in the community.

The main objectives of MDT are:

- To ensure early detection of the cases.
- To interrupt the transmission of infection.
- To prevent drug resistance, relapse and reaction.

The advantages of MDT over dapsone monotherapy are:

1. Shorter duration of treatment,
2. Better patient compliance,
3. High cure rate,
4. Cost-effectiveness and
5. Ease in health delivery system.

There are two types of MDT regimens used depending on the symptoms and signs shown by the patients - Paucibacillary (PB) and Multibacillary (MB). Recommended Regimens are discussed below [3, 5–7]:

i. Multibacillary leprosy:

MDT is recommended for following groups of patients:

- All smear positive cases.
- Skin lesions more than five in number.
- More than one nerve trunk thickening.
- All cases of relapse/reactivation and all cases who have been treated with Dapsone monotherapy earlier.

The drugs used in Multibacillary MDT and dosages are:

Rifampicin: 600 mg once monthly, supervised.
Dapsone: 100 mg daily, self administered.
Clofazimine: 300 mg once monthly, supervised and 50 mg daily, self administered.

Duration of treatment for Multibacillary leprosy is 12 months, can be extended to 18 months and continued where possible up to smear negativity. Sometimes LL/BL patients with high bacilli may need 2–3 years or more of MDT for achieving bacteriological negativity.

ii. Paucibacillary leprosy:

The drugs and dose schedule is:
Rifampicin 600 mg once a month for 6 months supervised.
Dapsone 100 mg daily for 6 months self administered.
Paucibacillary leprosy is treated for 6 months.

MDT is not contraindicated in patients with HIV infection.
Each MDT blister pack contains tablets for 4 weeks treatment. For easy identification color coding of the blister pack is done, that is, with different colors for multibacillary and paucibacillary cases both in adults and children.

The treatment in both PB and MB cases varies depending on the age of the patient. The patients between 10 to 14 years are treated as paediatric cases, while >14 years are considered adult. The standard treatment regimen for MB leprosy in adults is given for 12 months. The drugs in each blister pack are (**Figure 3**):

Two capsules of Rifampicin of 300 mg (600 mg once a month) to be taken as single dose under supervision.
Clofazimine 3 capsules of 100 mg each to be consumed once a month as single dose under supervision and 50 mg daily for next 28 days.
Dapsone 100 mg as single dose and then daily once for 1 month.

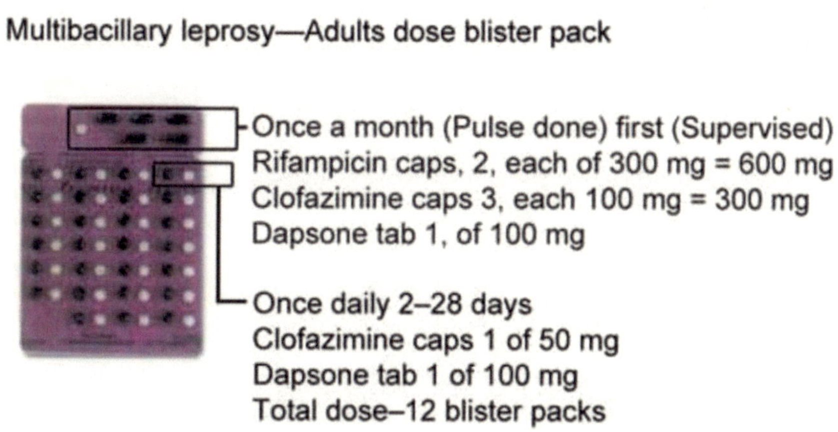

Figure 3.
MDT for adult MB type of leprosy [2, 7].

The standard adult treatment regimen for PB leprosy is (**Figure 4**):

Rifampicin: 600 mg once a month.
Dapsone: 100 mg daily.
Duration: 6 months (6 blister packs of 28 days each).

Treatment regimen for MB leprosy in children (ages 10–14 years) is (**Figure 5**):

Rifampicin: 450 mg once a month.
Clofazimine: 150 mg once a month, and 50 mg every other day.

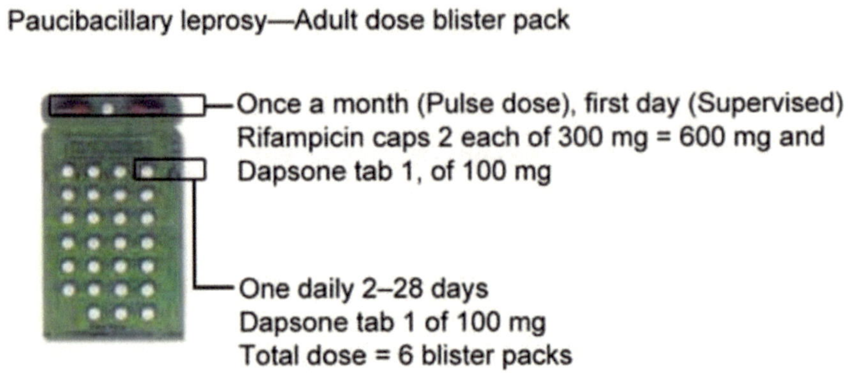

Figure 4.
MDT for adult PB type of leprosy [2, 7].

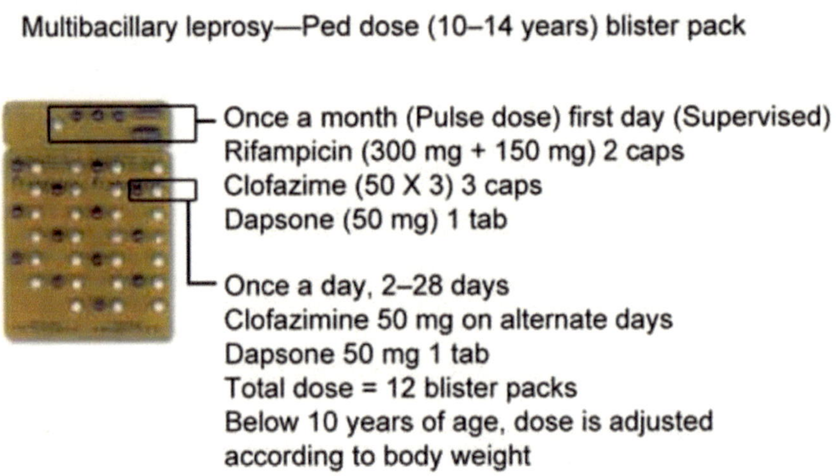

Figure 5.
MDT for pediatric MB type of leprosy [2, 7].

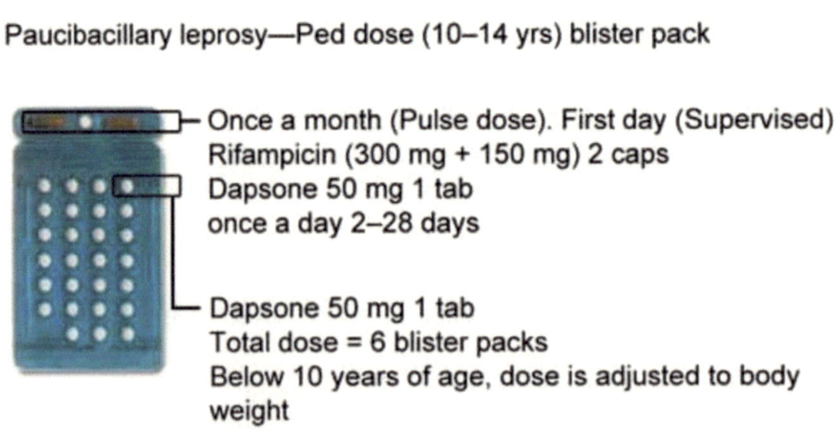

Figure 6.
MDT for pediatric PB type of leprosy [2, 7].

Dapsone: 50 mg daily.
Duration: 12 months (12 blister packs of 28 days each).
Treatment regimen for PB leprosy in children (ages 10–14 years) is (**Figure 6**):

Rifampicin: 450 mg once a month.
Dapsone: 50 mg daily.
Duration: 6 months (6 blister packs of 28 days each).

MDT is provided free-of-charge globally through an agreement between a pharmaceutical company and WHO. WHO manages distribution of MDT to countries in coordination with national leprosy programs.

5. Surveillance

Clinical surveillance of the patients after completion of treatment is an important part of MDT to ensure complete cure. For paucibacillary cases follow up for at least once a year for 2 years after completion of treatment and for multibacillary cases at least once a year for 5 years [3–5].

6. Immunoprophylaxis

Early diagnosis of cases, aggressive treatment and proactive measures to avoid complications and disabilities is the backbone for the success of any comprehensive program. In addition to accurate reporting and control measures, effective preventions will be needed to achieve elimination. Search for an effective vaccine either to be used alone or in combination with a drug has been going for a long time.

Presently BCG (Bacillus Calmette-Guerin) is the only vaccine that has shown some protection against *M. leprae* bacillus. A single dose of BCG gives 50 percent or higher protection against the disease. It is the most widely used vaccine in the world, yet the degree of protection it confers is not yet confirmed. The meta-analysis of many experimental studies concludes that the vaccine gives approximately 26% protection against leprosy. But the protection level decreases with time. To overcome this problem more than one dose of vaccine is advised.

Other variants of vaccination are also suggested.

a. **Adding killed *M. leprae* to BCG:** Various modifications have been suggested, such as the addition of killed *M. leprae* to BCG. This method almost doubles the vaccine efficacy in some populations as concluded by few studies. But the same cannot be said for patients below 15 years.

b. **Vaccination with *M. indicus pranii*** *(Mycobacterium W)*: This strain discovered in India. Testing of the MIP vaccine took place in 2005 and showed that it was effective for seven to 8 years, after which a booster dose would be needed to maintain the immunity. Recently the vaccine was approved by the Drug Controller General of India to be rolled out in a project involving five districts in the states of Bihar and Gujarat, where there are high rates of leprosy. Leprosy patients and their close contacts will benefit from this project, making India the first country in the world to have a large-scale leprosy vaccination initiative [8].

Another milestone in prevention of leprosy is the discovery of the vaccine candidate, called LepVax. Scientists at Infectious Disease Research Institute (IDRI), along with national and international collaborators including the

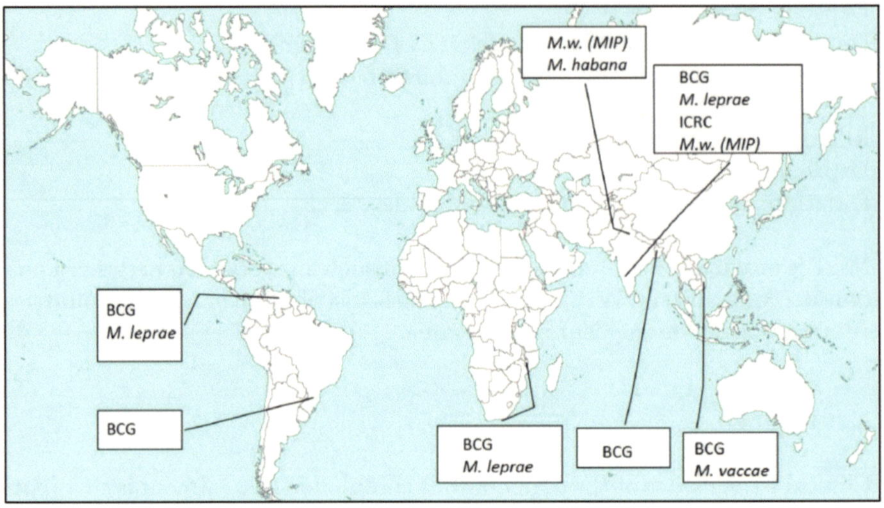

Figure 7.
Locations of leprosy vaccine testing.

National Hansen's Disease Program and the National Institute of Allergy and Infectious Diseases (NIAID), part of the National Institutes of Health, with financial support from American Leprosy Missions, have developed this leprosy vaccine. Based on the preclinical studies, the LepVax, has progressed to Phase I clinical testing in the United States, the first stage of safety testing in human volunteers. The clinical trial is focused not only on safety but also evaluates the immune response of the individual to the vaccine.

c. **Indian cancer research center (ICRC) bacilli:** Another variant belonging to the *M. avium intracellulare* group, the ICRC bacilli are thought to induce lepromin conversion in lepromatous leprosy patients and in lepromin-negative leprosy-free individuals. Its efficacy was reported to be 65.5 percent [8].

d. ***M. vaccae:*** The studies with this soil-dwelling mycobacterial species combined with BCG showed to provide greater protection against leprosy, but a Vietnamese trial contradicted the results [8].

e. ***M. Habana:*** This bacilli has been reported to induce lepromin conversion when used as a live vaccine in monkeys, and protected mice against the development of leprosy [8].

Chemoprophylaxis alone provides two-year protective window while effective immunization will provide a much broader protective window. Thus many studies and research is going on to provide both chemoprophylaxis and immunization for immediate and short-term protection and longer-term protection respectively. This strategy could have better impact and distinct appeal in controlling and preventing leprosy. Such trials could also provide a gateway for the assessment and implementation of new emerging vaccines (**Figure** 7).

7. Chemoprophylaxis (post-exposure prophylaxis)

Chemoprohylaxis using effective antibiotics focuses on providing protection to people at risk such as close contacts – family members, neighbors, co-workers, health care providers for lepers etc. Due to the stigma of disease the leprosy cases are found in clusters in all endemic regions, rather than being evenly dispersed over the whole area. Thus these high risk people can be identified and prophylaxis provided along with secondary prevention strategies. The process includes focused surveillance, contact tracing, early diagnosis and treatment. This helps in reducing the incidence and breaking the chain of transmission.

Chemoprophylaxis, as recommended by WHO Guideline Development Group (GDG), is done using single dose rifampicin (SDR) for contacts of leprosy patients both in adults and children of 2 years of age and above. Before starting the drug leprosy and TB disease are to be excluded. There should be no contraindications also for the use of rifampicin.

Other important considerations for the implementation of this chemoprophylaxis by programs are:

i. Adequate management of contacts.

ii. Consent of the index case to disclose his/her disease.

An RCT found that SDR reduces risk of leprosy over 5–6 years in leprosy contacts. For every 1000 contacts treated with SDR, there were four leprosy cases prevented after 1–2 years and three cases prevented after 5–6 years.

Recommended dosage schedules for SDR are given in **Table 1**.

The limitations of this approach are:

a. The protection is approximately for only 2 years.

b. High bacillary load cannot be eliminated using single dose.

c. Specific screening test needed to distinguish between contacts with high and low bacillary load.

Age/weight	Rifampicin single dose
Adults (≥15 years)	600 mg
10–14 years	450 mg
Children 6–9 years (weight ≥ 20 kg)	300 mg
Children <20 kg (≥2 years)	10–15 mg/kg

Table 1.
Rifampicin dose for chemoprophylaxis [3].

8. Deformity prevention and rehabilitation

Among communicable diseases, leprosy remains a leading cause of peripheral neuropathy and disability in the world, despite extensive efforts to reduce the disease burden. It is an important aspect of leprosy control. It means the medical, surgical, social, educational, and vocational restoration as far as possible of treated patients to normal activity so that they resume their place in the home, in society and industry [5–7]. Early treatment helps in disability limitation.

Rehabilitation: WHO has defined rehabilitation as "the combined and coordinated use of medical, social, educational and vocational measures for training and retraining the individual to the highest possible level of functional ability."

Preventive rehabilitation consists of prevention of development of disabilities in a leprosy patient by early diagnosis and prompt treatment. But once the patient becomes handicapped and suffers from the damage caused, should be trained and retrained to the maximum functional ability so that the patient becomes useful to self, to the family and to community at large by various measures such as medical (physical), surgical, psychological, vocational and social rehabilitation (Flow chart 20.10).

9. Health education

Health education is given to the patient, to the family and to the community at large about leprosy. The education should be directed to ensure general public and patients help them develop their own actions and efforts to change the perception about the disease and seeking professional help whenever required. Early recognition of symptoms, prompt diagnosis, health seeking behavior, personal care, treatment adherence and rehabilitation are important aspects of health education. The key messages included are about the cause of disease and the complete cure available to encourage people for early diagnosis and treatment. It also aims at helping people to change their attitude and behavior by removing the misunderstandings and misconceptions. Mass Health education also helps to eradicate social stigma, social ostracism and social prejudice associated with leprosy which is the biggest hindrance for the eradication of disease.

10. Social and financial support

The complications of the disease cause disfigurement and disabilities which in turn gives way to the stigma and strong discrimination of these patients. This results not only in physical and social isolation also financial dependency, ultimately forcing the leprosy patients to beg on streets for their survival. To address this issue WHO introduced the strategy of community-based rehabilitation (CBR). This intended to enhance the quality of life for lepers with disabilities through community initiatives. Community participation and using local resources to support the rehabilitation of people with disabilities within their own communities is the foundation of this concept [9, 10].

11. Programmatic measures

11.1 Prevention of leprosy globally

11.1.1 The enhanced global strategy for further reducing the disease burden due to leprosy 2011–2015

"Enhanced Global Strategy for Further Reducing the Disease Burden due to Leprosy for 2011–2015" was launched in 2009 by the World Health Organization. The target of the program was to reduce Grade 2 Disability rate (G2DR) in leprosy patients by at least 35% by the end of 2015 (G2DR is the number of new cases with grade 2 disability per 100,000 population). Since the elimination of leprosy in 2005, the prevalence is very less and thus G2DR has been proposed as an indicator. The advantage of G2DR as indicator is that, it is less susceptible to operational factors such as detection delay and is a more robust marker for mapping cases of leprosy in any country. This will also help the program implementers to focus on interventions that reduce visible deformities by enhancing early detection and treatment of leprosy patients and ultimately reduce the number of new leprosy cases in the population. However by the end of 2015, only Thailand was able to achieve this target [11].

11.1.2 Global leprosy strategy 2016–2020: accelerating towards a leprosy-free world

In 2016, WHO launched the "Global Leprosy Strategy 2016–2020: Accelerating towards a leprosy-free world" [9].

The program aims to reinvigorate efforts to control leprosy and avert disabilities, especially among children still affected by the disease in endemic countries.

The strategy is built around three major pillars:

i. Strengthen government ownership and partnerships;

ii. Stop leprosy and its complications; and

iii. Stop discrimination and promote inclusion.

The strategy of this program is:

- To sustain expertise and increase the number of skilled leprosy staff;
- To improve the participation of affected persons in leprosy services;
- To reduce visible deformities and stigma associated with the disease;
- To call for renewed political commitment and enhanced coordination among partners;
- To highlight the importance of research and improved data collection and analysis.

The key interventions needed to achieve these targets include:

- Early case detection especially in children before visible disabilities occur thus reduce transmission;
- In highly endemic areas or communities detection of disease among higher risk groups through campaigns;
- Improving health care coverage and access for marginalized populations such as poor patients, patients in the difficult to reach areas and the areas of conflicts.

Customization of the strategic interventions in endemic countries is permitted to suit the national plans to meet the new targets. E.g. Screening all close contacts of persons affected by leprosy; initiating a shorter and uniform treatment regimen; and incorporating specific interventions against stigmatization and discrimination.

Its ultimate goal of this program is to further reduce the global and local leprosy burden, that is, (a) zero disabilities in children with leprosy-affected, (b) G2DR less than one per million population and (c) repeal of laws that discriminate leprosy patients of their rights.

Conflict of interest

Author declares no conflict of interest.

Author details

Vaseem Anjum
Department of Community Medicine, Deccan College of Medical Sciences, Hyderabad, Telangana, India

*Address all correspondence to: vaseemanjum8@gmail.com

References

[1] World Health Organization. Global leprosy burden. Weekly Epidemiological Record. 2005;**13**:118-124

[2] Guide to eliminate leprosy as a Public Health Problem. Leprosy Elimination Group World Health Organisation CH-1211 Geneva 27 Switzerland. 2000. Available from: www.who.int/lep, WHO/CDS/CPE/CEE/2000.14

[3] Guidelines for the diagnosis, treatment and prevention of leprosy. New Delhi: World Health Organization, Regional Office for South-East Asia; 2017. Licence: CC BY-NC-SA 3.0 IGO

[4] World Health Organization, Department of Control of Neglected Tropical Diseases. Global leprosy update, 2017: Reducing the disease burden due to leprosy. Weekly Epidemiological Record. 2018;**93**(35):445-456

[5] Park K. Park Textbook of Preventive and Social Medicine. 24th ed. Banaras: Bhanott; 2014. pp. 332-347

[6] Bharadwaj R. Textbook of Public Health and Community Medicine. 1st ed. Pune: Department of Community Medicine, Armed Forces Medical College; 2009. pp. 1173-1176

[7] Suryakantha AH. Community Medicine with Recent Advances. 3rd ed. New Delhi: Jaypee Brothers Medical Publishers (P) Ltd; 2014. pp. 325-341

[8] Steven GR, Malcolm SD. The International Textbook of Leprosy, Part II, Section 6, Chapter 6.4. Vaccines for Prevention of Leprosy, Infectious Disease Research Institute; 2016

[9] World Health Organization, Regional Office for South-East Asia, Global Leprosy Programme. Global Leprosy Strategy 2016-2020: Accelerating Towards a Leprosy-Free World. New Delhi: WHO Regional Office for South-East Asia; 2016. Available from: http://apps.who.int/iris/bitstream/handle/10665/208824/9789290225096_en.pdf [Accessed: 09 July 2019]

[10] WHO/ILEP Technical Guide on Community-Based Rehabilitation and Leprosy: Meeting the Rehabilitation Needs of People Affected by Leprosy and Promoting Quality of Life. Geneva: World Health Organization; 2007

[11] Alberts CJ et al. Potential effect of the World Health Organization's 2011-2015 global leprosy strategy on the prevalence of grade 2 disability: A trend analysis. Bulletin of the World Health Organization. 2011;**89**(7):487-495. DOI: 10.2471/BLT.10.085662

Chapter 10

Laser Applications in Periodontology

Sura Dakhil Jassim

Abstract

Laser have various periodontal applications including calculus removal (erbium yttrium scandium gallium garnet and erbium yttrium aluminum garnet lasers), decontamination of root and implant surfaces and bio stimulation, incision and ablation, osseous surgery, excision of the soft tissue, and bacterial reduction. This chapter analyzes the most important occasions in which lasers are used in implant and periodontal field practices. There is a strong evidence that laser is used for surgical and nonsurgical periodontal therapies including root bio modification, bacterial decline and decontamination of infected implant surface (in peri-implantitis), and removal of the pocket epithelium. This chapter also highlights the most common disadvantages as well as the advantages of using lasers in periodontal therapy. Waterlase® and Periowave™ systems are recent devices that have further revolutionized the laser technology for its favorable clinical applications; however, the procedural cost with the laser device constitutes an obstacle for its routine application.

Keywords: erbium yttrium scandium gallium garnet laser, erbium yttrium aluminum garnet laser, periodontal therapy, peri-implantitis, bacterial reduction

1. Introduction

LASER, an abbreviation of light amplification by stimulated emission of radiation, was first established by Maiman in 1960 [1], a scientist of the Hughes Aircraft Company. Based on the theory originally proposed by Albert Einstein, Maiman used the ruby crystal that produces a coherent radiant light when activated by energy. Goldman et al. [2], a dermatologist experimenting laser for tattoo removal, showed painless surface crazing of enamel after focusing two pulses of red light beam from ruby crystal. Following experiments by Stern and Sognnaes [3], pendulum shifted from ruby laser to CO_2 and Nd:YAG lasers for better interactions with dental hard tissues. The 1970s and 1980s sought use of lasers for soft tissue surgical procedures, and Lenz et al. [4] were among the pioneers to report oral surgical application of CO_2 laser, together with Frame [5], Pecaro [6], and Pick [7] who used the same for oral soft tissue lesions and periodontal procedures. Myers and Myers [8] described the use of modified ophthalmic Nd:YAG laser for removal of dental caries and received the US FDA's permission for selling Nd:YAG laser device in 1989 [9]. After Myers's suggested use in soft tissue surgery [10], Nd:YAG laser was eventually used in periodontal procedures [11, 12], and since then lasers have been used largely by researchers and clinical periodontal practitioners.

Lasers can be used in a focused beam (for excisions and incisions) and in an unfocused beam (for ablation and coagulation). Some evidence suggests that lasers used as an adjunct to scaling and root planning (SRP) may provide additional benefits [13]. It had been shown that using lasers in periodontal treatment had a beneficial role in controlling of bacteremia, bacterial reduction, effective subgingival calculus elimination (using Er:YAG lasers), improved eradication of the pocket epithelium in pockets involving teeth, and enhancement of periodontal regeneration in humans and animals without a destructive effect on the neighboring pulp tissues and bone [14–21]. In India the capability of using laser device at laboratories and institutes offers a huge chance to the researchers and scientists concerned in the field of free electron lasers, semiconductor lasers, solid-state lasers, and gas lasers [22]. So because of the importance of the subject and the wide use of laser in India, this chapter focuses on the most important types of laser used in the India as well as in Iraq.

2. Types of laser

In dental field, lasers can be categorized by different ways: according to the type of the affected tissue, soft tissue and hard tissue lasers; according to the medium of laser used, like solid laser and gas laser; and finally according to wavelength of laser that is being used.

2.1 Neodymium yttrium aluminum garnet laser

The neodymium yttrium aluminum garnet laser (Nd:YAG) wavelength is strongly absorbed by the pigmented tissue. There has been research on using the Nd:YAG laser for nonsurgical sulcular debridement in periodontal disease control [23]. Neodymium yttrium aluminum garnet laser is a very effective surgical laser for coagulating and cutting periodontal soft tissues, with good hemostasis [24]. In addition Nd:YAG laser is used in laser-assisted new attachment procedure (LANAP) [25].

2.2 Carbon dioxide laser

The CO_2 laser has the advantage of rapid soft tissue elimination and hemostasis with a very shallow depth of penetration, and this advantage is due to its wavelength which has a great affinity for water. Carbon dioxide laser has the highest absorbance of any laser [26], but it is associated with several disadvantages including its high cost, relative large size, and its interactive destruction to the hard tissue.

2.3 Diode laser

Diode wavelengths are absorbed mainly by hemoglobin and pigmented tissue (melanin). On the other hand, they are poorly absorbed by the enamel and hydroxyapatite. Laser wavelengths, ranging from 810 to 980 nm, are produced from the active medium of the diode laser which is a solid-state semiconductor made of gallium, aluminum, arsenide, and infrequently indium. Diode laser is used in particular procedures including soft tissue crown lengthening, aesthetic gingival (gingivoplasty), removal of inflamed soft tissue, exposure of soft tissue impacted teeth, frenectomies, and photostimulation of the herpetic and aphthous lesions [27].

2.4 Erbium laser

The erbium wavelengths have the highest absorption of water in any dental laser wavelengths and have a great affinity for hydroxyapatite. Two distinct wavelengths of erbium lasers had been developed, including Er:YAG (yttrium aluminum garnet) lasers and Er,Cr:YSGG (yttrium scandium gallium garnet) lasers. Because of its great affinity for hydroxyapatite, it is the laser of choice for dealing with dental hard tissues [28], and because of its high absorption of water, erbium lasers can be used for periodontal soft tissue ablation, as dental soft tissue is composed of a high proportion of water [29].

3. Laser applications in periodontology

1. Soft tissue surgical applications
2. Removal of the pocket epithelium
3. Laser root conditioning
4. Bacterial reduction
5. Implant therapy

3.1 Soft tissue surgical applications

Lasers such as diode, CO_2,Nd:YAG, Er:YAG, and Er,Cr:YSGG are being extensively used in periodontal treatments including gingival soft tissue procedures such as gingivoplasty, gingivectomy, frenectomy, benign tumors or epulis elimination [30], irradiation of aphthous ulcers, gingival depigmentation, coagulation of free graft donor sites, second-stage exposure of dental implants [13], and crown lengthening procedures [30]. This diversity of laser use is due to its superior properties over conventional scalpel procedures which include bacteremia reduction, ease of soft tissue ablation, hemostasis [30], slight wound contraction and slight scarring, immediate sterilization, edema reduction, mechanical trauma reduction, no or little operative and postoperative pain [13, 31, 32], improved patient acceptance [13], more rapid healing, little need for suturing, much easier technique, and necessitating no topical anesthesia [33].

The penetration depth of lasers differs, and therefore their performance differs, and lasers possibly cause a hazardous effect on the underlying tissues by thermal injury. Laser light is absorbed in the superficial layers in Er:YAG,CO_2 and Er,Cr:YSGG lasers, and hence it has the advantage of being simple and rapidly vaporized from soft tissues, while other type of laser such as diode lasers and deeply penetrating Nd:YAG associate with more thermal influences, which consequently lead to formation of thick coagulation zone on the treated surface [21, 29, 30] and hence used similar to electrosurgical procedures [30]. Finkbeiner [34] has suggested the usefulness of argon laser in soft tissue welding and soldering compared to conventional tissue closure method. Epithelial exclusion using CO_2 laser had been suggested to retard its downward growth, and studies have shown effective removal of epithelium from gingival tissues without damaging the underlying connective tissues [35, 36].

3.2 Removal of the pocket epithelium

Lasers are also used for soft tissue periodontal applications. The Nd:YAG was the first laser wavelength to be compared to the scalpel for treating periodontal pockets [16] and controlling bacteremia and gingival bleeding [16, 18]. The probing pocket depth and bleeding index scores were reduced using the pulsed Nd:YAG laser. Furthermore, clinical evaluation of soft tissue biopsies taken from human subjects using the Nd:YAG laser versus a curette presented a complete removal of the epithelium of the pocket after use of the pulsed Nd:YAG laser compared to the curette [15]. Similar effects presented in pig jaws (in vitro) after the use of a 980 nm diode laser with 2–4 W power settings and continuous wave compared to the conventional curette [37]. There are advantages in the postsurgical outcomes with the removal of pocket epithelium. A recent clinical study in India showed that the modified Widman flap with removal of the pocket epithelium was more effective in reducing mean probing depth than access flap with intrasulcular incision. It showed greater gain of clinical attachment and demonstrated less gingival recession [38]. When deep periodontal pockets are present, removal of the pocket epithelium using a fiber-optic glass laser offers benefits. With or without flap elevation and a conventional periodontal access flap procedure, the pocket epithelium will be removed from the inner and the outer part of the pocket. Depending on how the patient heals, the epithelium can later be ablated every 7–10 days from the outer part of the pocket, usually under the use of topical anesthesia, in order to control apical migration. This can result in long-term, stable connective tissue attachment, without gingival recession. The principle underlying this approach is guided tissue regeneration; it has been called "laser-assisted guided tissue regeneration" [39]. This approach should be evaluated in different prospective clinical studies involving many patients and following exactly the same protocol in order to establish that it is a technological improvement that should be incorporated routinely in daily practice. Both clinical case series and clinical research have shown the potential of this application using the CO_2 laser, since the noncontact handpiece is able to ablate tissues very quickly, controlling the epithelial cell proliferation and further apical migration of a long junctional epithelium. Israel et al. [20] were able to demonstrate histologically the effects of this de-epithelialization technique in humans. The technique involves using the CO_2 laser to remove (ablate) the inner part of flap after conventional periodontal flap elevation and then using the same method in the outer part of the flap to achieve epithelial retardation. Case series in patients with generalized advanced periodontal disease have shown that the laser de-epithelialization technique leads to good results without the need for multiple membrane therapy [40, 41].

3.3 Laser root conditioning

The use of CO_2 lasers to decontaminate root surfaces has been investigated, providing more information about the exact power settings and parameters required to avoid root damage. Barone et al. [42] showed that a defocused, pulsed CO_2 laser is able to create smooth and clean root surfaces compared to a focused, continuous wave; the latter leads to melting and root surface damage. Later studies using the same parameters for CO_2 lasers reported root conditioning with a better fibroblastic activity, cellular proliferation, and greater fibroblast attachment [43]. Different clinical case reports have demonstrated these advantages of CO_2 laser de-epithelialization [44]. This technique has also been used in clinical studies and has shown that coronal flap advancement in conjunction with CO_2 laser root conditioning leads to improvements in clinical parameters and long-term tissue stability after 15 years, compared to the modified Widman periodontal flap procedure [45]. The authors concluded that this laser technique seemed to have greater effects and should be used in treating deep periodontal pockets (more than 7 mm deep).

3.4 Bacterial reduction

A laser application that has been especially promoted in the past is for the reduction of bacteria in pockets, due to the high absorption of specific laser wavelengths by the chromophores. Initially, the use of an Nd:YAG laser was shown to reduce the load of *Porphyromonas gingivalis* and *Prevotella intermedia* [46]. A study by Assaf et al. [47] is of special interest. Using a diode laser in conjunction with ultrasonic scaling for treatment of gingivitis, they were able to show a significantly lower incidence of bacteremia in the diode + ultrasonic group (36%) than the ultrasonic only group (68%). They suggested that diode lasers should be used to prevent bacteremia, especially in immunocompromised patients. Using a 980 nm diode laser to reduce periodonto-pathogenic bacteria in patients with aggressive periodontitis has also been investigated. Kamma et al. [48] confirmed that it was possible to reduce the total bacterial load in pockets without the use of any systemic antibiotic therapy. Clinical case series with 10 patients using in the same patient (in a randomized protocol) SRP in conjunction with 980 nm diode laser, SRP and an Nd:YAG laser, and SRP with photodynamic therapy (PDT) showed that the PDT was able to reduce significantly the bacteria in the pockets and provide a predictable clinical outcome for 3 months. In contrast to that, the use of Nd:YAG laser was not very beneficial and was similar to the control (SRP) group [49]. Due to the bacteria reduction and the reduced bleeding on probing provided by the PDT, the PDT was recommended for periodontal patients especially for the maintenance appointments.

3.5 Laser applications in implant dentistry

In the previous years the important role of laser in dental implant treatment has been discussed widely [50]. Because of the lack of comparable test and control sites, it is difficult nowadays to know if lasers, with their different types, can be used to treat peri-implantitis using randomized clinical trials [51]. Removal of peri-implant soft tissues and bacterial reduction, uses of laser in second-stage surgery [52], and decontamination of failing implants [53] are the most important applications for lasers in implant dentistry. However there are a lot of limitations of using laser in implant dentistry including the serious alarms about the overheating of the implant and the concern about the melting of the implant surface [54, 55], as well as the fears regarding missing of the re-osseointegration after peri-implantitis treatment with lasers. In recent years a lot of reviews have concentrated on these limitations and gave additional facts about re-stabilization and re-osseointegration of the implants subsequent to the laser decontamination of the implant surface [56]. Deppe et al. [57] showed that CO_2 laser decontamination of the surface of implants placed in dogs allowed new bone to grow and be in contact with the implant surface (re-osseointegration). In vitro studies of osteoblasts have confirmed these effects for CO_2 and Er,Cr:YSGG lasers [58]. Previous clinical case series were able to demonstrate new bone fill and long-term success of failing implants that were decontaminated with a CO_2 laser [59, 60]. The main advantage of using CO_2 laser irradiation on implant surfaces is that this wavelength does not pose the risk of overheating [61], unlike other wavelengths, such as that of diode, Nd:YAG, and Er:YAG lasers [62, 63]. A significant increase of the implant surface temperature has been demonstrated when irradiating implant surfaces with a diode laser in vitro for more than 10 s [62–64]. It is possible that authors have presented unsuccessful and nonpredictable clinical results from their studies because of overheating resulting from inconsistent power settings [65]. Limited facts available regarding laser-assisted decontamination of implant surfaces, with a limited number of included studies, as well as the great heterogeneity of the results had been pointed out by a recent systematic review. Nevertheless, even though data is incomplete regarding the clinical use of CO_2 (10.6 nm) lasers in the surgical treatment of peri-implantitis, its use appears promising [66].

The following summary of advantages and disadvantages of using lasers for periodontal therapy is based on the literature and the author's experience.

4. Advantages of using lasers in the periodontal therapy

Less pain. Less need for anesthetics (an advantage for medically compromised patients). No risk of bacteremia. Excellent wound healing. No scar tissue formation. Bleeding control (dependent on the wavelength and power settings). Usually no need for sutures. Use of fewer instruments and materials and no need for autoclaving (economic advantages). Ability to remove both hard and soft tissues. Lasers can be used in combination with scalpels (however, the laser is a tool and not a panacea) [67].

5. Disadvantages of using lasers in periodontal therapy

Relatively high cost of the devices. A need for additional education (especially in basic physics). Lasers do not eliminate the need for anesthesia. Every wavelength has different properties. The need for implementation of safety measures (i.e., goggle use, etc.) [68].

6. Healing following laser therapy

Despite apparent benefits of lasers regarding patient compliance and clinical observation, there are no enough data to support that laser is associated with reduced scarring, which itself appears to be different according to the wavelength and extremely related to the energy density, and there are no enough data to support quicker healing associated with laser therapy [13]. Limited experimental animal studies [68, 69] involving CO_2,Nd:YAG, diode lasers, or Er:YAG have evaluated the histological and immunohistochemical patterns of periodontal tissue healing following surgical and nonsurgical periodontal therapy. Sculean et al. [70] and Yukna et al. [71] reported healing response of intrabony defects after open flap surgery or treatment using a laser-assisted new attachment procedure in humans using Er:YAG and Nd:YAG lasers, respectively. Lippert et al. [72] claimed that CO_2 laser-induced wounds in oral and oropharyngeal mucosa healed significantly faster (in 32.8 ± 9.2 days) than those created by Nd:YAG laser (in 40.4 ± 9.2). However, in contrast to conventional scalpel surgery, the histological findings showed that the beginning of wound healing was delayed after laser surgery, and it depends on the size of the initial defect. Due to the more pronounced zone of necrosis at the base of the wound ground, this effect is more evident using the Nd:YAG laser [72]. Although, as compared to conventional treatment, overall [72] as well as initial periodontal wound healing laser application [73] has been shown to be delayed, few studies have reported that laser-induced wounds show a reduced propensity of contraction of the scar in comparison to the usual surgeries of scalpel [13]. Low-level laser treatment by GaAIAs radiation in milliwatt range has been shown to be effective in recent studies, as it absolutely affects proliferation of fibroblasts in gingiva or periodontal ligament, so it consequently maintains peri-implant and periodontal wound healing [73].

7. Latest advances

Waterlase® system is a revolutionary dental device that uses laser-energized water to cut or ablate soft and hard tissues and provide periodontists with the opportunity to perform more procedures in fewer appointments with less need for anesthesia, scalpels, and drill [74]. Periowave™, a photodynamic disinfection system, utilizes nontoxic dye (photosensitizer) in combination with a low-intensity laser, enabling singlet oxygen molecules to destroy bacteria [75]. After applying a light-sensitive drug (photosensitizer), low-intensity laser is directed on the area treated with the drug resulting in phototoxic reactions. Although the use of photosensitizers for complete suppression of the anaerobic perio-pathogens has been suggested, the same is not true for facultative anaerobes [76].

8. Cost and safety

Laser safety officer (LSO) is an elected, well-trained individual who guides safety of laser performs and confirms a harmless surroundings for exhausting it, as an important part of giving dental treatment with laser device is protection and safety. All clinicians must be aware and take care of the prevention of accidental and hazardous irradiation. The patient, clinician, and assistant must wear a protective eyewear particular for the wavelength and the type of laser in use. Additionally, the clinician should follow laser safety rules and join certificate courses by dental laser organizations; however the size and the cost of laser device still create a difficulty and a struggle for its practical application [77].

9. Conclusion

Lasers have been suggested as an adjunctive or alternative to conventional techniques for various periodontal procedures and considered superior in respect to easy ablation, decontamination, and hemostasis besides less postoperative pain and less operative pain. Application of lasers with their different types in implant dentistry and the recent laser practical modalities had revolutionized the outcome of periodontal therapy with patient acceptance. But, procedural cost and patient risk should be kept in mind and completely assumed before laser use.

Author details

Sura Dakhil Jassim
College of Dentistry, University of Babylon, Iraq

*Address all correspondence to: suradak85@yahoo.com

References

[1] Maiman TH. Stimulated optical radiation in ruby. Nature. 1960;**187**:493-494

[2] Goldman L, Gray JA, Goldman B, Meyer R. Effects of laser: Impact on teeth. Journal of the American Dental Association (1939). 1965;**70**:601-606

[3] Stern RH, Sognnaes RF. Laser inhibition of dental caries suggested by first tests in vivo. Journal of the American Dental Association (1939). 1972;**85**:1087-1090

[4] Jesse J, Desai S, Oshita P. The evolution of lasers in dentistry: Ruby to YSGG. 4-Continuing Dental Education Units

[5] Frame JW. Carbon dioxide laser surgery for benign oral lesions. British Dental Journal. 1985;**158**:125-128

[6] Pecaro BC, Garehime WJ. The CO_2 laser in oral and maxillofacial surgery. Journal of Oral and Maxillofacial Surgery. 1983;**41**:725-728

[7] Pick RM, Pecaro BC, Silberman CJ. The laser gingivectomy. Journal of Periodontology. 1985;**56**:492-494

[8] Myers TD, Myers WD. In vivo caries removal utilising the YAG laser. The Journal of the Michigan Dental Association. 1985;**67**:66-69

[9] Myers TD, Myers ED, Stone RM. First soft tissue study utilising a pulsed Nd:YAG dental laser. Northwest Dentistry. 1989;**68**:14-17

[10] Myers TD. What lasers can do for dentistry and you. Dental Management. 1989;**29**:26-28

[11] Midda M, Renton-harper P. Lasers in dentistry. British Dental Journal. 1991;**170**:343-346

[12] Midda M. The use of lasers in periodontology. Current Opinion in Dentistry. 1992;**2**:104-108

[13] Cobb CM. Lasers in periodontics: A review of the literature. Journal of Periodontology. 2006;**77**:545-564

[14] Pinero J. Nd:YAG-assisted periodontal curettage to prevent bacteria before cardiovascular surgery. Dentistry Today. 1998;**17**:84-87

[15] Gold SI, Vilardi MA. Pulsed laser beam effects on gingiva. Journal of Clinical Periodontology. 1994;**21**:391-396

[16] Romanos GE. Clinical applications of the Nd:YAG laser in oral soft tissue surgery and periodontology. Journal of Clinical Laser Medicine & Surgery. 1994;**12**:103-108

[17] Ben Hatit Y, Blum R, Severin C, Maquin M, Jabro MH. The effects of a pulsed Nd:YAG laser on subgingival bacterial flora and on cementum: An in vivo study. Journal of Clinical Laser Medicine & Surgery. 1996;**14**:137-143

[18] Yaneva B, Firkova E, Karaslavova E, Romanos GE. Bactericidal effects of using a fiber-less Er: YAG laser system for treatment of moderate chronic periodontitis: Preliminary results. Quintessence International. 2014;**45**:489-497

[19] Eberhard J, Ehlers H, Falk W, Açil Y, Albers HK, Jepsen S. Efficacy of subgingival calculus removal with Er: YAG laser compared to mechanical debridement: An in situ study. Journal of Clinical Periodontology. 2003;**30**:511-518

[20] Israel M, Rossmann JA, Froum SJ. Use of the carbon dioxide laser in retarding epithelial migration: A pilot histological human study utilizing case

reports. Journal of Periodontology. 1995;**66**:197-204

[21] Mizutani K, Aoki A, Takasaki AA, Kinoshita A, Hayashi C, Oda S, et al. Periodontal tissue healing following flap surgery using an Er: YAG laser in dogs. Lasers in Surgery and Medicine. 2006;**38**:314-324

[22] Shrivastava SK. Status of laser technology in India. International Journal of Innovative Research and Advanced Studies. 2016;**3**(10):181-185

[23] Aoki A, Mizutani K, Takasaki AA, Sasaki KM, Nagai S, Schwarz F, et al. Current status of clinical laser applications in periodontal therapy. General Dentistry. 2008;**56**:674-687

[24] Fornaini C, Rocca JP, Bertrand MF, Merigo E, Nammour S, Vescovi P. Nd: YAG and diode lasers in the surgical management of soft tissues related to orthodontic treatment. Photomedicine and Laser Surgery. 2007;**25**:381-392

[25] Slot DE, Kranendonk AA, Paraskevas S, Van der, Weijden F. The effect of a pulsed Nd: YAG laser in non-surgical periodontal therapy. Journal of Periodontology. 2009;**80**:1041-1056

[26] Fujiyama K, Deguchi T, Murakami T, Fujii A, Kushima K, Takano-Yamamoto T. Clinical effect of CO_2 laser in reducing pain in orthodontics. The Angle Orthodontist. 2008;**78**:299-303

[27] Hilgers JJ, Tracey SG. Clinical uses of diode lasers in orthodontics. Journal of Clinical Orthodontics. 2004;**38**:266-273

[28] Harashima T, Kinoshita J, Kimura Y, Brugnera A, Zanin F, Pecora JD, et al. Morphological comparative study on ablation of dental hard tissue at cavity preparation by Er: YAG and Er, CR: YSGG lasers. Photomedicine and Laser Surgery. 2005;**23**:52-55

[29] Ishikawa I, Aoki A, Takasaki AA. Clinical application of erbium: YAG laser in periodontology. Journal of the International Academy of Periodontology. 2008;**10**:22-30

[30] Ishikawa I, Aoki A, Takasaki AA, Mizutani K, Sasaki KM, Izumi Y. Application of lasers in periodontics: True innovation or myth? Periodontology 2000. 2009;**50**:90-126

[31] Wigdor H, Walsh J, Featherstone JDB, Virsuri S, et al. Lasers in dentistry. Lasers in Surgery and Medicine. 1995;**16**:103-133

[32] Luomanen M, Meurman JH, Lehto VP. Extracellular matrix in healing CO_2 laser incision wound. Journal of Oral Pathology. 1987;**16**:322-331

[33] White JM, Goodis HE, Rose CL. Use of pulsed Nd:YAG laser for intraoral soft tissue surgery. Lasers in Surgery and Medicine. 1991;**11**:455-461

[34] Finkbeiner RL. Free autogenous soft tissue graft with argon laser. Lasers in Surgery and Medicine. 1994;**15**:168-175

[35] Rossman J, McQuade M, Turunen D. Retardation of epithelial migration in monkeys using a carbon dioxide laser. Journal of Periodontology. 1992;**63**:902

[36] Rossmann J, Israel M. Laser deepithelialisation for enhanced guided tissue regeneration: A paradigm shift? Dental Clinics of North America. 2000;**44**:793-809

[37] Romanos GE, Henze M, Banihashemi S, Parsanejad HR, Winckler J, Nentwig GH. Removal of epithelium in periodontal pockets following diode (980 nm) laser application in the animal model: An in vitro study. Photomedicine and Laser Surgery. 2004;**22**:177-183

[38] Reddy S, Bhowmik N, Prasad MG, Kaul S, Rao V, Singh S. Evaluation of

postsurgical clinical outcomes with/without removal of pocket epithelium: A split mouth randomized trial. Journal of Indian Society of Periodontology. 2014;**18**:749-759

[39] Romanos GE. Advanced Laser Surgery in Dentistry. Chicago: Quintessence Publishing; 2015

[40] Israel M, Rossmann JA. An epithelial exclusion technique using the CO_2 laser for the treatment of periodontal defects. The Compendium of Continuing Education in Dentistry. 1998;**19**:86-88, 90, 92

[41] Rossmann JA, Israel M. Laser de-epithelialization for enhanced guided tissue regeneration. A paradigm shift? Dental Clinics of North America. 2000;**44**:793-809

[42] Barone A, Covani U, Crespi R, Romanos GE. Root surface morphological changes after focused versus defocused CO_2 laser irradiation: A scanning electron microscopy analysis. Journal of Periodontology. 2002;**73**:370-373

[43] Crespi R, Barone A, Covani U, Ciaglia RN, Romanos GE. Effects of CO_2 laser treatment on fibroblast attachment to root surfaces. A scanning electron microscopy analysis. Journal of Periodontology. 2002;**73**:1308-1312

[44] Crespi R, Covani U, Romanos GE, Barone A. CO_2 laser effects on root surfaces in periodontal treatment: Case reports. Journal of Oral Laser Applications. 2004;**4**:109-117

[45] Crespi R, Cappare P, Gherlone E, Romanos GE. Comparison of modified widman and coronally advanced flap surgery combined with CO_2 laser root irradiation in periodontal therapy: A 15-year follow-up. The International Journal of Periodontics & Restorative Dentistry. 2011;**31**:641-651

[46] Neill ME, Mellonig JT. Clinical efficacy of the Nd: YAG laser for combination periodontitis therapy. Practical Periodontics and Aesthetic Dentistry. 1997;**9**(6 Suppl):1-5

[47] Assaf M, Yilmaz S, Kuru B, Ipci SD, Noyun U, Kadir T. Effect of the diode laser on bacteremia associated with dental ultrasonic scaling: A clinical and microbiological study. Photomedicine and Laser Surgery. 2007;**25**:250-256

[48] Kamma JJ, Vasdekis VG, Romanos GE. The effect of diode laser (980 nm) treatment on aggressive periodontitis: Evaluation of microbial and clinical parameters. Photomedicine and Laser Surgery. 2009;**27**:11-19

[49] Romanos GE, Brink B. Photodynamic therapy in periodontal therapy: Microbiological observations from a private practice. General Dentistry. 2010;**58**:e68-e73

[50] Romanos GE, Gutknecht N, Dieter S, Schwarz F, Crespi R, Sculean A. Laser wavelengths and oral implantology. Lasers in Medical Science. 2009;**24**:961-970

[51] Romanos GE, Weitz D. Therapy of peri-implant diseases. Where is the evidence? The Journal of Evidence-Based Dental Practice. 2012;**12**:204-208

[52] Arnabat-Dominguez J, Espana-Tost AJ, Berini-Aytes L, Gay-Escoda C. Erbium: YAG laser application in the second phase of implant surgery: A pilot study in 20 patients. The International Journal of Oral & Maxillofacial Implants. 2003;**18**:104-112

[53] Romanos GE, Javed F, Delgado-Ruiz RA, Calvo-Guirado JL. Peri-implant diseases: A review of treatment interventions. Dental Clinics of North America. 2015;**59**:157-178

[54] Block CM, Mayo JA, Evans GH. Effects of the Nd: YAG dental laser on

plasma-sprayed and hydroxyapatite-coated titanium dental implants: Surface alteration and attempted sterilization. The International Journal of Oral & Maxillofacial Implants. 1992;**7**:441-449

[55] Romanos GE, Everts H, Nentwig GH. Effects of diode and Nd: YAG laser irradiation on titanium discs: A scanning electron microscope examination. Journal of Periodontology. 2000;**71**:810-815

[56] Javed F, Hussain HA, Romanos GE. Re-stability of dental implants following treatment of peri-implantitis. Interventional Medicine & Applied Science. 2013;**5**:116-121

[57] Deppe H, Horch HH, Henke J, Donath K. Peri-implant care of ailing implants with the carbon dioxide laser. The International Journal of Oral & Maxillofacial Implants. 2001;**16**:659-667

[58] Romanos G, Crespi R, Barone A, Covani U. Osteoblast attachment on titanium disks after laser irradiation. The International Journal of Oral & Maxillofacial Implants. 2006;**21**:232-236

[59] Romanos GE. Laser surgical tools in implant dentistry for the long-term prognosis of oral implants. In: Ishikawa I, Frame J, Aoki A, editors. Lasers in Dentistry. Amsterdam: International Congress Series, Elsevier Science BV; 2003. pp. 109-114

[60] Romanos G, Ko HH, Froum S, Tarnow D. The use of CO_2 laser in the treatment of peri-implantitis. Photomedicine and Laser Surgery. 2009;**27**:381-386

[61] Oyster DK, Parker WB, Gher ME. CO_2 lasers and temperature changes of titanium implants. Journal of Periodontology. 1995;**66**:1017-1024

[62] Geminiani A, Caton JG, Romanos GE. Temperature increase during CO_2 and Er: YAG irradiation on implant surfaces. Implant Dentistry. 2011;**20**:379-382

[63] Geminiani A, Caton JG, Romanos GE. Temperature change during non-contact diode laser irradiation of implant surfaces. Lasers in Medical Science. 2012;**27**:339-342

[64] Leja C, Geminiani A, Caton J, Romanos GE. Thermodynamic effects of laser irradiation of implants placed in bone: An in vitro study. Lasers in Medical Science. 2013;**28**:1435-1440

[65] Schwarz F, Sahm N, Iglhaut G, Becker J. Impact of the method of surface debridement and decontamination on the clinical outcome following combined surgical therapy of peri-implantitis: A randomized controlled clinical study. Journal of Clinical Periodontology. 2011;**38**:276-284

[66] Kotsakis GA, Konstantinidis I, Karoussis IK, Ma X, Chu H. Systematic review and meta-analysis of the effect of various laser wavelengths in the treatment of peri-implantitis. Journal of Periodontology. 2014;**85**:1203-1213

[67] Mitchell M. Laser use in dentistry. [Accessed: 15 October 2011]

[68] Arcoria CJ, Steele RE, Vitasek BA, Wagner MJ. Effects of coaxial CO_2/Nd:YAG irradiation on periodontal wound healing. Lasers in Surgery and Medicine. 1992;**12**:401-409

[69] Schwarz F, Jepsen S, Herten M, Aoki A, Sculean A, Becker J. Immunohistochemical characterization of periodontal wound healing following nonsurgical treatment with fluorescence controlled Er:YAG laser radiation in dogs. Lasers in Surgery and Medicine. 2007;**39**:428-440

[70] Sculean A, Schwarz F, Berakdar M, Windisch P, Arweiler NB, Romanos GE. Healing of intrabony

defects following surgical treatment with or without an Er:YAG laser. Journal of Clinical Periodontology. 2004;**31**:604-608

[71] Yukna RA, Carr RL, Evans GH. Histologic evaluation of an Nd:YAG laser-assisted new attachment procedure in humans. The International Journal of Periodontics & Restorative Dentistry. 2007;**27**:577-587

[72] Lippert BM, Teymoortash A, Folz BJ, Werner JA. Wound healing after laser treatment of oral and oropharyngeal cancer. Lasers in Medical Science. 2003;**18**:36-42

[73] Schwarz F, Aoki A, Sculean A, Becker J. The impact of laser application on periodontal and peri-implant wound healing. Periodontology 2000. 2009;**51**:79-108

[74] Mohan R, Bains VK. Waterlase in periodontics. Journal of Indian Society of Periodontology. 2006;**10**:316-321

[75] Thomas B, Saatian S, Saeidi R, Petrescu S, Okera H, Rakhshanfar S, et al. Photodynamic therapy: Is it more effective than current standard of care? An evidenced based study of literature. Available from: http://laws.justice.gc.ca/en/F-27/SOR-98-282/text.html

[76] Lee D. Application of laser in periodontics: A new approach in periodontal therapy. Dental Bulletin. 2007;**12**:23-25

[77] Piccione PJ. Dental laser safety. Dental Clinics of North America. 2004;**48**:795-807

Chapter 11

Development of a Rough Terrain Wheelchair Design

Ignatio Madanhire, Loice Gudukeya and Roy Mushonga

Abstract

Conventional wheelchairs do not cope well in less-resourced rural areas as they are not stable and can topple easily. This chapter seeks to develop a wheelchair design that offers optimum stability and comfort for people in rural areas where there is rough and uneven terrain environment. The design development process entailed the generation of three possible wheelchair design concepts. Wide rear wheel design was further developed to come up with a detailed design with a maximum tipping angle of 43.17 degrees. This could be considered to be a great improvement compared to the conventional wheelchair configuration. The design was made to function using a ratchet lever bar to push the rear wheels forward to initiate motion. It was established that fabrication of the prototype could be done easily at a lower cost cap of USD200 using locally available materials. The proposed wheelchair design would improve the mobility and consequent living conditions of those disabled individuals living in rough terrain rural set up environments.

Keywords: wheelchair, stability, rough terrain, off-road, uneven ground, design, rural

1. Introduction

Wheelchairs may take a variety of forms to meet particular needs of users. Such configurations may entail specialized seating set up, individualized controlling mechanisms, and in some cases specific to certain activities, as is the case with sports and beach wheelchairs [1]. The commonly known distinction among wheelchairs is between powered wheelchairs, where mobility is powered by batteries and electric motors, and manual propulsion, where the propulsive force is provided by the user pushing the wheelchair by hand, or by having someone pushing from the rear [2].

The user of a standard wheelchair, when utilizing the wheelchair on rough terrain, is confronted with a plenty of difficulties. The most exceedingly awful being, the unsteadiness brought about by a high position of gravity point from the wheel contact with the ground [3]. In this manner wheelchair may topple over in reverse during negotiating steep slanted territory. When horizontally navigating a steep grade, the wheelchair is probably going to tip sideways [4]. During descending a slope, the operator may risk sliding out of the seat or having the seat unstable and having a forward pitch [5].

Most wheelchair designs are not conducive for use in rough terrain (**Figure 1**) found in the rural country side, nonetheless this should not discourage those who are

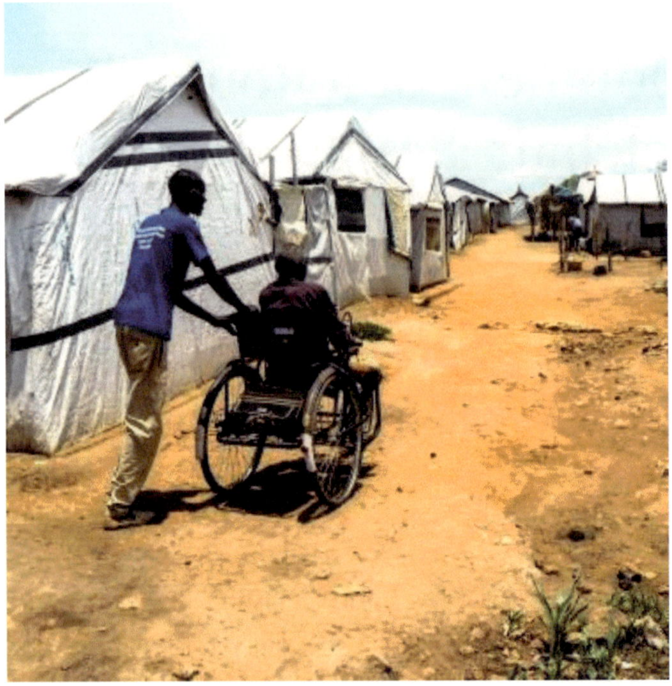

Figure 1.
Rough terrain [5].

unable to walk to work for themselves and earn a living [6]. It is in this regard that some effort has been made to improve the mobility of wheelchair users so that they are able to move from one point to the other despite how rough the terrain maybe.

2. Background

Users of wheelchairs continue to encounter some difficulties as they seek to navigate from one point to the other on rough terrain due to lack of stability when using rural off-road environment pathways [4]. Most existing wheelchairs are not suitable for use on extremely rough terrain thereby compromising the safety of the occupant [7]. Hence the objective of this chapter to design a wheelchair frame that offers optimum stability on rough terrain and does not readily overturn.

Effort to navigate extreme rugged pathways in a rural setting could be a challenge, such that even a great modern wheelchair may be found to be of limited usefulness [8]. What could be needed is an off-road design that is easy to manufacture and repair compared to designs done for a city environment where there are sidewalks. All terrain wheelchairs can increase the mobility range and access by taking occupant where one always wanted to go but were not able [9]. All terrain wheelchairs could be in various shapes and sizes, powered, manual and sometimes with a lever drive. Some have specific advantages such as the ability to maneuver on loose terrain covered by sand or gravel, in snow, over hilly terrain or on hills [10].

It is the unstable nature of existing wheelchair frames that demands for a wheelchair design modification to ensure increased increase stability on "non-ideal" terrain surfaces. Such rugged terrain may entail (but are not limited to): gravel, grass, dirt, and cracked asphalt or concrete. A wheelchair design modification is required for successful traversing of the adverse terrain while keeping four points of contact between the wheels and ground as well as maintaining the required stability and comfort for the operator [11]. It is the intention of this chapter to improve the current design within a reasonable cost range that most users within the rural area and other low-income earners category can afford to buy.

3. Wheelchair literature review

3.1 Design and standards

The intended mandate is come with a design with improved performance that provides requisite seating and postural support without compromising strength, durability and safety [12]. The International Organization for Standardization (ISO) formulated international standards for wheelchair frames, the ISO 7176 series (1). The series specify the relevant terminology and testing processes to evaluate wheelchair parameters such as performance, size, strength, durability and safety. In some cases, the required conditions in the ISO 7176 series may not capture all typical requirements in less-resourced environment, as some of the requirements were meant to simulate the conditions in city environs with smooth tarred roads. It is therefore necessary to consider varied environments when formulating national standards, by looking at key parameters such as the weights and sizes of users, typical uses, and the available wheelchair designs and associated technologies within the country [13].

3.2 General considerations

Wheelchair configuration should afford users to partake in whatever number life exercises as could be allowed. As a base prerequisite, a wheelchair ought to allow the operator to lead an increasingly dynamic existence without having any antagonistic impact on one's well-being or security. Solace and well-being comprise the two significant perspectives that influence the personal satisfaction of happy wheelchair users [14]. The well-being and security of operators ought not to be undermined so as to lessen costs during structure improvement. In spite of the fact that it might be contended that any wheelchair is superior to no wheelchair, this cannot be correct when the wheelchair turns into the reason of well-being dangers. It is in this respect a wheelchair ought to be intended to guarantee the client's improved great well-being and convenience [15].

3.3 Common wheelchair limitations

The basic difficulties that a standard wheelchair faces involve challenges while crossing lopsided surfaces or negotiating hindrances in the pathway. Such problems may be the failure to continue any further when a wheel gets stuck in a downturn, with the end result that when the user endeavors to free oneself, the seat may get agitated and topples [7]. A comparative issue, with similar results, may happen when endeavoring to cross obstructions, for example, rocks, logs or curbs the pathway (**Figure 2**). A surface not smooth, covered with scrub and stones, may likewise be considered as uneven or unpredictable consequently imposing difficulties to mobility.

There are also cases where the user may be unable to generate enough sustained human power to climb steep grades. Thus, the conventional wheelchair has limited capability to traverse steep inclines [7]. The standard wheelchair typically uses narrow width pneumatic tires which can easily get punctured by branches, rocks and the like. When utilized in sandy, loose and unstable soil, the wheels sink and the occupant may get stuck in the process [16].

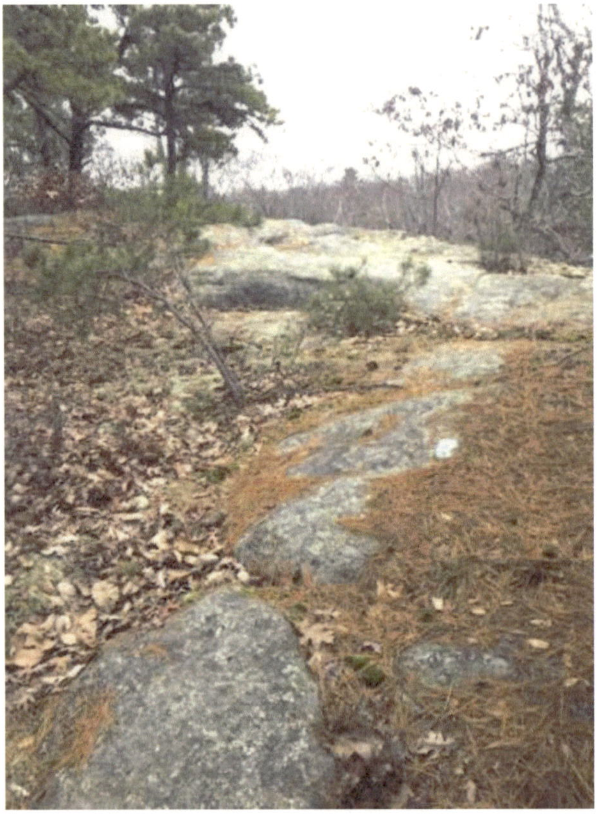

Figure 2.
Rock obstructions [7].

3.4 Mechanisms to negotiate uneven terrain

The system should allow for significantly more maneuverability on uneven (off-camber) terrain than the standard wheelchair. The suspension would manage the off-camber surfaces through autonomous adjustments (**Figure 3**), when the user

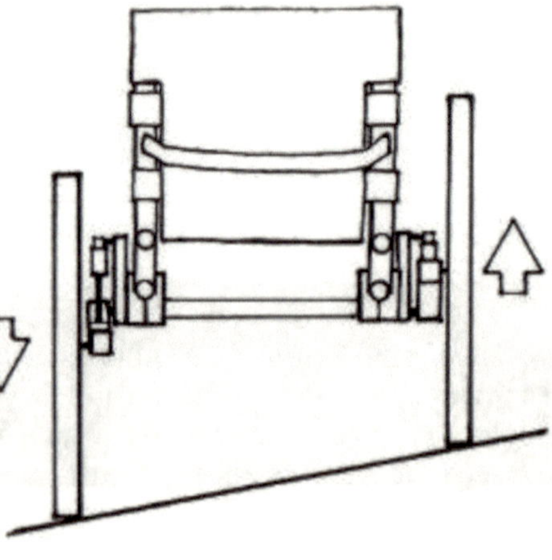

Figure 3.
Independent suspension travel [18].

is on an incline of around 10 degrees. As the right shock compresses and the left relaxes, consequently enabling the seat to level itself, offering greater stability to the wheelchair structure seat. The determination of shocks ought to take into consideration autonomous control of spring rate and damping ratio, consequently enabling the system work even in a stationary situation as well [17].

Different obstacles may require the suspension to work autonomously, for instance, a block of wood or a crack in the walkway can be effectively explored with the same suspension framework. As given in **Figure 4**, the right side of the wheelchair must articulate upwards so as to keep up all the four wheels in contact with the ground surface, as the wheelchair moves over the obstructions. The right rear shock compresses, while the others adjust to equilibrium, allowing for all four wheels to have some type of contact, and a resulting good stability is achieved [18].

The operators explore obstructions in their everyday life. A number of these snags require autonomous wheel articulation, while others may require the shocks to work in unison. A typical impediment that wheelchair clients face everyday (or avoid) is the street curb. Assuming the user is moving on a path perpendicular to the curb, the wheels will act in unison as the back end of the chair rolls off of the curb, with the suspension absorbing the force. This is not a navigation that could be safely done in a conventional wheelchair [18].

In some cases, there can be need to attach a set of wide auxiliary wheels or wheel extensions to the standard wheelchair for it to be stable when used off road on sandy, loose or unstable terrain. Of late, a couple of expansive tire-like plastic or elastomeric treads are connected and fitted onto the back wheels of the wheelchair to give a substitute handhold grip to the user in a way similar to mounted standard wheels arrangement above [19]. The treads are additionally marginally recessed inward from the original tire, being of a smaller diameter than the back wheel, to allow the wheelchair to ride exclusively on the tire on hard surfaces and make drive on such surfaces equivalent to one would typically anticipate. The treads act together with a second pair of lightweight plastic wheels which are adjusted to fit on either side of every one of the two stanchion mounted front wheels, the combination acting to give an broad bearing surface to better steadiness, load bearing capacity and simpler controlling of said vehicle when utilized on said sandy, loose or shaky landscapes. The wheelchair may likewise be fitted with an anti-tip over mechanical assembly to prevent flipping in reverse when navigating difficult landscape and to allow the wheelchair to be moved in an upward angled position which puts the most substantial portion of the weight on the back wheel, increasing grip on the shaky terrain [19].

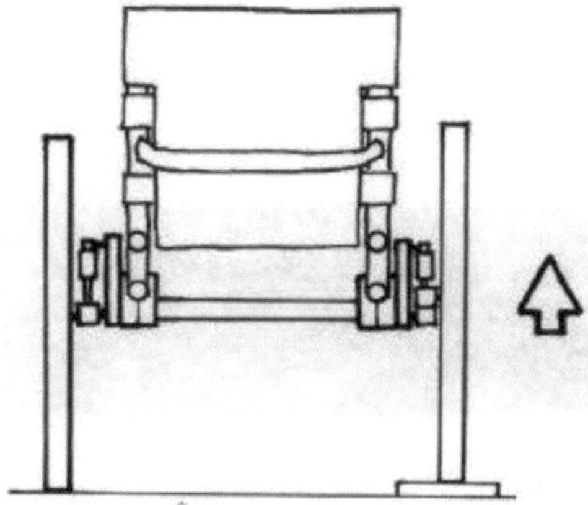

Figure 4.
Independent pass over obstacle [18].

Push-bar outfitted gadget permits structures that allow people of varying physical strength to move the wheelchair along a wide scope of landscapes, including delicately tricky terrain. The push-bar enable the users to initiate mobility without hand to wheel system. The unique design drives the chair forward with a forward movement of the drive bars while pulling back on the push-bars effects the braking mechanism. Turning is accomplished with a forward movement on one push-bar and a backward movement on the other push-bar. The off-road seat of this design offers the operator a multi-speed equipped favorable advantage over traditional wheelchairs. Changing into lower gears for very adverse terrain such as sandy environment, gives the operators the opportunity to go where they have not had the option to go with conventional wheelchairs. Just changing into higher gears considers allows for movement on pavement and other hard surfaces. The push-bars are removable and may consequently be put away with so that the wheelchair might be moved utilizing traditional hand-to-wheel pushing [20]. This component enables the user to deal with a wide range of landscapes and conditions that are normally restrictive to operators of ordinary wheelchairs and power wheelchairs to be used particularly in open air situations and elements for example forest floors, uneven and harsh terrain. Further, it very well may be utilized to conquer numerous every day snags, for example, curbs and high thresholds [21]. It is advantageous for people with less upper body and arm strength. Accordingly, it accommodates more independent participation in open air exercises, such as hunting, chasing, and so forth.

The review above points toward one thing that current rough terrain wheelchairs do not provide total stability ("not ideal"). Thus, there is still a need to come up with a wheelchair that will prevent the user either toppling backward, forward or sideways.

4. Materials and methods

The design development process entailed coming up with a design that improves the wheelchair stability mechanism, safety precautions as well as reduce powering requirements. Some investigations were done on existing all-terrain stability mechanisms, including the possibility of redesigning the wheels and adjusting the center of gravity for improved stability. The safety of the operator, the machine and influence to the nearby environment were considered among other key parameters. Some effort was made to ensure that the final framework of the wheelchair would address the issues of user safety.

The researchers carried out a study on current wheelchair powering methods as well as noting their efficiencies. Power transmission mechanism was fundamental in achieving speed and power. Some engagement with different disability organizations was done to acquire first hand expectations of users.

The generated design concepts were evaluated and analyzed for suitability for adoption. The chosen concept was further developed to come up with dimensions of the wheelchair, sizing of the wheelchair parts, material selection and detailed drawing of the final design. The detailed drawings were drawn using AutoCAD (2007) and Autodesk Inventor (2017) was used to simulate the strength of the wheelchair frame. The bill of materials was drawn up and the cost estimate and the feasibility of fabricating the prototype unit in the local workshop were done.

5. Design concept generation

The concepts were formulated based on the ability of the design to meet the objective criteria which were: reliability, maintainability, efficiency, robustness, machinability, stability, safety, cost, ease of operation, and weight. Three possible design solutions were generated for the off road wheelchair as explained in the following sections.

5.1 Cambered rear wheels concept

The wheelchair is operated like a normal conventional wheelchair, by pushing the wheels forward. Sideways stability is affected by wheelchair width (**Figure 5**). The rear wheels are tilted inwards to increase the base width thus stabilizing the chair. A back-caster wheel is fitted to prevent the wheelchair from falling backwards.

The further out to the side of the wheelchair base, the more the chair l resists tipping over sideways. The camber pushes the wheels nearer to the wheelchair user and more in accordance with the operator's forward push stroke, therefore making it simpler to push. This can be particularly useful for ladies, who normally have smaller shoulders yet more extensive hips than men. Additionally, with cambering, traction is improved when navigating slopes. The wheelchair provides more stability, comfortable seating and it is better for overweight people. On the other hand, a wide wheelchair is more difficult to get through narrow pathways as camber increases the width of the wheelchair. Most anti-tip designs restrict the wheelchair's ability to travel over uneven surfaces (such as kerbs or dips). It is also hard to push.

5.2 Extended front caster wheels concept

The user propels the wheelchair forward by pushing the rear wheels to the front. A back-caster wheel is fitted to prevent the wheelchair from tipping backwards.

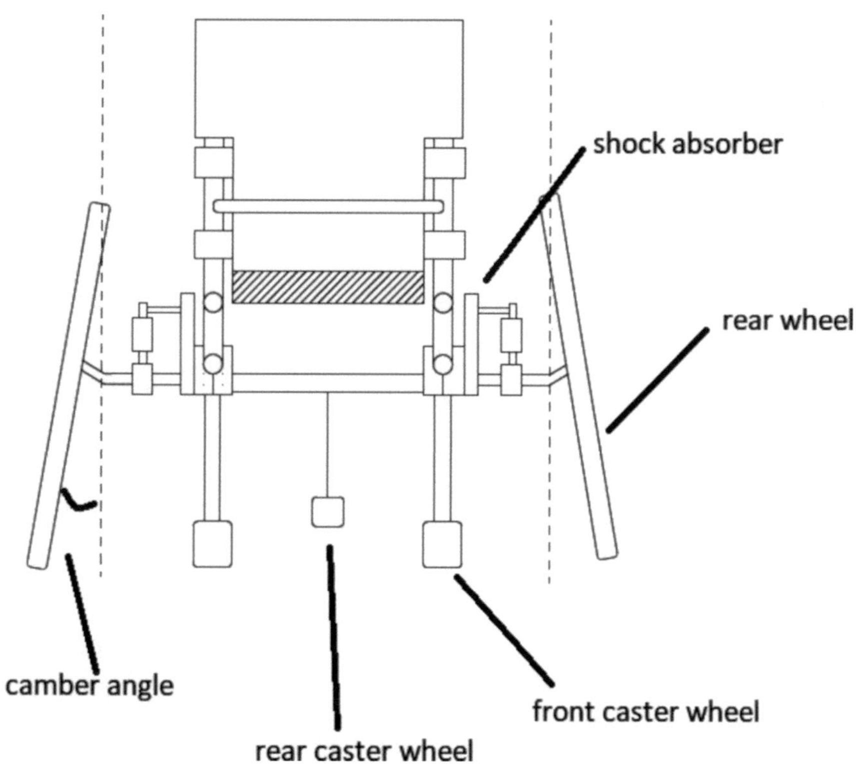

Figure 5.
Cambered rear wheels.

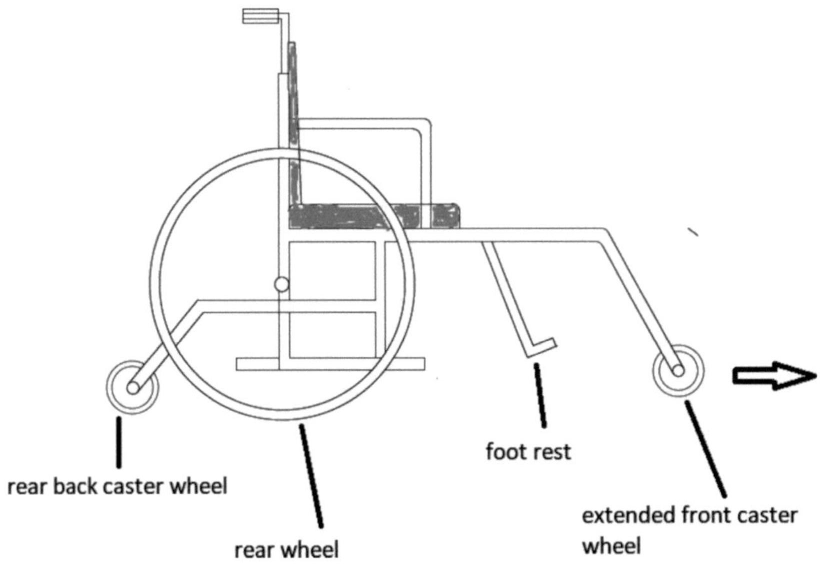

Figure 6.
Extended front caster wheels.

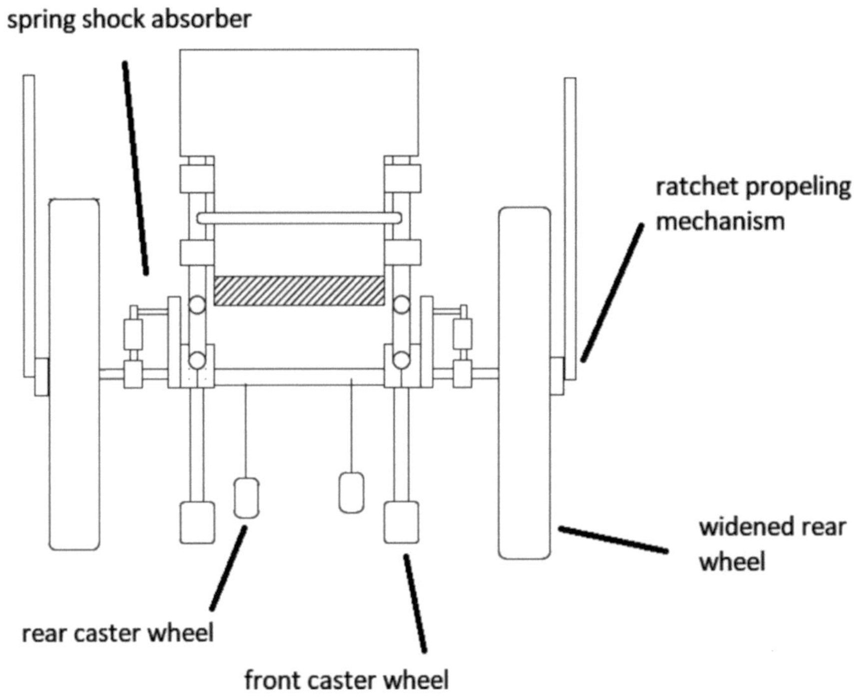

Figure 7.
Widened rear wheels [12].

Forward stability is affected by the size and position of the front castor wheel in relation to the operator's center of gravity. The front caster wheels of the above wheelchair in **Figure 6** are extended to the front to provide forward stability.

The wheelchair resists tipping forward when the castor wheels are stopped suddenly by an object they cannot roll over. Less weight on the front wheels will reduce the rolling resistance of the front wheels, allowing the wheelchair to roll more easily. More of the user's weight on the rear wheels will provide more traction on the rear wheels to drive through soft ground. On the downside, overall wheelchair length is longer, making it harder to maneuver in confined spaces.

5.3 Widened rear wheels concept

Sideways stability is affected by wheelchair width, thus the need for wide rear wheels. A ratchet arm assembly is operatively connected to each of the rear wheels to enable the operator to propel the wheelchair by that method, should the person so choose. Shock absorbers are fitted to the rear wheels to provide independent wheel articulation, such that if one wheel is to go over an obstacle the other one remains on the ground (**Figure 7**).

The further out to the side of the wheelchair the front and rear wheels touch the ground, the more the chair will resist tipping over sideways. The width of the rear wheels increases their bearing ability such that when utilized in sandy, loose or unstable terrain they do not sink into the underlying terrain and loose traction resulting in the occupant being left stuck. The wheelchair becomes easy to push and there is increased stability. On the downside a wide wheelchair is more difficult to get through narrow pathways. Side way stability is limited due to vertical wheels.

Using the binary dominance matrix method, widened rear wheels concept was chosen for further development. The mechanical design of this concept was developed into the final design in the next section of this chapter.

6. Detailed wheelchair design

The widened rear wheels design concept was further designed in detail. The parts making up the system were sized and materials for the parts selected according to the design standards for mechanical parts. The designed parts were tested to configure if they could withstand the operating stresses and adjustments if any were taken in order to minimize failure of the parts during operation. The main parts are the widened rear wheels, ratchet bar, spring shock absorbers, rear caster wheels and front caster wheels given in **Figure 8**.

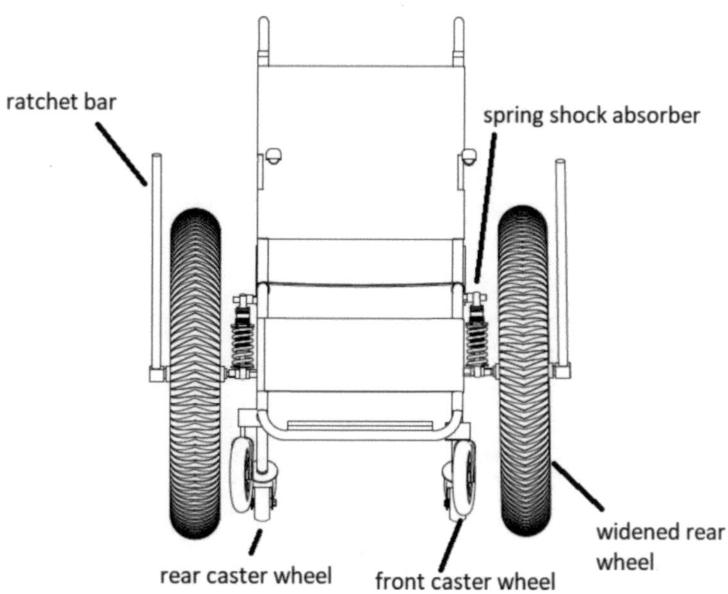

Figure 8.
Detailed design assembly.

6.1 Center of gravity

The center of gravity (CG) is the focal point of a body's weight appropriation, where the force of gravity can be considered to act. It is the point in any object about which it is in perfect balance regardless of how it is turned or pivoted around that point. For a limited arrangement of point masses, CG might be characterized as the normal of positions weighted by mass. For its figuring a few parameters were viewed as, for example, the thickness of the material, the volume of the piece and the good ways from the origin arrange around the focal point of the piece. This is critical for the stability of the wheel chair. Thus considering x, y and z axis the center of gravity of the point masses will be given, and to find the center of gravity of composite bodies this was considered in the detailed design.

6.2 Calculations of stress and failure

Forces on a wheelchair casters and wheels, when the assumption is that the operator weighs 100 kg (**Figures 9–12**) (Eqs. (1)–(3)).

$$\text{Considering: } Fperson = Fp = 981N\ (100\ kg) \tag{1}$$

$$Lcaster = Lc = 315.81\ mm \tag{2}$$

$$Ltotal = Lc + Lw = 448.11\ mm \tag{3}$$

The findings are that each rear wheel will take a weight force of 345 N. While the caster wheel takes 144.815 N.

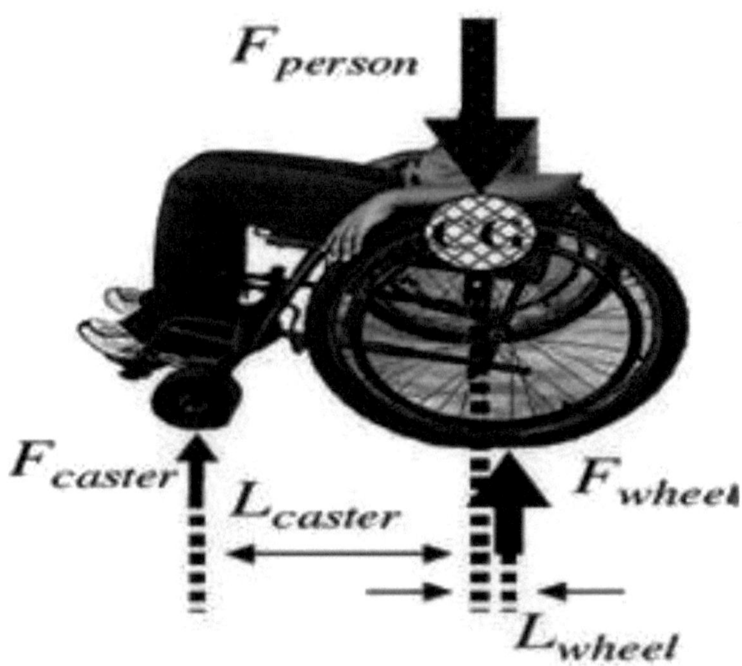

Figure 9.
Force analysis [3, 13].

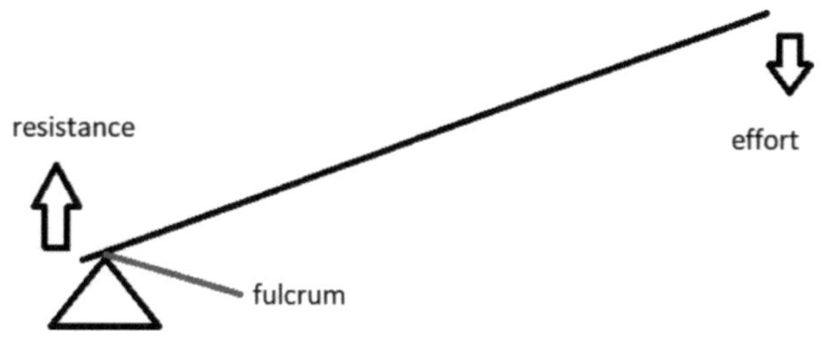

Figure 10.
Ratchet set up [13].

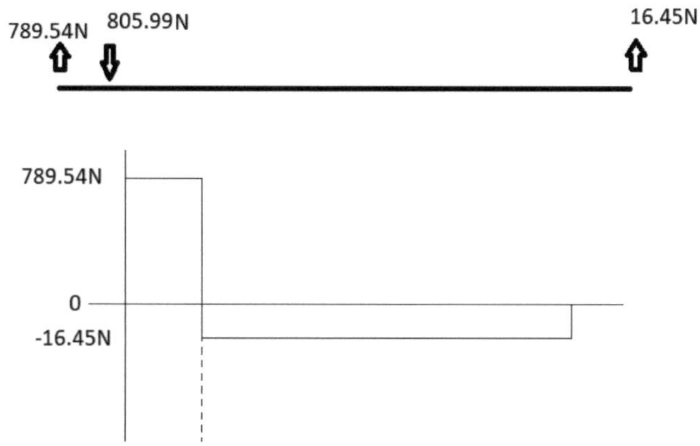

Figure 11.
Shear force diagram on the ratchet lever [13].

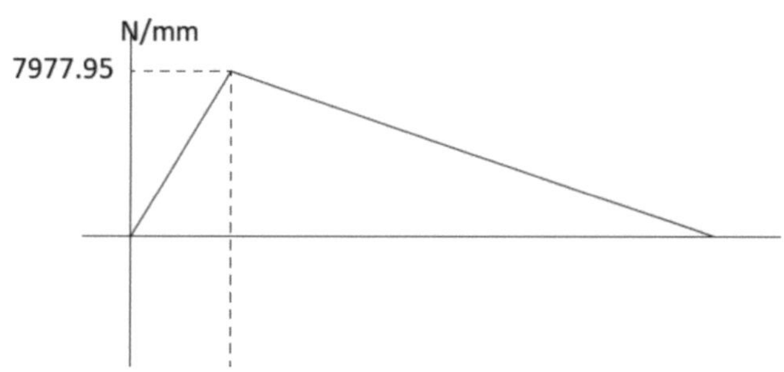

Figure 12.
Bending moment diagram [13].

6.3 Internal moments and forces in a wheelchair axle

The forces and moments acting on the back hub of a wheelchair were determined a similar path as above. The greatest moment exits where the hub is welded to the frame. There are vertical forces applied on the wheel starting from the ground, there likewise might be horizontal forces that act on the wheel when the wheelchair tips over, these forces cause moments on the axle. Von Mises stresses were analyzed for the axle to take note of the critical points.

6.4 Bending stress in a wheelchair axle

At the point when a section is twisted the applied moment creates stresses in the material. On one side of the part the material is extended and in this way has tensile stresses. On the opposite side the material is compressed by compressive loading. The maximum bending moment was found to be 62.125 MPa.

6.5 Stress and failure

Shear stress is the stress that attempts to tear something separate. It is characterized as the shear force divided by the area over which the force is acting. In a wheelchair hub, its value is low and is rather higher in the X-brace pivot of a wheelchair. The modulus of elasticity (E) is a material property that tells how much a material make an effort not to distort when it is under stress. Strain is the proportion of how a lot of a material twists when under pressure.

Looking at the most extreme bending stress in a wheelchair axle with the limit elastic of the material used, it is possible to know whether the hub is sufficiently strong enough to hold up under the individual user's weight and other external forces applied on it. The weight of the person should not exceed 212.33 kg.

6.6 Shock absorber spring

The material of the spring should have high fatigue strength, high ductility, high resilience and it should be creep resistant, hence carbon steel was chosen. The free length of 100 mm and the spring wire diameter was determined to be 5 mm.

6.7 Ratchet bar

The ratchet is used to turn the wheels by the operator. The effort by the operator was determined to be 16.45 N, at the top of the lever assuming the frictionless movements.

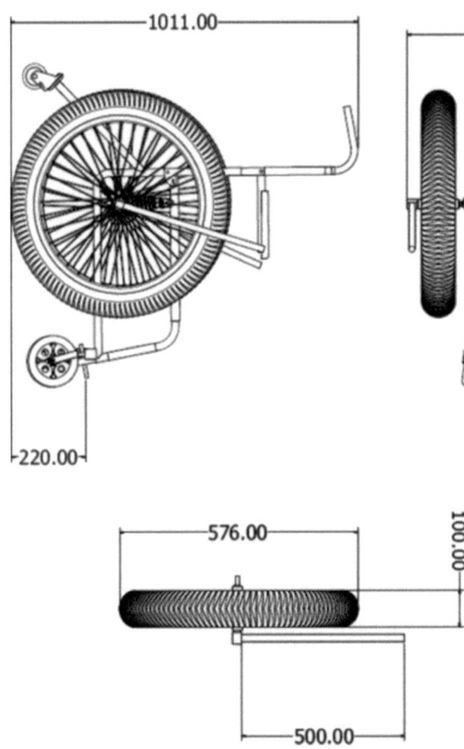

Figure 13.
Side and top view of sized design, and the sized rear wheel.

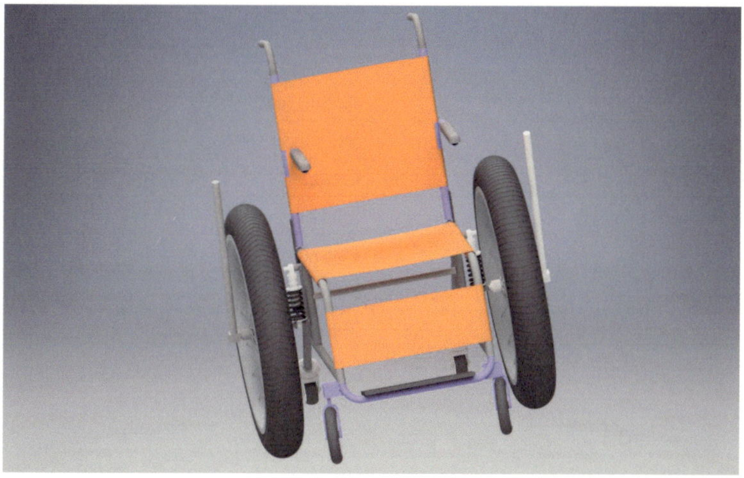

Figure 14.
Final wide wheel design.

If this results in a reaction on the fulcrum of 789.54 N, the force and bending moment distribution acting in the lever is described by the shear force diagram and bending moment diagram as shown below.

For a bending moment of 7922 Nm, the material for the lever, is designed to be mild steel selected from tables to be Fe 310 steel of tensile strength 310 Nmm^2, yield stress 180 Nmm^2 and minimum elongation of 26.

Designing for a factor of safety of 3, the resulting allowable working stress is 60 Nmm^2.

6.8 Tipping angle

The widened rear wheels design was found that it could sustain a tipping angle of about 43.17 degrees from the calculations.

6.9 Designed wide rear wheels

Figure 13 gives the sized views of the resulting design, as well as the recommended the rear wheel size.

The final 3D view of the resulting wheelchair is given by **Figure 14** below.

7. Economic analysis

Some costing was done for components that are going to be manufactured from workshop and others standardized components which are going to be bought. **Table 1** gives the major components the materials they would be made from.

The bill of quantities are given by **Table 2** as well as the costing of a prototype.

The cost of fabricating a prototype is estimated to be USD 186 including components cost and labor, which is within a maximum cap of USD200. This could vary depending on the manufacturer's requirements and specifications.

Component	Material
Wheelchair frame	Mild steel
Spring	Carbon steel
Ratchet bar	Mild steel
Seating material	Cotton
Rear wheel axle	Mild steel
Caster wheel bearing	Mild steel
Rear wheel rim	Mild steel
Footrest	Mild steel

Table 1.
Components and material specifications.

Component	Quantity	Total cost (USD)
Frame	16 × 500 mm	30
Rear wheel	2	28
Caster wheels	4	16
Ratchet	2	32
Shock absorber	2	60
Labor	—	20
	Total	186

Table 2.
Bill of quantities.

8. Recommendations

The wheelchair design is still limited when it comes to very steep inclines, in which case an incorporation of a motor to assist the hand effort will be required. There is also need to have adjustable rear wheels that can be pushed in or outwards from the chair so that it is not hindered when passing through narrow pathways of the rural terrain.

The operator has to always lock the brakes before getting in and out of the wheelchair. They have to also avoid putting heavy loads on the back of a wheelchair, as this may result in a shift in the position of center of gravity. This could cause the chair to tip over backwards.

The operator of the chair can keep it maintained by being knowledgeable about the wheelchair, and having a handy list of providers that one can rely on for repairs, parts, and maintenance. The user may not be able to perform the basic daily and weekly cleaning and upkeep but can set up a routine that can be followed by caregivers, family members or others to monitor the chair for problems. Assemble and store a set of tools that you will need to have on hand for maintenance and emergencies. There is need to keep the wheelchair clean to help keep the operator healthy and free of infections, this will also make it easier to identify equipment problems as they arise. The casters (front wheels) can present a safety hazard when they are worn out. One has to always check your casters for cracks in the spokes that may eventually cause the caster to collapse.

9. Conclusion

The chapter investigated the development of a rough terrain wheelchair design which is capable to withstand tipping angles up to 43.17 degrees, which is relatively higher as compared to conventional wheelchairs. The wheelchair counters toppling in almost every direction due to the wide wheels and back caster wheels for anti-tipping. This wheelchair is intended to improve the mobility of those operators living in rural uneven terrain by reducing wheelchair related accidents. The incorporation of the spring shock absorber will also contribute to the comfortable sitting of the user. The overall cost of the design was estimated to be USD 186, if local raw materials are used for manufacturing of the wheelchair.

Acknowledgements

We would like to thank the University of Zimbabwe (UZ), Mechanical Workshop team for working with this team of researchers in fabricating the prototype which gave the study a practical form result. We also acknowledge Danhiko Rehabilitation Centre for allowing us to access their facilities and also their input on wheelchair operator expectations. Also, we do really appreciate the solicited guidance offered by colleagues we work with at the University of Zimbabwe. Finally, we wish to thank all those who are implementing measures that help to protect the disabled from any injuries.

Author details

Ignatio Madanhire*, Loice Gudukeya and Roy Mushonga
University of Zimbabwe, Harare, Zimbabwe

*Address all correspondence to: imadanhire@gmail.com

References

[1] Andrew M, Kwarciak MS. Determining the general considerations in needs and requirements of the wheelchair users from MHD and HHD countries. Journal of Rehabilitation Research and Development. 2014;**1**(2):1-2

[2] Philipa C, Angela C. Fact sheet on wheelchairs. 2007;**1**:1-4

[3] Winter A, Hotchkiss R, Durban M. Mechanical principles of wheelchair design. 2010

[4] Forkenbrock DJ. Comparison of external costs of rail and truck freight transportation. Transportation Research Part A: Policy and Practice. 2001;**35**(4):321-337. DOI: 10.1016/S0965-8564(99)00061-0

[5] Devillard X et al. Validation of a new ergometer adapted to all types of manual wheelchair. European Journal of Applied Physiology. 2005;**85**:479-485. DOI: 10.1007/s004210100407

[6] Devillard X et al. Validation of a new ergometer adapted to all types of manual wheelchair. World Health Organization; 2001

[7] Landerman LR, Shipp KM. Activity restriction among wheelchair users. Journal of the American Geriatrics Society. 2003:1244-1251

[8] Chakwiriza J, Nhemachena C. Rural travel and disability in Leroro and Moremela Villages South Africa; 2010

[9] Cooper RA, Cooper R, Boninger ML. Trends and Issues in Wheelchair Technologies. Assistive Technology. 2008;**20**(2):61-72

[10] Db M. Guidance on the Stability of Wheelchairs BULLETIN, 2004(March); 2004

[11] Jones ML, Sanford JA. People with mobility impairments in the United States today and in 2010. Assistive Technology. 1996;**8**(1):43-53

[12] Di Marco A, Russell M, Masters M. In Practice Standards for Wheelchair Prescription. Physical Medicine and Rehabilitation; 2003. pp. 30-39

[13] Wirth DA. The International Organization for Standardization: Private Voluntary Standards as Swords and Shields. Massachusetts institute of Technology; 2009. pp. 79-102

[14] Adventures A. All-Terrain Wheelchair System; 2011

[15] Rory A, Ken J, Stewart JK, David P, VanSickle DP. Evaluation of Methods for Determining Static Stability of Manual Wheelchairs. Sacramento: California State University; 2011

[16] Trudel G et al. Effects of rear-wheel camber on wheelchair stability. Archives of Physical Medicine and Rehabilitation. 1997;**78**(January):78-81

[17] Van der Woude L, Dallmeijer A, Janssen T. Alternative modes of manual wheelchair ambulation: An overview. American Journal of Physical Medicine and Rehabilitation. 2001b;**80**:765-777

[18] Winter A. Mechanical Principle of Wheelchair Design. USA: Massachusetts Institute of Technology; 2010

[19] Hill PEJ. United States Patent (19) 11 Patent Number: US. Patent June 27, 1995(19); 1995

[20] Examiner A, Stabley MR, Chris A. (12) United States Patent (10) Patent No.: 1(12); 2011

[21] Paquet V, Feathers D. An anthropometric study of manual and powered wheelchair users. International Journal of Industrial Ergonomics. 2004;**33**:191-204. DOI: 10.1016/j.ergon.2003.10.003

Section 2

Case Studies and Country-Specific Issues in Public Health

Chapter 12

Temporal Trend and Inequality in Immunization Coverage in India

Basant Kumar Panda

Abstract

Since 1978, India through its various health policies target to achieve the universal immunization, but profound progress is yet to be seen. This paper examine the trend in immunization coverage and differential access among the population subgroups. Data for the analysis was extracted from the two recent rounds of the National Family Health Survey (NFHS) conducted in 2005–2006 and 2015–2016. Descriptive statistics were used to understand the level of coverage, whereas the ratio method and concentration index was used to understand the inequality. The study identified immunization coverage had improved from 44 percent in 2005–2006 to 62 percent in 2015–2016. However, considerable variation was observed among the regions and various wealth quintiles. In the Southern region, 63 percent of children from the poorest wealth quintile were fully immunized compared to 36 percent in North Eastern region. The coverage of full immunization among richest children was found to be 1.5 times higher than that of the poorest. The concentration index remains positive showing the pro-rich inequality. A positive result was found in the Northern and Northeastern region, where the poorest were showing an impeccable improvement over the period. Moreover, the study found the gap by place of residence and gender was close to convergence. The study suggests that the immunization programs have to be inclusive, with widespread reach, leaving no stones unturned. These steps can be beneficial in diminishing inequalities, acting as an essential ingredient in achieving the sustainable development goals.

Keywords: inequality, immunization, India, NFHS, temporal

1. Introduction

Socioeconomic inequalities in a child health is a major policy concern to achieve the Sustainable Development Goals (SDGs) framed by the United Nations in 2015 [1]. However, progress toward reducing these inequalities in child health indicators is not noteworthy among and between the countries [2]. Irrespective of the continued global effort to reduce the infant and child mortality rates, the targets of Millennium Development Goals (MDG) remained unattainable in many developing countries [3]. Nearly, 5.6 million of under-five death occurs worldwide [4], out of which quarter of death are due to vaccine-preventable diseases. Moreover, an estimated 19.9 million infants worldwide stay absent for routine immunization services. Around 60 percent of these children live in 10 countries, mainly from Africa and South Asia including India [5]. Though the Global Vaccine Action Plan (GVAP) has been endorsed by 194 countries in 2012, to ensure the equitable access to immunization by the year 2020, profound progress is yet to be seen [6].

Immunization coverage is given high priority globally and nationally especially for developing countries like India. The Indian immunization program started in 1978 after the Alma-Ata declaration aimed at immunizing all children [7]. To accelerate this, appropriate policy measures were put in place during those times, but the task of attaining these were quite arduous. The Government of India recently launched the *Mission Indradhanush* (UIP) in 2014 with the target of achieving universal immunization coverage https://www.nhp.gov.in/mission-indradhanush1_pg. Irrespective of these attempts, nearly one-third of the children remain to be far away from vaccinations in India [8–12].

India, known for its multifaceted society and social hierarchy, dealt with higher social, economic, and regional inequality. A growing number of studies in India examined inequalities in child health status including full immunization coverage [9, 13, 14]. The studies found significant gap in wealth-related, rural–urban, and gender-related inequality in immunization coverage [15–18]. Some studies also observed large differentials among the economic groups, caste, and religion of the household [11, 19, 20]. Among the other factors, maternal education, proximity to a health facility, place of delivery, and pre- and postnatal checkup of mothers are among the leading factors affecting immunization coverage in India [21–24]. Apart from that, appropriateness of the timing of the vaccination is lagging in India and many states [25]. In order to reduce the disparity in immunization coverage, countries must adopt proequity programs aimed at reducing the gap in immunization coverage.

The present study is conceptualized under the following rationale. Firstly, in terms of immunization, India is one of the major contributor of unimmunized children in the world [5]. So, it is essential to understand the pattern of full immunization coverage in general and specific vaccinations in particular among various geographies of India. Secondly, many literatures suggest the pervasiveness of economic inequality among children in various health indicators. Therefore, it becomes imperative to study the pattern of inequality among the better off and worse off population subgroups. Thirdly, the WHO Commission on social determinants of health positioned strategically to reduce health inequalities and considers gender as one of the main determinants. It is widely established that pronounced gender bias still exists in India, favoring males over females. In this concern, understanding gender segregation in immunization practices is critical for policy formulation. In the same line, this study is a revisit to understand the temporal variation and inequality in immunization coverage among the regions of India. The present study will deliver the dynamic pattern of inequality in regions of India and provide guidance to frame policy as per the present challenges at hand.

The main objective of this paper was to document pattern and inequalities in immunization coverage in India over two periods of time (2005–2006 and 2015–2016). Further, this paper was an attempt to understand inequality patterns in immunization coverage by the wealth quintile at the regional level. We have investigated inequalities in full immunization coverage using various inequality indexes that are related to three characteristics, namely economic status, place of residence, and sex of the child.

2. Data and methods

2.1 Data

In an attempt to understand the variation in immunization among children, data from the third and fourth rounds of National Family Health Surveys (NFHSs) were used. These surveys were conducted in 2005–2006 and 2015–2016 by International Institute for Population Sciences (IIPS) under the stewardship of the Ministry of Health and Family Welfare (MoHFW), Government of India, with technical support from ICF International. The survey is designed in line with Demographic and Health Surveys (DHS) conducted worldwide. Both the surveys were large-scale surveys that provide state- and national-level estimates on fertility, infant mortality and child mortality, and other family welfare and health indicators. The survey uses a multi-stage stratified random sampling to select the households. Using the appropriate sampling weight, the survey provides estimates for various geographical regions. More about the survey design, sampling procedure, and questionnaire are provided in the national report [8].

The unit of our analysis is the regions of India. The two rounds of National Family Health Survey have followed a uniform pattern in segregating the states qualifying them for a particular region. In our study, the composition of regions based on the state is guided by the NFHS report. As uniformity is maintained in framing the geographical region, it is comparable over time.

3. Methods

Full immunization among children aged 12–23 months is the primary outcome variable in this study. Children are considered as fully immunized only when they receive vaccination against tuberculosis (BCG), three doses of diphtheria, pertussis (whooping cough), and tetanus (DPT) vaccine; three doses of poliomyelitis (Polio) vaccine; and one dose of the measles vaccine by the age of 12 months. In India, BCG should be given at birth or first clinical contact; DPT and polio require three vaccinations at approximately 4, 8, and 12 weeks of age; and the measles vaccine should be given at age 12 months or sooner after reaching 9 months of age. Information on vaccination coverage was collected from the child's health card and direct reporting from the mother. We have used the kid's file for analysis; the survey has selected only those households that had childbirths in the last 5 years prior to the survey. The sample size of the children is 49,284 in 2015–2016 and 9559 in 2005–2006.

3.1 Measuring inequality in immunization coverage

This study used two summary indexes to measure inequality in immunization coverage. The first measure is a simple ratio of the threshold of the population characteristics. The ratio measure is considered as a crude measure as it does not consider the estimates except the threshold. Despite its limitation, the measure is considered as a crucial relative measure of inequality and provides a clear idea of discrepancy in health indicators among the population subgroup. Wealth inequality ratio (WIR), rural–urban inequality ratio (RUIR), and gender-related inequality ratio (GIR) were calculated to quantify the inequality based on these attributes. The formula for these measures as guided by the other studies [26, 27] are as follows:

$$\text{Rich} - \text{Poor Inequality Ratio} = \left(\frac{\%\text{of fully immunized children in the richest wealth class}}{\%\text{of fully immunized children in the poorest wealth class}}\right) * 100$$

$$\text{Urban} - \text{Rural Inequality Ratio} = \left(\frac{\%\text{of fully immunized urban children}}{\%\text{of fully immunized rural children}}\right) * 100$$

$$\text{Gender Inequality Ratio} = \left(\frac{\%\text{of fully immunized boys}}{\%\text{of fully immunized girls}}\right) * 100$$

The second summary measure used here was the concentration index, which is one of the widely used inequality measures in public health research. This is a wealth-based inequality measure that provides the concentration of health indicators at a different economic level in the various subgroups of the population. The concentration index is defined as twice the area between the concentration curve and the line of equality (the 45-degree line). So, in some cases, when there is no socioeconomic-related inequality, the concentration index is found to be zero. The thumb rule is that the index takes a negative value when the curve lies above the line of equality, indicating unbalanced concentration of the health variable (in this case immunization coverage) among the poor, and a positive value when it lies below the line of equality indicating disproportionate concentration of the health variable (in this case immunization coverage) among the poor. The formula for finding the concentration index is as follows:

$$\text{Concentration Index} : C = \frac{2}{\mu}\sum_{i=1}^{n} covw\left(y_i, R_i\right)$$

where y_i is the full immunization coverage of the ith child; Ri is the fractional rank of the ith child (for weighted data) in terms of the index of household economic status; μ is the (weighted) unconditional mean of the full immunization coverage of the sample; and cov_w denotes the weighted covariance. All the analyses are performed in Stata 14.

4. Results

Figure 1 presents the pattern and trend in immunization coverage in India and the regions for 2005–2006 and 2015–2016. The full immunization coverage in India had gone up by 18 percent from 44 percent in 2005–2006 to 62 percent in 2015–2016. Several vaccinations such as DPT, BCG, and measles and full immunization had shown a significant improvement in the same period except for the polio vaccination.

Table 1 shows full immunization coverage across different wealth classes at two time periods (2005–2006 and 2015–2016). It is clearly evident that the coverage of all vaccines was higher among wealthier classes of the society. The full immunization coverage across the different wealth quintile had grown over the years, and

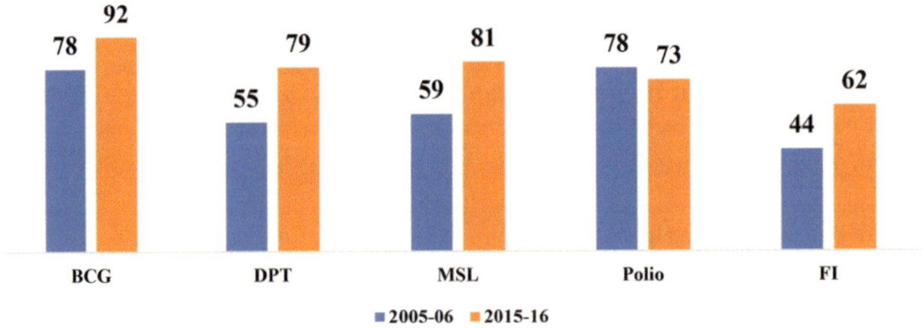

Figure 1.
Coverage of various components of immunization in India in NFHS-3 (2005–2006) and NFHS-4 (2015–2016).

Vaccination component	NFHS-3 (2005–2006)				NFHS-4 (2015–2016)			
	Poorest	Richest	Ratio	CI*	Poorest	Richest	Ratio	CI*
BCG	64.00	95.60	1.49	0.08	86.99	95.42	1.10	0.02
DPT	33.90	81.90	2.42	0.17	70.40	85.66	1.22	0.04
POLIO	40.00	85.20	2.13	0.04	66.74	78.35	1.17	0.03
MSL	69.90	87.37	1.25	0.16	73.18	88.79	1.21	0.04
FI	24.45	71.02	2.90	0.21	53.42	70.25	1.32	0.06

**CI stands for concentration index.*

Table 1.
Level of various vaccinations and full immunization coverage and inequality measures among the wealth quintile in India in 2005–2006 and 2015–2016.

ratio among the richest and poorest has narrowed much. For instance, wealth inequality ratio (WIR) was found to be 2.42 in 2005–2006, which reduced to almost half (1.22) in 2015–2016.

The concentration index for all the vaccinations was found to be positive, which signifies the prorich inequality. The concentration curve for full immunization coverage (**Figure 2**) for both the periods lies below the line of equality indicating higher level of coverage among the higher wealth quintile. The curve for 2015–2016 is closer to the line of equality than that of 2005–2006 representing the decreasing wealth-based inequality over time.

Table 2 exhibits region-wise differential in immunization coverage among the poorest and richest wealth quintile across regions of India. Immunization coverage remained higher in the Southern region, both for the poorest and richest during both the periods. The immunization coverage for the Northeastern region was found to be 11.4 percent, lowest among the poorest wealth quintile in 2005–2006, while the Western region accounted for the lowest with 40.23 percent in 2015–2016. The ratio for both the periods was highest in the Northeastern region with 5.47 in 2005–2006 and 1.85 in 2015–2016. On the contrary, the ratio for the Southern region occupied the bottom position. An interesting pattern was observed with a

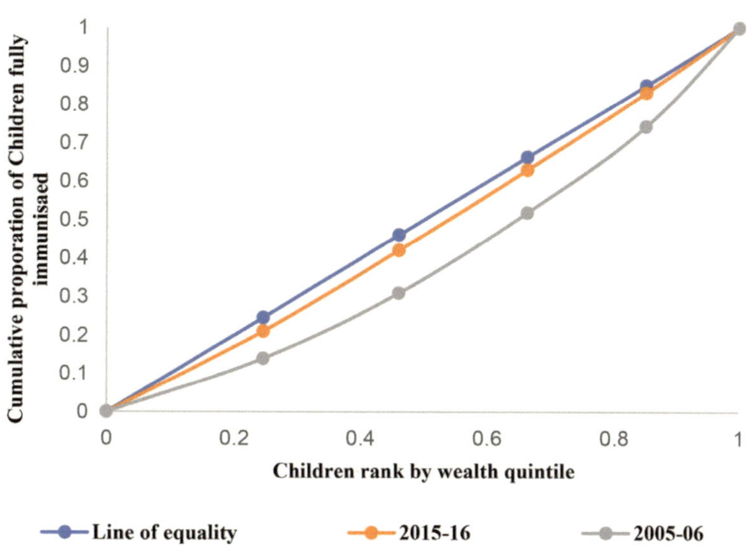

Figure 2.
Concentration curve of full immunization coverage by wealth quintal in 2005–2006 and 2015–2016.

	NFHS-3 (2005–2006)				NFHS-4 (2015–2016)			
Region	**Poorest**	**Richest**	**Ratio**	**CI***	**Poorest**	**Richest**	**Ratio**	**CI***
East	30.31	76.30	2.51	0.18	63.51	71.04	1.12	0.06
West	29.94	69.86	2.33	0.16	40.23	62.20	1.55	0.07
North	13.63	72.13	5.29	0.26	41.41	75.71	1.83	0.10
South	40.42	78.95	1.95	0.11	63.35	71.73	1.13	0.02
Central	18.40	60.34	3.27	0.23	43.85	68.20	1.56	0.10
North East	11.40	62.43	5.47	0.25	36.60	67.66	1.85	0.12

**CI stands for concentration Index.*

Table 2.
Level of full immunization coverage and inequality measure among the wealth quintile in India in 2005–2006 and 2015–2016.

drastic decline in the WIR from 5.29 to 1.83 in the Northern region and 5.47 to 1.85 in the Northeastern region. This is accompanied by an increase in immunization coverage among the poorest wealth quintile from 13.63 and 11.40 percent in 2005–2006 to 41.41 and 36.60 percent in 2015–2016 in the North and Northeastern region, respectively. Splitting the full immunization rates according to the mother's education and wealth group, we found a gap among the two thresholds favoring the richest and highly educated (**Figure 3**). The same inspected across regions manifested a significant role of education in enhancing immunization coverage.

Table 3 explains the urban–rural differentials in immunization coverage and describes the urban–rural gap in immunization coverage across the regions of India. It was clear from the table that the coverage in full immunization at the national level for both rural and urban has improved. However, rural areas had fared well in comparison to the urban areas, shrinking the gap between them, as indicated in the latest round. However, the Southern region had excelled in immunization coverage leaving behind other regions and India as well. Another very striking finding can be seen from the Northeastern region, where the figures had shown improvements in a decade, with the urban coverage increasing from 40 to 67.09 percent in 2015–2016. Moreover, the rural areas of the Central region have shown an upward trend from 24.68 to 52.97 percent in 2015–2016. Over the years, immunization coverage had

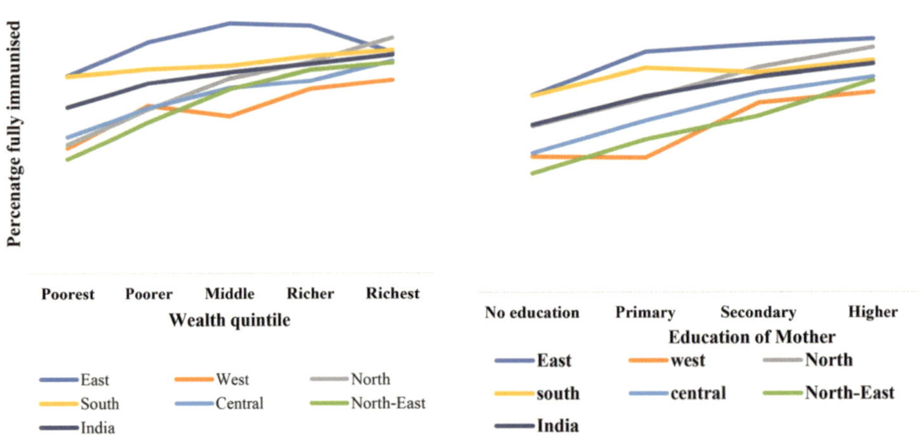

Figure 3.
Percentage of children fully immunized by household wealth and education status of mothers in India, 2015–2016.

increased significantly in both urban as well as rural areas and interestingly the increase was more profound in rural areas.

Table 4 presents results of gender differentials in full immunization across the various regions of India. It can be noted that in almost all the regions of the country, the percentage of children receiving full immunization had improved over time both for male and female. There were no differentials in immunization among the male and female found in 2015–2016 depicting the gender inequality ratio closer to one. This reflects an improvement in immunization practices and reduction of the gap between males and females.

To make the result more tangible over time, we have calculated the predicted probability of full immunization coverage using the binary logistics regression and presented in **Table 5**. The predicated probability was 69 percent among the richest compared to 54 percent among the poorest. Wealth-related inequality ratio is 1.27 in 2015–2016, which declined from 1.77 in 2005–2006. Among all the regions, we found a significant gap among these two optimum groups. The highest adjusted wealth-related inequality ratio was observed in Northeastern and Northern region. Considering all other variable constants, the predicted probability for full immuni-

Region	NFHS-3 (2005–2006)			NFHS-4 (2015–2016)		
	Urban	Rural	URIR*	Urban	Rural	URIR*
East	56.36	42.52	1.33	71.92	70.47	1.02
West	64.66	46.23	1.40	54.71	54.94	1.00
North	60.12	40.77	1.47	67.59	62.36	1.08
South	64.63	57.19	1.13	68.35	68.37	1.00
Central	44.68	24.68	1.81	59.11	52.97	1.12
North East	39.39	33.56	1.17	67.09	47.86	1.40
India	57.69	38.72	1.49	64.24	61.72	1.04

**URIR stands for urban–rural inequality ratio.*

Table 3.
Level of full immunization coverage by place of residence and urban–rural inequality ratio among the regions of India in 2005–2006 and 2015–2016.

Region	NFHS-3 (2005–2006)			NFHS-4 (2015–2016)		
	Male	Female	GIR*	Male	Female	GIR*
East	45.85	43.50	1.05	71.32	70.08	0.98
West	57.37	50.69	1.13	53.39	56.39	1.06
North	47.48	44.36	1.07	61.97	66.60	1.07
South	62.77	56.92	1.10	68.35	68.38	1.00
Central	30.53	26.81	1.14	55.99	52.56	0.94
North East	33.96	34.99	0.97	51.33	50.04	0.97
India	45.48	41.62	1.09	62.30	62.50	1.00

**GIR stands for gender inequality ratio.*

Table 4.
Level of full immunization coverage among male and female and gender inequality ratio by regions of India in 2005–2006 and 2015–2016.

zation as nearly equivalent in case of rural and urban as well as for male and female. Considering education-related inequality, we found that the predicative probability of full immunization among the mothers belonging to higher education group is 67

NFHS-3 (2005–2006)	India	East	West	North	South	Central	North-East
Wealth status of household							
Poorest	0.35	0.38	0.39	0.29	0.56	0.27	0.15
Poorer	0.39	0.48	0.45	0.45	0.56	0.29	0.25
Middle	0.49	0.50	0.55	0.57	0.67	0.33	0.41
Richer	0.53	0.59	0.64	0.62	0.64	0.35	0.41
Richest	0.61	0.57	0.72	0.66	0.71	0.43	0.61
Education of mothers							
No education	0.37	0.38	0.51	0.44	0.49	0.24	0.27
Primary	0.47	0.49	0.59	0.50	0.67	0.37	0.32
Secondary	0.57	0.60	0.64	0.68	0.66	0.46	0.43
Higher	0.65	0.69	0.71	0.74	0.82	0.55	0.45
Place of residence							
Urban	0.46	0.41	0.62	0.52	0.64	0.37	0.33
Rural	0.49	0.51	0.61	0.59	0.66	0.30	0.38
Sex of the child							
Male	0.49	0.47	0.63	0.57	0.67	0.33	0.37
Female	0.48	0.48	0.60	0.57	0.63	0.31	0.35
NFHS-4 (2015–2016)							
Wealth status of household							
Poorest	0.54	0.66	0.42	0.54	0.71	0.48	0.40
Poorer	0.61	0.73	0.55	0.62	0.66	0.55	0.52
Middle	0.65	0.76	0.55	0.69	0.68	0.59	0.58
Richer	0.67	0.74	0.63	0.68	0.71	0.61	0.58
Richest	0.69	0.71	0.66	0.73	0.73	0.64	0.57
Education of mothers							
No education	0.56	0.65	0.48	0.62	0.66	0.49	0.41
Primary	0.62	0.74	0.52	0.65	0.73	0.57	0.53
Secondary	0.65	0.73	0.61	0.69	0.70	0.60	0.56
Higher	0.67	0.72	0.58	0.72	0.71	0.62	0.60
Place of residence							
Urban	0.61	0.64	0.54	0.65	0.70	0.55	0.52
Rural	0.63	0.71	0.60	0.68	0.70	0.56	0.53
Sex of the child							
Male	0.62	0.70	0.57	0.65	0.69	0.57	0.52
Female	0.63	0.70	0.59	0.69	0.71	0.54	0.54

Table 5.
Predicated probabilities of full immunization coverage by wealth status, education of mother, place of residence, and sex of the child in India and its region in 2005–2006 and 2015–2016.

percent compared to 56 percent among uneducated mothers in India. Like other two characteristics, education of mother also exhibits significant disparity among these two threshold levels. Almost all of the regions show the pattern of declining trend of education-related disparity, but there continues to be a gap that cannot be ignored.

5. Discussion

The present study has made an effort to revisit the temporal change and differential access in immunization coverage in regions of India. In the line of previous literature, the present study using the last two rounds of NFHS studied the rich-poor inequality, rural–urban inequality, and gender-related inequality to understand the equity gap in immunization among regions of India. The latest round of NFHS found that there was a substantial increase of 18 percent in coverage of full immunization as compared to earlier rounds. Expect the polio vaccine, all other vaccines had improved over time. The full immunization coverage, as well as DPT and measles vaccines, had improved for more than 40 percent in the period 2005–2016. The improvement in the immunization program can be attributable to the national immunization policies in India.

In India, immunizations are provided free of cost in public health facilities. Irrespective of this, 91% of children were vaccinated against BCG, while DPT and measles are lower compared to it. By convention, a newborn is immediately vaccinated by a dose of BCG, after his entry into this world, whereas, at a later point in time, it becomes little difficult for some parents to let their child receive the doses further signifying the importance of getting immunized at birth. A study found that 40 percent of children in India are left out before completing the series of DPT [17]. The burden of work on mothers, commuting to the public health facility, can be attributed for witnessing an increase in dropouts in further doses of vaccinations. However, a very astonishing picture gets reflected from the observed decline in polio vaccination. Though it is cost-free and has widespread coverage, the figures fell a little from 78 to 73 percent in a decade. The reasons may be ascertained that the present population does not consider polio as a severe and threatening disease [28].

The findings show that inequality in specific vaccination coverage as well as in full immunization coverage had shown substantial prorich inequality. The inequality in full immunization coverage was found to be higher among the richer classes also followed to be in the regions. The result was consistent with other studies in India and abroad [18, 26]. But the temporal variation in each vaccination witnessed a significant decline in the gap among the poorest and richest wealth quintile. The ratio in full immunization coverage almost halved over the intersurvey period. This can be thought of as an improvement in the coverage of vaccination among children from the poorest wealth quintile. DPT coverage among children from the poorest wealth quintile doubled, while measles improved 1.5 times over the period, which is instrumental in doubling the full immunization coverage. A positive pattern can be witnessed in the Northern and Northeastern region, where the poorest are showing an impeccable improvement over the period. This can be accredited to advancement in the coverage of immunization, dedicated, well-trained, and sensitive ASHA workers, or community health workers.

Children from urban areas were reported to be better immunized as compared to their rural counterparts. These findings were in tune with studies done in the regional context. In 2015–2016, we found a very marginal rural–urban gap among the regions except for the Northeastern region. The reasons can be due to low urbanization and inadequate or unfit health facilities. The previous literature has highlighted the male advantages in obtaining the vaccination [13, 27]. This study found that the gap in immunization was close to convergence. These achievements can be attributed to an increase in female education, effective gender sensitization programs, and improved communication between health workers and the community.

This study is an attempt in understanding the changes in coverage and inequality among the regions of India dealt with some limitation. The sample size of the children in the NFHS-3 was very less, so it is misleading to find the estimates by different wealth quintiles among the smaller states. Estimates of vaccination coverage in India are based on the vaccination card or the parental recall, but the accuracy and validity of the response are critical. In India, vaccination card is not universal, and the use of parental recall against the absence of vaccination card can sometimes be incomplete or inaccurate.

6. Conclusion and policy implications

Our analysis shows that a significant variation can be observed in the region-wise distribution of a child's immunization. With an aim to increase the immunization coverage among children, the government has initiated several programs, targeted at achieving universal immunization. Though the initiation of new programs gets underway, the achievement of desired targets to be met is often confronted with the lack of community health workers, inadequate infrastructure and human resource, and majorly political will. The study suggests that the immunization programs have to be inclusive, with widespread reach, leaving no stones unturned. These steps can be beneficial in diminishing inequalities, acting as an important ingredient in achieving the Sustainable Development Goals.

Acknowledgements

The author likes to thank the editor of the book as well as the reviewer.

Competing interests

The author declared that he does not have any competing interest.

Funding

The author had not received any funding for this work.

Ethics approval and consent to participate

As the study is based on the secondary data and available in public domain, it needs no prior approval.

Author details

Basant Kumar Panda
International Institute for Population Sciences, Mumbai, India

*Address all correspondence to: basantpanda99@gmail.com

References

[1] UN. Final list of proposed Sustainable Development Goal indicators. 2015. https://sustainabledevelopment.un.org/content/documents/11803Official-List-of-Proposed-SDG-Indicators.pdf

[2] WHO. State of Inequality: Reproductive Maternal Newborn and Child Health: Interactive Visualization of Health Data. Geneva, Switzerland: World Health Organization; 2015

[3] Victora C, Requejo J, Boerma T, et al. Countdown to 2030 for reproductive, maternal, newborn, child, and adolescent health and nutrition. The Lancet Global Health. 2016;**4**(11):e775-ee76. DOI: 10.1016/S2214-109X(16)30204-2

[4] Wang H, Liddell CA, Coates MM, et al. Global, regional, and national levels of neonatal, infant, and under-5 mortality during 1990–2013: A systematic analysis for the global burden of disease study 2013. The Lancet. 2014;**384**(9947):957-979

[5] Feldstein LR, Mariat S, Gacic-Dobo M, et al. Global routine vaccination coverage, 2016. MMWR. Morbidity and Mortality Weekly Report. 2017;**66**(45):1252

[6] Berkley S, Chan M, Elias C, et al. Global Vaccine Action Plan 2011–2020. World Health Organization, Geneva, Switzerland. 2013

[7] Bhatnagar P, Gupta S, Kumar R, et al. Estimation of child vaccination coverage at state and national levels in India. Bulletin of the World Health Organization. 2016;**94**(10):728

[8] IIPS and ICF. Natinal Family Health Survey (NFHS-4), 2015–16: Government of India, New Delhi, India. 2017

[9] Khan J, Shil A, Prakash R. Exploring the spatial heterogeneity in different doses of vaccination coverage in India. PLoS One. 2018;**13**(11):e0207209. DOI: 10.1371/journal.pone.0207209

[10] Rammohan A, Awofeso N. District-level variations in childhood immunizations in India: The role of socio-economic factors and health infrastructure. Social Science & Medicine. 2015;**145**:163-172. DOI: 10.1016/j.socscimed.2015.05.004

[11] Raushan R. Social disparity in child immunization: Factors explaining gap in rural India. Journal of Social Inclusion Studies. 2015;**2**(1):59-74

[12] Shrivastwa N, Gillespie BW, Kolenic GE, et al. Predictors of vaccination in India for children aged 12-36 months. American Journal of Preventive Medicine. 2015;**49**(6 Suppl 4):S435-S444. DOI: 10.1016/j.amepre.2015.05.008

[13] Pande RP. Selective gender differences in childhood nutrition and immunization in rural India: The role of siblings. Demography. 2003;**40**(3):395-418. DOI: 10.1353/dem.2003.0029

[14] Sissoko D, Trottier H, Malvy D, et al. The influence of compositional and contextual factors on non-receipt of basic vaccines among children of 12-23-month old in India: A multilevel analysis. PLoS One. 2014;**9**(9):e106528. DOI: 10.1371/journal.pone.0106528

[15] Kumar A, Mohanty SK. Socio-economic differentials in childhood immunization in India, 1992–2006. Journal of Population Research. 2011;**28**(4):301-324. DOI: 10.1007/s12546-011-9069-y

[16] Prusty RK, Kumar A. Socioeconomic dynamics of gender

disparity in childhood immunization in India, 1992-2006. PLoS One. 2014;**9**(8): e104598. DOI: 10.1371/journal.pone.0104598

[17] Sahoo H. Coverage of child immunisation and its determinants in India. Social Change. 2012;**42**(2): 187-202. DOI: 10.1177/004908571204200203

[18] Singh PK. Trends in child immunization across geographical regions in India: Focus on urban-rural and gender differentials. PLoS One. 2013;**8**(9):e73102. DOI: 10.1371/journal.pone.0073102

[19] Baru R, Acharya A, Acharya S, et al. Inequities in access to health services in India: Caste, class and region. Economic and Political Weekly. 2010;XLV(38): 49-58

[20] Panda BK, Mohanty SK. Progress and prospects of health-related sustainable development goals in india. Journal of biosocial science. 2019;**51**(3): 335-352

[21] Debnath A, Bhattacharjee N. Wealth-based inequality in child immunization in India: A decomposition approach. Journal of Biosocial Science. 2018;**50**(3):312-325. DOI: 10.1017/S0021932017000402

[22] Lauridsen J, Pradhan J. Socio-economic inequality of immunization coverage in India. Health Economics Review. 2011;**1**(1):11. DOI: 10.1186/2191-1991-1-11

[23] Vikram K, Vanneman R, Desai S. Linkages between maternal education and childhood immunization in India. Social Science & Medicine. 2012;**75**(2): 331-339. DOI: 10.1016/j.socscimed.2012.02.043

[24] Rammohan A, Awofeso N, Fernandez RC. Paternal education status significantly influences infants' measles vaccination uptake, independent of maternal education status. BMC Public Health. 2012;**12**:336. DOI: 10.1186/1471-2458-12-336

[25] Awofeso N, Rammohan A, Iqbal K. Age-appropriate vaccination against measles and DPT-3 in India–Closing the gaps. BMC Public Health. 2013;**13**:1-7. Available from: http://www.biomedcentral.com/1471-2458/13/358

[26] Restrepo-Mendez MC, Barros AJ, Wong KL, et al. Inequalities in full immunization coverage: Trends in low- and middle-income countries. Bulletin of the World Health Organization. 2016; **94**(11):794-805B. DOI: 10.2471/BLT.15.162172

[27] Singh A. Gender based within-household inequality in childhood immunization in India: Changes over time and across regions. PLoS One. 2012;**7**(4):e35045. DOI: 10.1371/journal.pone.0035045

[28] Kc A, Nelin V, Raaijmakers H, et al. Increased immunization coverage addresses the equity gap in Nepal. Bulletin of the World Health Organization. 2017;**95**(4):261-269. DOI: 10.2471/BLT.16.178327

Chapter 13

Social and Institutional Support in Breast Cancer Management among Elderly Women in Nigeria

Kenechukwu N. Anugwom

Abstract

The focus of the study was on the social and institutional support available in Nigeria for the management of breast cancer among elderly women. It examined the occurrence and sociocultural factors implicated in breast cancer among elderly women in Nigeria. It discovered that there is increasing incidence of breast cancer among elderly women in Nigeria with an equally increasing mortality rate due largely to low awareness of this menace among women who are past childbearing age. In addition to a low level of awareness are other sociocultural factors such as age, income, education, and the belief systems of the people that the study identified as drivers of increasing menace of breast cancer among elderly women. The above are compounded by the scarcity and inaccessibility of cancer treatment and management facilities in Nigeria. Incidentally, counseling services from such professions as social work and clinical psychology are hardly in existence, leaving the burden of management and care entirely to the families of those affected by the ailment. This calls for a rethink of the sociocultural and support context of public health management in Nigeria. This paper examines the availability and adequacy of existing social and institutional support for breast cancer in Nigeria.

Keywords: breast, cancer, social, support, institutional, management, elderly, women

1. Introduction

The paper using information obtained through a survey examines the social and institutional support mechanisms in breast cancer management in Nigeria. Its main assumption is that despite what may be considered an alarming incidence of occurrence nowadays, breast cancer in management in Nigeria seems bedeviled by inadequate support. In other words, in spite of a significant incidence of breast cancer in Nigeria, the public health system has not responded commensurately, while social support has been affected by wrong notions of causes and stereotypes with severe implications for health of those affected and coping capacity of families [1]. In other words, the quality and access of women to reproductive health services are important in confronting these health problems. In spite of the above, women can only seek them out when the need arises if they are aware of their existence and where they can be received. In other words, awareness and access are critical in obtaining breast cancer services in Nigeria. Consequently, the extent to which members of the society hold the informed perception about the nature and care of breast cancer is crucial in accessing health provisions and services targeted at the disease.

Given that reproductive health-care provisioning has to do with the availability of health-care services to individuals in the society with regard to their reproductive well-being, societal perception of the causes, nature and management of breast cancer can be seen as making a major difference in whether aged women afflicted by breast cancer survive or not [2]. Among women, older women, i.e. those beyond childbearing age, may be seen as particularly disadvantaged. This is especially the case of Nigeria where the health needs of elderly women are not totally covered given the lack of a clearly conceptualized social policy on health care of elderly members of the Nigerian population [3]. Therefore, the survival and meaningful existence of women may not only depend on the health-care services available but also on the conviction of elderly their families and the larger society of the need to spend both time and money on the reproductive health needs of these women even as they have passed the stages of conception and childbearing. Breast cancer is without doubt largely a reproduction health problem much like cervical cancer. In this sense, both ailments can be addressed through reproductive health provisioning in the public health sector. Irrespective of the attitude of family members to the reproductive health of elderly women, there is also a crucial need for women as they age to become sensitive of the likelihood of reproductive health challenges they may encounter especially breast cancer and adopt right attitudes to such issues. Actually, a general consensus which appears true is that early detection makes a big difference in both the treatment and management of breast cancer. Conceding to this opinion, [4] asserted that the high mortality associated with the disease has been ascribed to late detection, lack of knowledge and inadequate medical response. In other words, knowledge and awareness by these women and the society at large are crucial. Hence, the poor attitude of society to women's health including breast cancer may be the product of misconception or lack of awareness of the reproductive health-care challenges women face as they age.

Even though it is contended that 85–90% of cancer incidence is attributable to lifestyle choices as diet and smoking and environmental factors, culture is however seen as the single most influential determinant of these life choices [5]. Culture in this sense refers to factors which exist in a given social environment that influence or inform health-seeking behaviors as well as support system. Thus, such things as perception of nature of illnesses, early access to and availability of health services, beliefs about one's susceptibility to a given illness, etc. are critical elements of one's cultural environment in this case. Therefore, the effort to nib the incidence of breast cancer in the bud must start from a good awareness and knowledge of the sociocultural factors that influence both cancer risk behaviors and attitudes to its prevention and control. Scholars of reproductive health diseases have suggested that there is what may be conceived as an emerging breast cancer epidemic in Africa and some scholars see the increase in breast cancer as ironically related to such things as increasing life expectancy in the general population, improved control of infectious diseases and changing life styles including diet and obstetric practices [1]. As Oluwatosin and Oladepo [4] and Adebamowo and Ajayi [6] observed, breast cancer has become the number one or commonest form of cancer among women with an increasing mortality rate; unfortunately, the mortality associated with the disease has been ascribed to late detection, lack of knowledge and inadequate medical response. In view of the above, the focus of a study on breast cancer among elderly women as a core reproductive health challenge in Nigeria can be seen as really imperative.

Actually it has been established that breast cancer mortality can be reduced by 30% for women aged 50–69 years with routine screening and mammography followed by appropriate treatment [7]. In other words, improved awareness of breast cancer and its appropriate perception and consequent behaviour modification are essential for prevention and control of the disease. Interestingly quite a good number of authors have identified socio-economic factors, adequacy or otherwise of the health-care system and cultural factors as the barriers to the utilization of such preventive practices as mammography, clinical breast examination and breast self-examination by women [8–10].

Perhaps, the challenges of the reproductive health care of the aged in Nigeria are underlined by the fact that nowadays, an increasing number of women are afflicted by diseases of the reproductive system long after ceasing childbearing. This problem is however not peculiar to Nigeria since there appears to be an observable steady increase in such diseases around the world [11]. But while a reproductive health disease like breast cancer may continue to affect elderly women, its early detection has often made a crucial difference between life and death.

This paper is therefore based on the study and findings from a study carried out in the Southeastern Nigeria which sought to reveal the dominant public perception and opinions regarding breast cancer among elderly women in Nigeria and how these affect social and institutional support in the management of the disease. The importance of the study is further enhanced by the fact that scholars are largely in agreement that breast cancer has been so far under-researched and dependence on small clinical and case studies has limited both social and medical responses to the disease [1].

2. Overview of literature

2.1 Sociocultural factors in the management of breast cancer

According to Oluwatosin and Oladepo [4], Adebamowo and Ajayi [6], Okobia et al. [12] and Adotey and Jebbin [13], awareness and knowledge of breast cancer is critical to its early detection and management because its treatment and management are affected by social factors which according to Kagawa-Singer [5] and Levi [14] affect the treatment and management of breast cancer. These factors which the authors classified as lifestyle choices emanate from cultural beliefs, values and practices and may in fact be consistent with the fact that just like values and beliefs, awareness of the impact of breast cancer especially the likelihood of fatality differs among cultural and social groups globally.

While acknowledging the tremendous progress made in the understanding of cell biology and the genetic changes involved in oncogenesis, a few authors have pointed out the relative lag in sociocultural and behaviour studies of cancer which has undermined the expected impact of these advances on cancer control. As Kagawa-Singer (5:2) asserted, positive change in prevention and control of cancer means that "first, greater resources must be directed towards social and behavioural research, and second, better strategies must be developed to study the effects of cultural differences on health behaviour". This sentiment is related to the earlier contention of DeVita et al. [15] in that currently only about 5–10% of cancer globally is known to be due to inherited genetic abnormalities, while the remaining 90% is attributable to lifestyle factors like smoking, diet and environmental factors which are largely determined or influenced by sociocultural contexts. Interestingly the above authors in spite of their medical backgrounds see studies of the social and behavioral factors impacting on awareness and knowledge of cancer as critical to its control and prevention.

2.2 Social and institutional support

When confronted with challenges, having people to turn to or share problems with usually gives some sort of solace or succor to those affected. These sources of succor can come in form of social or institutional pillars aimed at giving readily available shoulders to lean on in times of distress. In the case of breast cancer, social support comes from interactions with people be they family, friends, co-workers or even the church community. Though it has not been established scientifically, this kind of support has been revealed to increase the quality of life and help promote recovery and patients who have some sort of social support have quicker recovery and better survival [16]. In another study on the importance of social support in the management of breast cancer, it was revealed that such support had a significant effect on emotional adjustment of the patients after surgery as this often comes in form of family and friends who talk to and help the patients with personal problems [17]. This can be explained by the fact that these patients from such relationships and interactions develop resilience against the diseases while nurturing the feeling that they are not alone in the fight.

Institutional support on the other hand can be described as the kind of support patients and their families receive from official bodies be it governmental or religious bodies. This institutional support more often than not comes from the church and herbal homes due to the belief that breast cancer is more spiritual than medical. In this kind of situation, the disease is viewed as caused by evil arrows from enemies and as such demands more for spiritual healing more than medical [17]. Unfortunately, when confronted with breast cancer, most women in Nigeria usually seek help from religious institutions more than medical attention, leading to late detection and a high mortality rate. According to Ololade et al. [18], they seek advice from an imam or a pastor, requesting for prayers for healing but do not seek anything else not just because of their faith in prayers but because they may not be able to afford treatment, thereby resigning to fate and hoping for the best.

In some cases, individuals receive institutional support for the treatment of breast cancer through their work places, and this makes it easier for both the patients and their families to maintain some level of emotional stability during the course of the treatment knowing that they do not have to bother about the financial implications of the disease. In a recent study by Mitchelle and Lorenz [19], it was revealed that those who have their employers paying for their medical bills are more likely to present early and seek orthodox treatment instead of running to churches and traditional healers. Therefore, whether social or institutional, there is no gainsaying the fact that cancer patients and their families (just like any other category of people in distress) cope better with their challenges when they receive some form of support be it from close relations or from formal institutions.

3. Findings

The findings of this study are discussed here under the following subheadings:

1. Sociocultural factors in the management of breast cancer

2. Public health institutions and breast cancer management in Nigeria

3. Social workers and breast cancer care and management in Nigeria

3.1 Sociocultural factors in the management of breast cancer

In line with the literature, it was discovered in the study that a number of factors influenced awareness and treatment of breast cancer in Nigeria. These factors ranges from sex, education, age to income, and social factors affect women's awareness of the disease and their use and access to breast cancer services. The results of the study showed that 17.3% of the respondents in the study stated the major factors that affect women's awareness and use and access to breast cancer-related services in the state as financial constraints. This is because even if the services are made available on women's doorsteps, using them would still be a problem as these women sometimes find it difficult to feed not to talk of being able to afford cancer treatments, which are usually very exorbitant. On the other hand, 9.8 and 18.7% argued that the factors that affect them the most are lack of awareness and illiteracy, respectively, because when one is either unaware of the availability of some services or completely uneducated, one's use of these services will be limited if not non-existent entirely.

Therefore income was observed as having a direct relationship with awareness of breast cancer occurrence among elderly women. Hence, while only 31% of the respondents who earn low monthly income were aware of the occurrence of breast cancer among elderly women, 61.6 and 72.9% of those who earn middle and high incomes, respectively, were aware of breast cancer among elderly women. This is not surprising since improved income is a product of improved social status which places the individual in a position to access relevant health information. In agreement with the preceding statement, one of the respondents in the IDI stated that:

> *"there is a relationship between income and awareness of breast cancer occurrence among elderly women because most rich people nowadays usually go for routine medical check-ups both within the country and abroad and this creates a lot of awareness on diseases such as breast cancer" [20]*

The above gained credibility from the opinion of Ashing-Giwa [21] that financial constraints can serve as a barrier to the use of breast cancer preventive and control measures like mammography as women who are living at or below the poverty level have to struggle with competing issues such as food, shelter, safety and employment that take precedence over their own health and well-being. Therefore, given that improved income often results from higher education, this impacts on one's awareness and knowledge generally.

From the foregoing therefore, it was not surprising when it was observed that the respondents with high education were more aware of the occurrence of breast cancer among elderly women than the others because the results showed that the higher the educational qualification, the higher the number of respondents who were aware of breast cancer occurrence among elderly women. Consequently, 71.7% of those with high educational qualification (from university first degree and above) were aware of the occurrence of breast cancer among elderly women, while only 22.6% of the respondents with low educational qualifications were aware of the occurrence of the disease among elderly women.

In the words of Adebamowo and Ajayi [6] and Ohanaka [22], the elderly in Nigeria who are illiterate and reside in the rural communities are usually not reached during public health campaigns, hence, the lack of awareness of breast cancer among those who are uneducated. Ohanaka goes on to contend that though screening and mammography remain the most effective means of detecting breast cancer in elderly women, the facility is not readily available in Nigeria therefore leaving health education on the use of BSE as the only option. The above is unsurprising since some of the respondents encountered in the interviews especially in Nsukka LGA were still totally uneducated with regard to breast cancer and as such had no ideas concerning its treatment and where they may be received. They were still confusing it with "mastitis" which is a disease of the mammary gland which inhibits the perfect flow of breast milk after child birth which in Nsukka dialect is referred to as "eshi era". In the words of a middle-aged woman in the area, she requested that the interviewers describe the nature of the disease to her as she understood breast cancer to be a new name for "eshi era".

3.2 Public health institutions and breast cancer management in Nigeria

Recent studies have revealed that the public health institutions played an insignificant role in the management and care of breast cancer among elderly women in Nigeria [20]. According to the study also, 26.1% of the respondents used in the study were of the opinion that most people affected by breast cancer in the state make use of the public health institutions in the state, while 73.9% were of a contrary opinion. According to some of the IDI respondents, depending on the public health institutions when afflicted by breast cancer can be equated to suicide. In the words of one respondent:

> *"How can someone afflicted with a disease as serious as breast cancer depend on the government hospitals for treatment and survival? Most times, if the doctors are not on strike, the nurses and other members of staff are on their own strike and worse still, sometimes, you are told that some of the drugs or equipment are either out of use or completely spoilt" [20]*

These sentiments capture the extent of distrust people have in the public health institutions in the state when it comes to such diseases as cancer treatment, and this distrust of the public health institutions to assist elderly women suffering from breast cancer is not peculiar to Nigeria since it has been reported that some doctors in public health institutions are reluctant to consider surgery and resort to "tamoxifen" (an effective anticancer drug) because it is easier to administer, but several studies have proven that the cancer will eventually grow and spread if a tumor is not first removed surgically, even if the patient continues to take the drug [23]. In their study, a group of scholars in their study of elderly Swiss women with breast cancer stated that the under treatment of elderly women with breast cancer is usually often based on the belief that they do not tolerate treatment and that among the Swiss many elderly women with breast cancer died because they did not receive full or appropriate treatment for their diseases; consequently, breast cancer patients over age 80 who did not receive adequate treatment had a much higher death rate from their cancer than women who did receive proper treatment [24].

According to Mitchelle and Lorenz [19] and Anugwom [25], it was also revealed that the respondents who said that public health institutions should not be trusted further stated that when afflicted by the disease, the best places to be visit would be private hospitals and chemists/pharmacists giving 27.2 and 25.2% of the respondents, respectively. This in some way underlines a gross lack of faith and trust of people in government hospitals as one of the IDI respondents supported these opinions saying:

> *"When you go to these big teaching hospitals, it takes you days, even weeks to see a doctor except you know someone who works there and sometimes before you get the chance to see a doctor, the patient in question either dies or his/her conditions gets out of hand. This is unlike the private hospitals where both the doctors and*

> *the nurses are usually friendly and treat their patients with utmost care in order to retain their patients and the reputations of their hospitals as their continued stay in the business and daily bread depend on these. Therefore, even though private hospitals are usually more expensive, people still prefer to use them for their treatments or where the patient comes from a wealthy family, she is flown out of the country to such countries as India, Germany and the US for treatment" [20]*

Interestingly also, another 47.6% of the respondents stated that people afflicted by breast cancer go to spiritual houses and herbalists, and this was buttressed by the fact that even key persons in the interview who were mostly doctors, public health officers and nurses were also of the opinion that sometimes, these diseases manifest as a result of charms and spells cast on people through evil means and given that God is omnipotent and can cure all sorts of diseases, He can also destroy the evil effects of the spell and heal the patients of their ailments.

3.3 Social workers and breast cancer care and management in Nigeria

Though social work and social workers through counseling and advocacy go a long way in helping patients and their families cope with ill health in developed countries, patients afflicted with cancer and their families in the southeastern parts of Nigeria do not experience this solace as social work faces the challenge of popularity and professionalization in the country as a whole [2].

While trying to ascertain how much assistance and which services social workers rendered to individuals afflicted with breast cancer, the respondents were asked about their knowledge of professional counseling services or intervention by professionals especially social workers in the case of breast cancer, and their responses were disheartening as they revealed a low level of knowledge of such services in the area. Most of the respondents did not even know what social work meant let alone knowing what social workers do, while those who claimed to know stated categorically that there were no social work services with regard to cancer detection, management, and treatment. It was just a few respondents in the high urban areas like Enugu North who stated that they knew of such services, and this also underlines the fact that those women in the rural or semiurban areas of the state are neglected not just by the government but also by individual bodies that rise up to the challenges of such deadly diseases as breast cancer.

In clearer terms, the results from the study showed that though 37.9% of the respondents used in the study argued social work services are available in the state to assist those affected by breast cancer, 62.1% of the respondents stated categorically that there are no such services in the state, and this shows that those who believed that there are no such help for women suffering from breast cancer are more in number than those who said there are such services, thereby confirming the opinions of one of two key persons in the in-depth interview, a senior nursing officer in a popular teaching hospital in Enugu and a public health officer, respectively; they opined that:

> *"though there are services going on in the state to help women detect cancer early enough to make treatment easier and more effective, these services are usually provided by some other groups or associations but there is none known to be organized and delivered by social workers"; "social workers though not totally new in the country any more, are yet to gain the same level of recognition they have in the western societies both from the Nigerian government and the individuals who need their services" [2, 20]*

This revelation challenges social workers in the state and Nigeria as a whole to get more involved and work towards meaningful intervention strategies in relation to public health and breast cancer in particular given that both cancer victims and their families need a lot of social support and counseling for their coping with cancer. This involvement of social workers can come in the form of creating more awareness on both the occurrence of breast cancer and ways of managing and treating it when it does occur. This opinion gains more substance by the results from the study where 76.4% of the respondents stated that people's awareness of breast cancer and its prevention, care and management can be improved by social workers in the state through rural-based workshops/seminars, while 12.5 and 11.1% stated that the awareness needed can be created through regular counseling for women with breast cancer and in-service training for medical practitioners respectively; this can be explained by the fact that people are usually more responsive to things they are familiar with and, obviously, a lot of people are familiar with workshops/seminars [20, 25].

4. Methodology

The area of the study is Enugu State, a state that goes by such nicknames as "Wawa State", "Coal" and "Ọrānke Amaichekù" which is a mainland state in southeastern Nigeria, and the study focused on three LGAs drawn from the state. Hence, the study was carried out in Nsukka, Udi and Enugu north local government areas [26]. These areas are within the same axis and made for easier data collection. Furthermore, these areas have similarities in their traditions and attitudes towards diseases because traditionally they believe that certain serious diseases occur in individuals' lives as a result of evil deeds by the individuals or evil manipulations by the individuals' enemies.

Enugu State has a population of 3, 267, and 837, and it was this population that formed the population of the study. The study sample was therefore drawn from the members of this population who are 18 years and above. Thirty respondents were selected for the in-depth interview (IDI) using the purposive sampling method, i.e. 10 respondents from each of the LGAs. The selection was guided by gender equity, age variation and different educational levels of the respondents in a bid to cover as much diversity as possible in the sample. In this case, the researcher used judgmental criteria in selecting respondents considered both knowledgeable in the subject of the study and also representative of the population. Thus, such factors as sex, age, and the need to spread respondents throughout the various quarters in each LGA were used in ensuring gender and socio-economic diversity or spread in the selection of the respondents for the IDIs.

The in-depth interview guide/schedule addressed such issues as reproductive health of elderly women; awareness of breast cancer; dominant perception of the public health system and the management of breast cancer among elderly women; sociocultural factors impacting on perception of breast cancer among elderly women; societal perception of factors associated with breast cancer; services and agencies of breast cancer management, etc. They also provided probing questions aimed at generating more in-depth views or opinions and aided the researcher in maintaining focus during the interviews and in garnering deeper insights into people's perceptions of the concerns of the study. In addition, the non-verbal gestures and communications of the interviewees were also noted. These IDIs were conducted by the researcher with the help of a research assistant who acted as a recorder and note taker. The interviews were conducted in locations and at times chosen by the respondents, and the interviews were also recorded in order to explicitly capture both verbal and non-verbal responses. Finally, the analysis of the IDIs focused on identifying common themes in the study and used them as a basis for comparing and contrasting opinions of respondents and how these are consistent or otherwise.

5. Discussions and conclusion

The goal of the study was to find out the dominant public perception of breast cancer among elderly women and the sociocultural factors that influence awareness, treatment and management of breast cancer using Enugu State which portends both urban and rural characteristics. Due to low socio-economic status, a good number of the women in this category are in this day and time still struggling to understand what the disease is all about and what exactly causes it. Low level of education/illiteracy served as a very strong negative influence in the awareness of the disease in the state, and in some cases, they argued based on their convictions that it is "mastitis" which is locally referred to as "eshi era" in areas like Nsukka as this only affects nursing mothers and implies a collection of breast milk even though it does not flow and inflict a lot of pain on the nursing mother. This however is handled by the intake of some local herbs and the bathing of the breasts with some concoctions to make the milk start flowing. In the case of breast cancer, the worry is that it affects everyone especially those who had exceeded the childbearing ages. It was also not surprising that they did not go for the regular medically advocated screening for breast cancer given that they do not even know what it means and what it is meant for.

Disheartening also was the discovery that most women died of breast cancers even after they had been detected because of their lack of access and use of the necessary health care needed for its treatment and management as a result of lack of funds and distance as they are often very far away from the places where these facilities can be accessed. Unfortunately, most public health centres that are easily accessible do not provide these women with the usual breast cancer screening and other related services needed for early detection. Even when they are eventually detected which are usually very late, financial constraints do not allow them to receive the necessary treatment to relieve their pains as the treatment is not subsidized by the government. Consequently, some of them refer to it as the *big man's disease* stating that when a poor person is affected by the disease, it simply means that her days are numbered. For a good number of the women, all they know about the disease is that it is a disease that affects the breasts and which can only be treated through surgery (i.e. the removal of the affected breasts). As a result of this poor knowledge about the disease, it was not surprising therefore that such terms as mammography, screening and staging were totally novel to them underlining the level of unawareness of breast cancer among women especially those from lower socio-economic status.

Social workers are, therefore, encouraged to help in the fight against breast cancer by creating awareness through seminars and workshops for women and the general public taking into consideration the educational level of the target audience. Consequently, posters, pictures and PowerPoint presentations should be used in getting the clear nature and symptoms of the disease across women as well as showing them the correct ways of carrying out the BSE, what mammography is all about and when to start seeking such services. Since there is an established distrust of public hospitals, government should also organize seminars focusing not only on women or the general public but also on the medical personnel especially those of them working in rural and semiurban-based public health centres in order to sensitize them to the kind of commitment needed in dealing with both cancer patients and their families bearing in mind that the disease poses a very serious challenge not only to the affected persons but to their entire family. These seminars should also aim at educating the people on the right ways to live to prevent cancers and the right ways to live and manage them when they do occur. They should also be aimed at purging their minds of any misconceptions or stigmas they may have attached to the disease and those who are affected by it.

Finally, with regard to the theoretical framework, the study showed that the basic assumptions of the theories are true judging by the fact that those who believed they would be susceptible to breast cancer tried to live out a particular life pattern going in line with the Health Belief Model (HBM), while those who had little or no knowledge about the disease attributed it to charms or spells cast on individuals by other evil people in the society and had no idea how to deal with the disease or where to get help when affected by the disease going in line with the assertions of the Health Communication Theory (HCT).

Author details

Kenechukwu N. Anugwom
Department of Social Work, Faculty of the Social Sciences, University of Nigeria, Nsukka, Enugu State, Nigeria

*Address all correspondence to: keneeder@yahoo.com

References

[1] Akarolo-Anthony SN, Ogundiran TO, Adebamowo CA. Emerging breast cancer epidemic: Evidence from Africa. Breast Cancer Research. 2010;**12**(4):3-9

[2] Anugwom KN. Perception of breast cancer among elderly women in Southeastern Nigeria: Implications for healthcare provisioning and care. In: CODESRIEA International Conference on Governance of Public Health in Africa; 19-20, November, 2015; Dakar. 2015

[3] Federal Ministry of Health. National Reproductive Health Policy and Strategy. Abuja: FMoH; 2001

[4] Oluwatosin OA, Oladepo O. Knowledge of breast cancer and its early detection measures among rural women in Akinyele local government area, Ibadan, Nigeria. BMC Cancer. 2010;**26**(6):271. DOI: 10.1186/1471-2407-6-271

[5] Kagawa-Singer M. A socio-cultural perspective on cancer control issues for Asian Americans. Asian American Pacific Island Journal of Health. 2000;**8**(1):12-17

[6] Adebamowo CA, Ajayi OO. Breast cancer in Nigeria. West African Journal of Medicine. 2000;**19**:179-191

[7] Morbidity and Mortality Weekly Report. Update: National breast and cervical cancer early detection program. MMWR. 1996;**45**(23):484-487

[8] Burns R, McCarthy E, Freund K, Maxwell S, Schwartz M, Ash A, et al. Black women receive less mammography even with similar use of primary care. Annals of Internal Medicine. 1996;**25**(3):173-182

[9] Millon-Underwood S, Sanders E, Davis M. Determinants of participation in state-of-the-art cancer prevention, early detection/screening, and treatment trials among African Americans. Cancer Nursing. 1993;**16**(1):25-33

[10] Price J, Desmond S, Slenker S, Smith D, Stewart P. Urban black women's perception of breast cancer and mammography. Journal of Community Health. 1992;**17**:191-204

[11] WHO (World Health Organization). "Breast Cancer: Prevention and Control." Cancer Facts and Figures for Minority Americans. Atlanta: American Cancer Society. Available from: www.who.int/cancer/detection/breastcancer/en; 1999 [Accessed: 11 July 2011]

[12] Okobia MN, Bunker CH, Okonofua FE, Osine U. Knowledge, attitude and practice of Nigerian women towards breast cancer: A cross-sectional survey. World Journal of Surgical Oncology. 2006;**4**:1-9

[13] Adotey JM, Jebbin NJ. Attitudes to knowledge and practice of breast self-examination (BSE) in Port Harcourt. Nigerian Journal of Medicine. 2004;**13**(2):166-170

[14] Levi F. Worldwide patterns of cancer mortality, 1990-1994. European Journal of Cancer Prevention. 1999;**8**(5):381-400

[15] DeVita V, Hellman S, Rosenberg SA. Cancer: Principles and Practice of Oncology. Philadelphia: J.B Lippincott; 1989

[16] Komen SG. Social Support and Breast Cancer Survival. 2017. Available from: https://ww5.komen.org/BreastCancer/Table53Socialsupportandbreastcancersurvival.html

[17] Oyewusi S. Social support as emotional adjustment determinant of breast cancer patients after surgery

in selected hospitals in Nigeria. In: Proceedings of the 107th Annual Meeting of the American Association for Cancer Research; New Orleans: Philadelphia (PA). 2016

[18] Ololade K, Adewumi A, Babatunde F, Adegboyega B. The "evil arrow" myths and misconceptions of the cancer at the Lagos University Teaching Hospital, Nigeria. South African Journal of Oncology. 2019;**3**(1):1-5

[19] Mitchelle B, Lorenz K. Collaboration Aims to Improve Cancer Care in Nigeria. Stanford School of Medicine; 2019

[20] Anugwom KN. Societal perception of breast cancer amongst elderly women in Enugu State [thesis]. Nsukka: Department of Social Work, University of Nigeria; 2016

[21] Ashing-Giwa K. Health behavior change models and their socio-cultural relevance for breast cancer screening in African American women. Women and Health. 1999;**28**(4):53-71

[22] Ohanaka CE. Breast cancer in the elderly. Journal of Medicine and Biomedical Research. 2002;**1**(1):39-42

[23] American Cancer Society. Adequate treatment of breast cancer deadly for elderly women. Journal of Clinical Oncology. 2009;**21**(19):3580-3587

[24] Bouchardy C, Rapiti E, Fioretti G, Paul L, Isabelle NC, Schäfer JK, et al. Under treatment strongly decreases prognosis of breast cancer in elderly women. Journal of Clinical Oncology. 2003;**21**:3580-3587

[25] Anugwom KN. Societal perceptions of breast cancer among elderly women in Nigeria. Southern African Journal of Social Work and Social Development. 2019;**31**(1):1-19. DOI: 10.25159/2415-5829/4202

[26] Anugwom EE. Starting out: The omugwo practice and instilling the rudiments of childrearing in mothers among the Igbo of Southeastern Nigeria. In: Liamputtong P, editor. Childrearing and Infant Care Issues: Across-Cultural Perspective. New York: Nova Science Publishers Inc; 2007. pp. 77-83

Chapter 14

The Health and Economic Costs of Violence against Women and Girls on Survivors, Their Families, and Communities in Ghana

Gina Alvarado Merino, Stacey Scriver, Jennifer L. Mueller, Lila O'Brien-Milne, Ama P. Fenny and Nata Duvvury

Abstract

Violence against women and girls (VAWG) is a worldwide phenomenon. Globally, 35% of women have experienced physical or sexual intimate partner violence (IPV) or non-partner sexual violence in their lives. VAWG is estimated to cost the global economy about US$ eight trillion. Most studies on violence in Ghana discuss domestic violence or some forms of sexual violence but lack a comprehensive view of VAWG and its costs and impacts on communities, businesses, and the national economy. Our international consortium undertook a mixed-methods study to estimate the economic and non-economic losses caused by VAWG. We surveyed 2002 women and 805 male and female employees and conducted 24 in-depth interviews (IDIs) and 8 focus group discussions (FGDs). The study finds that costs of VAWG are high and multi-fold. It estimates costs to health, social relationships, and productivity for individuals, their families, and communities. Individual well-being and capabilities are impacted through absenteeism or missed care work and mental health issues. VAWG deepens household poverty by out-of-pocket expenditures that arise to address medical and legal issues that result from violence. Additionally, VAWG affects the vibrancy of communities as women's participation and leadership decline. These costs accumulate to have profound effects on the Ghanaian economy and society.

Keywords: violence against women, intimate partner violence, costs of violence

1. Introduction

Violence against women and girls (VAWG) is a critical public health, societal, and economic problem affecting 35% of women globally [1]. Women from all countries, socio-economic status, culture and religion can be affected by violence perpetrated by spouses, other family members, authority figures, work colleagues, acquaintances and strangers. The impacts of such violence are widespread and long lasting, ranging from physical injuries, to functional disorders, to reduced capabilities [1]. Countries in the continent of Africa are not exempt from such experiences. In this chapter we focus on evidence of the impacts of VAWG in Ghana.

Ghana is a middle income country that has made progress in improving the status of women, currently ranking 59th out of 144 countries in the Global Gender Gap Index and 11th in Africa [2]. Nevertheless, VAWG has persisted as a problem affecting approximately one third of women during their lifetime [3, 4]. While there are a wide range of forms of violence that women in Ghana may experience, the most common form of violence reported across multiple studies, is intimate partner violence (IPV). Other forms of violence reported in Ghana include sexual violence by non-partners, violence by other family members, sexual harassment, forced and early marriage, female genital mutilation and other forms of harmful cultural practices [5–7].

Increasing the political will to invest in the prevention of VAWG is an ongoing task that many organisations in Ghana are undertaking. We aim to contribute to such efforts by providing evidence that VAWG affects the health and well-being of those who experience it directly, as well as their families and communities, creating costs that undermine personal capacity, family and community stability, and ultimately the economy as a whole. In this study, we focus on IPV, as well as violence against women by other family members in the home, violence in the workplace, educational institute and/or public space and consider the impact of physical, sexual, economic and psychological violence.

Our study examines the economic losses caused by VAWG and the non-economic costs of violence that impact economic growth, development, and social stability. The project was supported by the UK Department for International Development (DFID) in recognition of the dearth of knowledge on the social and economic costs of VAWG. The study presented in this chapter is part of a larger project that the National University of Ireland, Galway with Ipsos-MORI and International Centre for Research on Women (ICRW), in collaboration with in-country partners, conducted in Ghana, Pakistan and South Sudan to estimate the economic losses caused by VAWG.

In this chapter we present evidence of the costs of violence as they impact on the health and wellbeing of women who experience violence in Ghana. We further consider the 'costs' to households and communities. Finally, we extrapolate some of these costs to the national level to consider how VAWG impacts the economy of Ghana. Importantly, these findings represent only a small proportion of the overall cost of VAWG, based on costs captured in the study that are tangible and quantifiable. The overall loss to Ghanaian society and economy due to VAWG is certain to be far higher than can be presented here.

2. Literature/state of knowledge

The literature about VAWG in Ghana provides a plethora of evidence about the depth and prevalence of the problem. The 2008 Ghana Demographic and Health Survey (GDHS) suggests that at least one out of every three ever-married women experienced some form of sexual, physical, and/or emotional violence from a husband or partner in their lifetime [3]. Similar findings were also identified in the recent Ghana Family Life and Health Survey (GFLHS) [4]. Here, the study found that 28% of women reported experiencing IPV (including physical, sexual, economic, social, and/or psychological violence) in the past 12 months. The study also highlighted the impact on daily life and wellbeing of survivors of IPV and their families [4].

Feminist contributions to understanding VAWG have identified that unequal gender power relations that are characteristic of patriarchy influence the forms and prevalence of VAWG in Ghana [5], as elsewhere on the African Continent [8], and globally [9]. Heise's ecological framework further develops the theory in relation to the aetiology of VAWG through recognition of the complex interplay between personal, situational and socio-cultural factors [10]. These contributions clearly situate the drivers of VAWG within social experiences, and thus importantly shift away from explanations of violence that are purely psychological (e.g. as a personality defect) or due to simplistic cause and effect (e.g. the woman burned the dinner so the man beat her). Such understandings have allowed the emergence of a wide-range of interventions and programmes targeted at ending, reducing or mitigating VAWG [11]; however, investment and uptake of these remains limited, in part due to failure to fully grasp the impacts of violence on economic stability, growth and development. Heise's application of the social and ecological framework to explain VAWG has been adopted internationally as a theoretical framework that calls attention to the interplay of factors at multiple levels, the individual, the household, the community and society as a whole. Our study uses this framework to discuss the impacts of VAWG at different societal levels as well [10].

A number of studies have demonstrated the pervasive effects of violence on the health of survivors. In 2016, in Ghana, a mixed methods nationally representative study found that 44% of women who had experienced domestic physical violence in the previous 12 months had been ill in the 30 days prior to the survey, compared to 31% of women who had not experienced this type of domestic violence [4]. In studies in northern Ghana, women reported feelings of worthlessness, suicidal ideation, hypertension, sleep disruption, genital sores, and premature termination of pregnancy as a result of the violence they experienced [12, 13]. The GFLHS study also identified strong correlations between exposure to IPV and serious mental illness. Relationships were further identified between IPV, health impacts and quality of life, with violence affecting women's ability to go to work, to school, complete domestic chores, and concentrate on activities as well as reducing their level of confidence [4].

In addition to physical and mental health impacts and their sequelae, a number of studies in Ghana have outlined pathways through which VAWG impacts individuals and households in Ghana. For instance, Essel finds evidence of women being prevented from working by intimate partners or who have their earnings taken by them [14]. Cantalupo et al. and Danso document costs to victims of VAWG, such as fees for doctors, that result in losses to household income [15, 16]. The children of women were also found to be affected by their mothers' experience of violence, including impacts on behaviour and education that results in long-term opportunity costs [4]. However, there is a dearth of studies that aim to assess the costs of violence beyond the individual or household, resulting in a fragmented understanding of the true impact of VAWG in Ghana.

Despite the high prevalence, there is still a gap between needs and service provision to women and girls who have experienced VAWG. The government of Ghana is a signatory of international treaties that convey a framework for actions to prevent and combat VAWG [17]. Ghana has a Domestic Violence Act, which aims to protect domestic violence victims [18], and approved a National Gender Policy in 2015 [19]. Its main instrument at the local level, the Domestic Violence Victims Services Unit (DOVVSU), has a key role in implementing the law and policy on GBV in Ghana despite having only nearly 180 inadequately resourced units [17]. Advocating for adequate investment in programmes aimed at reducing the prevalence of VAWG or mitigating the impact of VAWG, in line with Government obligations, is facilitated by adequate information about the costs of violence.

Understanding the broad range of impacts of VAWG is still a key gap in the literature. Such evidence is particularly compelling to incentivise government investments in programmes and services for survivors. Identifying and quantifying, where possible, the costs of violence is thus an important contribution towards understanding and addressing VAWG in Ghana.

3. Methodology

This chapter discusses the impacts of VAWG and its health, social and economic effects on the families and communities of the survivors. We argue that the impact of VAWG goes beyond individual health effects. VAWG affects individual women and girls, their families, their communities and larger societal and economic structures (See **Figure 1** for the conceptual framework of the study). Using this framework, this study measures the impact of intimate partner violence (IPV) and sexual violence by non-intimate partner (NPSV) on the health and wellbeing of the women and girls who experience violence. It also estimates the social and economic costs of VAWG by analysing the direct and indirect tangible and intangible costs by looking at the impact on both the individual and society.

For this, a mixed method study consisting of both quantitative surveys with women and with households and qualitative interviews was implemented. For the quantitative study, the team used a household questionnaire to collect data about the general household and individuals within the household and a women's questionnaire applied only to women between 18 and 60 years of age. A multidisciplinary team surveyed 2002 women and 1917 households in 10 regions in Ghana.

The surveyors requested consent to a follow up qualitative interview to all participants in the women's survey. The team selected women and men to participate in in-depth interviews (IDIs), key informant interviews (KIIs) and focus group discussions (FGDs) conducted in Ga and Twi. The team conducted 28 IDIs and 8 FGDs with between 6 and 10 women and men and 10 KIIs (**Table 1**).

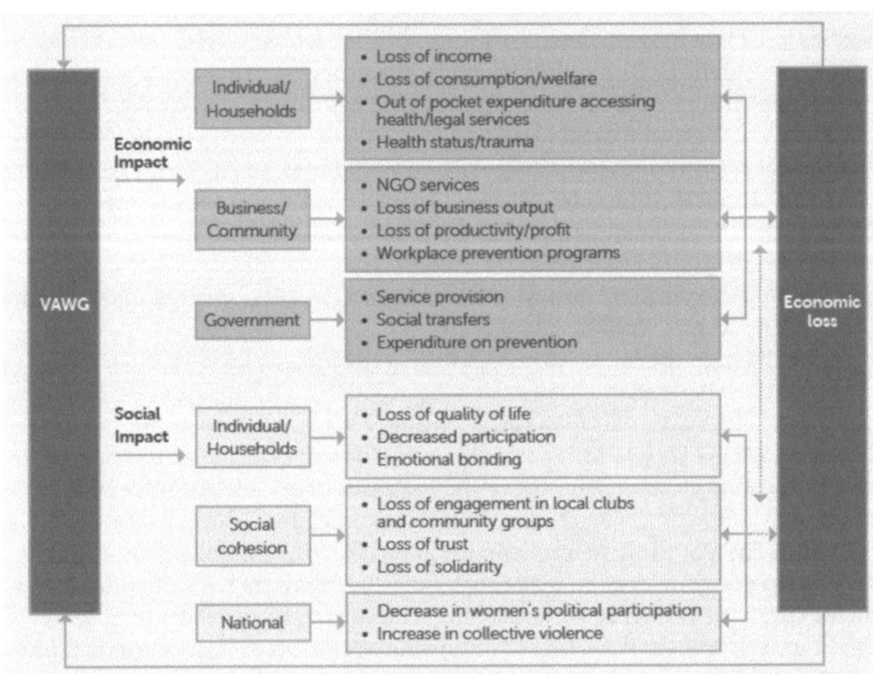

Figure 1.
Conceptual framework of social and economic impacts of VAWG and economic loss.

	Urban areas	Rural areas	Total
Quantitative survey (female)	1046	956	2002
In-depth interviews (female)	15	13	28
Focus group discussions (male, 6–10 participants in each group)	15	13	28
Focus group discussions (female, 6–10 participants in each group)	16	19	35
Key informant interviews (female/male)	5	5	10

Table 1.
Number of participants by type of data collection activity.

Researchers used Stata and/or SPSS for the quantitative analysis and NVivo to analyse qualitative data. During the analysis, the team created quality of life measures to establish health effects of IPV on the woman involved, her partner and her children. The authors used econometric modelling to establish implications, including economic, social and health, of experiences of violence. The analysis included violence at the household level and at the workplace, educational institutes and in public spaces. At the household level, the analysis included the type and nature of injuries suffered, and the impact of IPV on reproductive, physical and mental health.

4. Findings and discussion

The study found, in-line with previous studies, that violence is a common experience for women in Ghana. An estimated 46% of the respondents of the women's survey reported having experienced physical, psychological, sexual or economic violence in the home, workplace, educational institution, or public space in the past 12 months. In the case of IPV, 43% of partnered women had suffered IPV in the last 12 months.

Incidents of violence ranged in severity. In relation to IPV, the study found that 38% of IPV survivors reported suffering severe violence. This means that they experienced economic or psychological violence in a frequency greater than 10 times, physical violence greater than three times and/or sexual violence during the last 12 months. Twenty-five percent of women reported moderate violence, defined as physical violence once or twice and economic and psychological violence 6–10 times. Finally 36% reported low violence, defined as economic or psychological violence up to five times in past 12 months.

Additionally, women reported VAWG in a range of locations, and violence by different types of perpetrators, not just their partners or relatives. About 4% of the total sample in this study reported experiencing violence in educational institutions. About 18% of female respondents reported having suffered some form of violence in a public space, such as the market, on public transportation or on streets. About 43% of female respondents who are married or have a partner and 47% of female respondents who are staying with other family members reported IPV and violence by other family members respectively. Twenty four percent of female respondents who were working reported workplace violence.

The evidence indicates that women in Ghana experience violence from a range of actors and locations. Notably, while violence occurs in workplaces, public spaces and in educational institutes, the home was identified as the place women are most likely to experience violence. The impact of these incidents of violence, on both physical and psychological well-being and on women's capabilities is critical to assess to gain a deeper understanding of the scope and depth of the problem of VAWG in Ghana.

4.1 Impacts on women's health, well-being, and capabilities

Impacts of VAWG can occur in a myriad of ways, often indirect, hence difficult to fully capture in a single study. However, the negative impact of VAWG on the health and well-being of survivors is clear. As is explored below, these impacts often have far-reaching consequences that go beyond the immediate injuries (whether physical or psychological) to constrain women's capabilities in relation to a number of functions, including working, learning, and socialising.

4.1.1 Physical, mental health, and reproductive impacts of IPV

In line with the literature, participants in this survey and qualitative study identified a number of different negative impacts due to VAWG. These included physical, reproductive, and mental health impacts, discussed further below.

Many participants highlighted physical injuries, chronic pain, and disability as a result of beating, hitting, slapping, or other physically violent acts. Drawing from data from the women's survey, a set of scores were constructed, including disability, illness, and depression scores, to identify the strength and significance of the relationship between these health outcomes and experience of IPV, the most commonly experienced form of VAWG in the study. The disability score was calculated based on the following elements: visual, auditory, mobility, cognitive, and articulation difficulties. The score was computed by summing up the level of difficulty of these elements as experienced by respondents. There was a weak but statistically significant relationship between experience of physical and/or sexual IPV and higher disability score.

Similarly, an acute illness score was constructed that identified particularly strong relationships between higher scores on the scale and experience of any form of IPV. The acute illness score was calculated based on: acute health problem, acute impairment, acute pain, consulting any health care worker, headache, loss of appetite, poor sleep, anxiety, difficulty in thinking clearly, mood, crying, loss of enjoyment, difficulty in making decisions, loss of productivity, loss of interest, worthlessness, and tiredness in past 4 weeks. The acute illness score was statistically significantly higher among women who experienced any of the forms of IPV considered (P-value <0.001).

Participants reported insomnia, feelings of anxiety, and varying degrees of depression. Women reported chronic fear after being raped; that fear was described as turning into intense and persistent worry that some women said "could lead one to lose [their] sanity". A depression score, calculated based on suicidal thoughts, loss of interest, mood, poor sleep, tiredness, loss of appetite, worthlessness, and difficulty in thinking clearly, found that women who had experienced any form of IPV scored statistically significantly higher than women who had not experienced IPV (P value <0.001) (**Table 2**).

Out of the total sample of 2002 women, about 52% of women who had experienced health problems in the last 4 weeks also reported experiencing IPV in the last 12 months. Nineteen percent of women who experienced IPV reported having had suicidal thoughts. Out of this number, 63% attempted suicide.

The survey data was used to identify sexual and reproductive health impacts of physical and sexual violence (PSV). The proportion of women who had miscarried and had suffered PSV (15%) is higher than the proportion of women who have miscarried and have not suffered PSV (14%). We did not find significant differences between women who had suffered PSV and those who had not suffered PSV in terms of abortions and still births.

	Economic		Psychological		Physical		Sexual	
	Yes	No	Yes	No	Yes	No	Yes	No
Disability score								
Mean	0.52	0.43	0.49	0.44	0.65	0.41	0.77	0.43
Mean difference	**0.09**		**0.05**		**0.24**		**0.34**	
95% CI	0.366; 0.682	0.344; 0.518	0.359; 0.614	0.343; 0.534	0.445; 0.845	0.324; 0.486	0.440; 1.094	0.348; 0.503
P value	**0.293**		**0.554**		**0.012**		**0.011**	
Acute illness score								
Mean	11.31	8.29	11.19	8.09	11.43	8.57	14.16	8.66
Mean difference	3.02		3.1		2.86		5.50	
95% CI	10.539; 12.081	7.746; 8.835	10.460; 11.914	7.536; 8.643	10.550; 12.308	8.040; 9.097	12.989; 15.331	8.195; 9.119
P value	**0.000**		**0.000**		**0.000**		**0.000**	
Depression score								
Mean	3.2	1.6	2.8	1.6	3.02	1.71	3.98	1.78
Mean difference	1.6		1.2		1.31		2.20	
95% CI	2.928; 3.495	1.415; 1.689	2.515; 3.013	1.423; 1.715	2.670; 3.361	1.575; 1.847	3.404; 4.561	1.652; 1.908
P value	**0.000**		**0.000**		**0.000**		**0.000**	

Table 2.
Physical and mental health outcome scores among partnered women in past 12 months [20].

IDI and FGD participants discussed the link between physical violence and sexual abuse and miscarriages and bleeding, and some mentioned contracting infectious diseases such as HIV and other STIs. Many participants linked VAWG experiences to fatal consequences indirectly as they discussed that depression could lead to suicide or fatal complications of unsafe abortions. Respondents discussed several instances of women who died, or were severely ill, from injuries suffered as a result of VAWG or unsafe abortions.

Notably, some participants also distinguished between acceptable and unacceptable levels of physical violence, based on the degree of harm to the victim, as explained by a participant below:

> *"...There are different kinds of beating; there is love beating and a beating which can lead to death. There are times your husband will beat, but that is love beating... This small one will not hurt you [reference to love beating]. Wicked beating can lead to death..." - Urban In-Depth Interview, Female*

4.1.2 Impacts on capabilities due to VAWG

The mental and physical health effects of VAWG can have secondary affects that impact on women's capabilities. Participants described how violence could impact women's mobility, as well as cause them to miss work and school due to physical injuries or psychological distress. VAWG can also create barriers to women's social and political participation as well as economic agency. Rural participants discussed feelings of shame, fear, and embarrassment associated with having experienced VAWG that kept them from going out in their community to do chores or do attend social events. Participants also discussed remaining at home out of fear of encountering their perpetrator(s) while out in public.

> *"...She will not be able to go there [market]. She will fear that the man will show up over there to disgrace her. It is a market where a lot of people are found. If he shows up over there, the woman will feel bad so she will not go there, so that she will save herself of the disgrace. If she wants something from the market, she will send someone..." - Rural In-Depth Interview, Female*

Women also reported missing work and being unable to conduct other daily activities given the physical and mental health effects, social stigma and reduced mobility that may result of experiencing VAWG. The women's survey asked respondents about missed work and schooling due to VAWG. The results show that about 6% of women experiencing IPV missed on an average 11 days of work from their economic activity in the prior 12 months. Approximately 4% of women experiencing another form of violence reported missing about 10 days of work in the 12 months. About 8% of women living with school going children reported children missing about 3 days annually due to IPV.

The withdrawal from social and work spaces due to VAWG places a constraint on women's capabilities that may translate over time to reduced social status and position, isolation and further vulnerabilities. Missed work is likely to result in lost wages and carries with it a significant opportunity cost. These impacts further expose women to poverty, itself a risk-factor for violence. Thus, VAWG significantly undermines women's potential—an impact that may be passed on to other family members and the next generation.

4.2 Impacts to households

Individual women survivors of VAWG are not the only ones affected by the experience of violence. Family members, including children, are also likely to suffer a range of costs due to VAWG. Below, we discuss the findings of the impacts of VAWG on the health and finances of the relatives of survivors and the impact on the children of survivors.

4.2.1 Health effects on the relatives of survivors

Participants identified several mental health effects of VAWG on relatives of survivors. Among these effects, they discussed depression and feelings of guilt. They also discussed anxiety caused by threats from the perpetrator, social stigma and isolation. This anxiety may affect direct victims but also their relatives, including parents or children of the women and girls affected by VAWG. Further, participants in the qualitative research described that victims of VAWG whose capacity to carry out chores and household duties was reduced, relied on family members for assistance. The time-burden of taking on such extra workloads by the relatives of survivors also contributes to a loss to households.

4.2.2 Economic costs

Families may experience increased expenses and/or loss of income or productivity due to VAWG. The lack of shelters and public support for VAWG survivors create financial hardship that may lead to household dissolution or homelessness in extreme cases. Some participants emphasised that these financial burdens fall onto the woman's family because there is a lack of formal social support for affected women and their families. Women described economic worries and concerns about their ability to take care of their children as a barrier to escaping VAWG. Families are burdened by hospital bills when survivors require medical care for physical injuries, pregnancies, STIs, or mental health care as a result of VAWG, in addition to the cost of caring for children of women who are no longer able to care for their children due to death or long-term injury.

The study also identified out of pocket expenditures incurred on health care, police, court, shelter and replacing property. For example, a participant described:

> *"...I was speaking to a woman about this yesterday, and she said when her husband gets angry at her, he just destroys things that belong to her...when she came back he had disconnected the light and spoilt her kettle..." - Rural In-Depth Interview, Female*

To estimate these economic costs to households of VAWG an accounting methodology was employed whereby costs were calculated for specific categories and added to calculate the total cost to households and/or society [21]. Tangible costs can be grouped into direct, from the use of goods and services and indirect, calculated using imputed monetary value such as lost income and reduced profits [22]. This approach was used to estimate the costs to households due to VAWG.

The calculations based on the accounting methodology described above were applied to the survey data. It was found that, on average, almost 11% of women experiencing IPV incurred costs of GH¢275.62 due to IPV. Among women experiencing any form of violence, 11% of women reported out of pocket expenditures equivalent to US$53 in the last 12 months, including on health-related expenditures, filing police reports, or replacement of furniture; this amount is equivalent to 10% of the annual per capita expenditure on non-food consumption in Ghana. This economic loss to households has the potential to result in further vulnerability, including poverty, or to the re-direction of funds away from long-term planning, such as children's education or building a business, towards immediate survival.

4.2.3 Impacts on the children of survivors

IPV does not only affect the victims' physical and psychological health and social wellbeing, but also the children in the home. Participants discussed direct effects on children, such as fear, anxiety, stigma, and pain; they also discussed how VAWG can lead to the loss of school days when homes are dissolved as a result of violence.

Evidence from the women's survey provides further support that children are negatively affected by the violence experienced by their mothers. Twenty-one percent of participants in the survey noted that their children felt scared after witnessing IPV. About 18% of them said their children felt confused and 14% reported that their children asked a lot of questions about the incident. An important finding was the children of women who experienced violence were more likely to miss school, due to their mother's being unable to bring them, or having to help care for their mothers after an incident. It was found that 3 days of school were lost on average per year, among those women with children who reported violence and responded to the question. When extrapolated to the national level, this indicates that nearly 300,000 school days are lost to children in Ghana annually—a significant drain on future potential.

Participants and key informants mentioned that VAWG may become normalised among children who witness it in the household. They were especially concerned about how witnessing violence could lead to male children perpetuating violence in the future and female children accepting violence as a normal part of relationships. While this intangible impact cannot be immediately monetized, the long-term cost to society would be immense and would ultimately translate into economic costs.

It is clear that the cost VAWG is not only an issue for the survivor. It has impacts that ripple beyond the individual to their children and other relatives. Indeed, as is explored below, they also affect whole communities.

4.3 Impacts to community and participation

4.3.1 Help-seeking behaviour and service usage

Studies suggest that the rate of help seeking for VAWG, and IPV in particular, is generally low. Stigma, fear and challenges in availability and access all create barriers to help-seeking. Our survey shows that only 3% of survivors of IPV reported any of the incidents to the police.

Among those who did seek help, participants mentioned seeking help from the Department of Social Welfare, police, and assemblymen as a source of legal aid and punishment for perpetrators; others sought help from local chiefs, traditional community elders, family elders, and religious leaders. However, many participants reported that women were unlikely to seek formal help, such as from police or legal institutions, preferring to seek advice from community or church elders, family members, or close friends, or to keep the issue secret. Reasons for this included normalisation ("this is just how marriage is"), that IPV is a personal issue, and love for their partners. One participant went further, to say that women who did report their husbands would be disparaged by the community:

> *"People insulted the woman that she was stupid and a foolish. How could she report a man who was the father of her children? Why did she not forgive the man for the sake of her children?" - Rural In-Depth Interview, Female*

The evidence suggests that family unity and even community cohesion were deemed as more important than individual wellbeing. Thus, reporting violence was seen as either a failure of the woman to maintain a peaceful household or a selfish act that sacrificed her family's reputation or wellbeing for her own interests. In such contexts, reporting of IPV is unlikely to occur, potentially reinforcing existing stigma against women who experience violence.

4.3.2 Women's participation in the community and leadership

Respondents discussed how experiencing VAWG impacted women's participation in community events and decision-making. They explained that a leader who experiences any type of VAWG would no longer be seen as having "the qualities of a leader" or as being "qualified" to give her opinion on issues in the community, as she would no longer be deemed a good role model. This affects the ability of survivors to take and keep leadership positions in their community. In communities where VAWG is common, the fear of experiencing violence may have an effect on women's and girls' mobility and leadership undermining their potential. Women and girls in the community who have not experienced violence themselves may reduce their mobility and participation in order to avoid the violence they have heard that others have experienced.

"... It depends. People may decide to vote against her, or ask her to step down because they think she might not be a good example to the younger ones. At other times too, they may decide to help her fight against the violence she may be experiencing from her partner..." - Urban In-Depth Interview, Female

When women reduce their participation and involvement, communities experience a loss of input that undermines genuine democratic functioning. Considering the high proportion of women in Ghana who experience violence, the potential consequences of even a small percentage of them reducing leadership activities and participation, is substantial.

4.4 Impacts on the economy

The economic implications of VAWG at individual, household and community levels impact the overall economy via productivity loss. Productivity loss emerged as an impact that women and households experience and discussed within the qualitative research. A participant in a focus group with young urban women remarked:

"[A woman who is abused by her husband] will not be able to focus on her work so her income level will reduce. If you are working for someone, and you always have a divided attention, you will not be able to meet your set target." -Urban Focus Group Discussion, Female

In the quantitative survey, productivity loss was probed through measuring absenteeism (missing work), tardiness (being late or leaving early by an hour), and presenteeism (being less productive or having less focus, low concentration, working slowly, stopping work or having an accident). The estimates of productivity loss due to IPV and VAWG more broadly were derived as the difference in means between working women experiencing violence and those not experiencing violence.

For women who experience IPV, the productivity loss was equivalent to 12 working days per woman in the past 12 months; nearly two-thirds of this loss is due to being less productive at work and the remaining one third is due to absenteeism (see **Table 3**). For women experiencing any form of violence across various locations, the total days of lost productivity is 26 days per woman in the past 12 months. This translates into nearly 65 million days at the national level or equivalent to 216,000 employed women not working, assuming women work 300 days in the year. Overall, the economy is estimated to lose output equivalent to 5% of its female workforce not working annually due to VAWG.

Category	Due to partner violence		Due to any violence	
	Mean days lost	Total days lost	Mean days lost	Total days lost
Absenteeism	4.1	4,714,811	15.14	37,042,551
Presenteeism	7.49	8,601,655	11.27	27,789,032
Total	**11.59**	**13,316,465**	**26.41**	**64,831,583**

Notes for calculation of mean and total days lost:
-The weighted IPV prevalence rate among working women = 24.13% (based on study survey).
-The weighted any violence prevalence rate among working women = 51.47% (based on study survey).
-Used estimated number of women aged 18–60 in Ghana as of 2016 = 7,377,138 (Ghana Statistical Service—GSS).
-Used the employment rate of women 15+ 2016 = 64.6% (Ghana Labour Force Survey).

Table 3.
National estimate of productivity loss due to violence [20].

The impact of annual loss of output combined with the ongoing negative consequences for the capability and participation of women establishes the systematic but unrecognised drain that violence against women and girls imposes on the economic prosperity and societal well-being of the nation.

5. Conclusion

In this mixed methods study, we found that VAWG is a persistent public health problem that affects women and girls who experience it, as well as their families and communities. Almost half of the women who participated in the women's survey reported having experienced physical, psychological, sexual, or economic violence in the home, workplace, educational institution, or public space in the past 12 months. The violence women and girls experience varies in severity. It also varies by type of perpetrator and place of experience. Women reported experiencing violence in educational institutions, in public spaces, such as the market, on public transportation or on streets, in their work places, and at home. Nevertheless, it was also found that the home was the most dangerous place for women in Ghana.

This study also found that there are clear negative impacts on the health and well-being of survivors of VAWG. The effects that we identified have far-reaching consequences that go beyond immediate injuries (whether physical or psychological) to affect women's ability to work, learn, and socialise. Participants in the study identified physical, reproductive, and mental health impacts. The study also found a statistically significant correlation between an illness score, a depression score, and experiencing any form of IPV.

The effects of VAWG on the health of women who have experienced violence affect other areas of their lives, creating a complex net of effects that goes beyond their individual health and well-being to affect their livelihood, through the impact of VAWG on the women and girls' capabilities, with economic costs that have to be covered by women and girls and their families. Family members' health may also be affected by VAWG. More subtle and difficult to notice are the costs that VAWG brings to the communities and countries.

VAWG also affects community cohesion and, according to the participants in our study, is often underestimated given that women and girls hardly ever report VAWG to formal authorities. The overall economy of Ghana is impacted due to the productivity loss that results from VAWG.

The study highlights the importance of research on costs/impacts of violence that recognise the social embeddedness of individuals and their locations within broader ecological systems. Such approaches go beyond simplistic accounts of immediate injuries and impacts but rather recognize how negative impacts ripple outwards—both through social networks as well as through time—thus creating much more substantive impacts with consequences for societies, economies and generations. While this study focused on Ghana, similar effects have been identified in South Sudan [23] and are likely to be replicated throughout countries in Africa. Further studies on the costs of VAWG are recommended, particularly longitudinal studies that can produce robust evidence of the long-term consequences of VAWG on capabilities in developing countries.

This study identifies the serious and long-lasting costs of VAWG to individuals, households, communities and economy through assessment of data from Ghana. The evidence generated by this study can be used by advocates across developing, low-to-middle income countries in Africa to influence policy makers and stakeholders, showing them the importance of investing funds in sustainable actions to prevent VAWG. Given the lack of funding for shelters and treatment for women and girls who experience violence, the authors suggest increasing the funding for support services, treatment and prevention initiatives. Such investments are sure to yield high returns—reducing the human and financial losses that impact on the health of populations and, ultimately, achieving development goals.

Acknowledgements

The project that forms the basis for this chapter was made possible by funding from the UK Department for International Development through the What Works to Prevent Violence against Women and Girls programme. We would also like to acknowledge the contributions of Felix Asante, University of Ghana, who oversaw the project in Ghana, Carol Ballantine, National University of Ireland, for her assistance with the literature review, and Mrinal Chadha for his work on quantitative analysis. We would also like to acknowledge the research team in Ghana who undertook data collection.

Conflict of interest

The authors declare no conflict of interest.

Notes/thanks/other declarations

We gratefully acknowledge the women who willingly gave their time to share their experiences and insights on the impacts of violence for them and their communities.

Author details

Gina Alvarado Merino[1], Stacey Scriver[2*], Jennifer L. Mueller[3], Lila O'Brien-Milne[3], Ama P. Fenny[4] and Nata Duvvury[2]

1 Landesa, Washington, District of Columbia, United States

2 Centre for Global Women's Studies, National University of Ireland Galway, Galway, Ireland

3 International Center for Research on Women, Washington, District of Columbia, United States

4 Institute of Statistical, Social and Economic Research, University of Ghana, Accra, Ghana

*Address all correspondence to: stacey.scriver@nuigalway.ie

References

[1] WHO, Department of Reproductive Health and Research, London School of Hygiene and Tropical Medicine, South African Medical Research Council. Global and Regional Estimates of Violence against Women: Prevalence and Health Effects of Intimate Partner Violence and Nonpartner Sexual Violence; 2013

[2] World Economic Forum. The Global Gender Gap Report; 2016

[3] Ghana Statistical Service, Ghana Health Service and Macro I. Ghana Demographic and Health Survey 2008. Accra, Ghana: GSS, GHS, and ICF Macro; 2009

[4] IDS, GSS and Associates. Domestic Violence in Ghana: Incidents, Attitudes, Determinants and Behaviours; 2016

[5] Amoakohene MI. Violence against women in Ghana: A look at women's perceptions and review of policy and social responses. Social Science & Medicine. 2004;**59**:2373-2385

[6] Committee on the Elimination of Discrimination against Women. Concluding Observations on the Combined Sixth and Seventh Periodic Reports of Ghana; 2014

[7] Ballantine C, Fenny A, Asante F, Duvvury N. Working Paper No. 4—Ghana: The Economic and Social Impact of Violence against Women and Girls (VAWG); 2017

[8] Bowman CG. Theories of domestic violence in the African context. Journal of Gender, Social Policy & the Law. 2003;**11**:847-863

[9] Hunnicutt G. Varieties of patriarchy and violence against women: Resurrecting "patriarchy" as a theoretical tool. Violence Against Women. 2009;**15**:553-573

[10] Heise L. Violence against women: An integrated, ecological framework. Violence Against Women. 1998;**4**:262-290

[11] Fulu F, Heise L. What Do we Know about Violence against Women and Girls and What More Do we Need to Know to Prevent it? A Summary of the Evidence; 2014

[12] Issahaku PA. Health implications of partner violence against women in Ghana. Violence and Victims. 2015;**30**:250-264

[13] Sedziafa AP, Tenkorang EY, Owusu AY. Kinship and intimate partner violence among married women in Ghana: A qualitative exploration. Journal of Interpersonal Violence. 2016;**33**:2197-2224

[14] Essel PI. Effects of Violence against Women on the Socio-Economic Growth of the Nation; WiLDAF Ghana; 2016

[15] Cantalupo NC, Martin LV, Pak K, Shin S. Domestic violence in Ghana: The open secret. The Georgetown Journal of Gender and the Law. 2006;**7**:10-56

[16] Danso J. State Must Support Domestic Violence Victims-Court. Ghana News Agency; 2017

[17] Ministry of Gender, Children and Social Protection. National Gender Policy. Theme/Ghana: Mainstreaming Gender Equality and Women's Empowerment into Ghana's Development Efforts; 2015

[18] Domestic Violence Act, c.732 Ghana; 2007. Available from: http://www.ilo.org/dyn/natlex/docs/ELECTRONIC/88525/101248/F503368907/GHA88525.pdf

[19] Government of Ghana. National Gender Policy; 2015. Available from:

http://www.ilo.org/dyn/natlex/docs/ELECTRONIC/103987/126660/F-515436150/GHA103987.pdf

[20] Asante F, Fenny A, Dzudzor M, Chadha M, Scriver S, Ballantine C, et al. Economic and Social Costs of Violence Against Women and Girls in Ghana: Country Technical Report. NUI Galway: Galway; 2019. p. 59

[21] Addo-Lartey A, Alangea D, Sikweyiya Y, Chirwa E, Coker-Appiah D, Jewkes R, et al. Rural response system to prevent violence against women: Methodology for a community randomised controlled trial in the central region of Ghana. Global Health Action. 2019;**12**:1. DOI: 10.1080/16549716.2019.1612604

[22] Duvvury N, Grown C, Redner J. Costs of Intimate Partner Violence at the Household and Community Levels: An Operational Framework for Developing Countries; ICRW. 2004.

[23] Elmusharaf K, Scriver S, Chadha M, Ballantine C, Sabir M, Raghavendra S, et al. Economic and Social Costs of Violence Against Women and Girls in South Sudan: Country Technical Report. NUI Galway: Galway; 2019. Available from: https://whatworks.co.za/resources/reports/item/594-economic-and-social-costs-of-violence-against-women-in-south-sudan-technical-report

Chapter 15

Obesity in School Children in India

Vangal Krishnaswamy Sashindran and Puja Dudeja

Abstract

The global prevalence of obesity has doubled from 1990 to 2015. Worryingly, the increase is more in children than in adults. In just three decades, the number of school-going children and adolescents with obesity has increased by 10-fold, and the International Association for the Study of Obesity (IASO) and International Obesity Task Force (IOTF) reckon that 200 million school children worldwide are either overweight or obese. The prevalence of obesity among 5- to 19-year-old Indian children, ranged between 3.6 and 11.7%. It is predicted that by 2025 there will be 17 million obese children in India. Urbanisation is the single most important factor linked to obesity in India. Epigenetic, dietary, familial, psychosocial, parental education and parental occupation are other important factors. About 50% of obese children will become obese adults. The prevalence of hypertension, type 2 diabetes dyslipidaemia and non-alcoholic fatty liver disease in children is also increasing parallelly. Prevention of childhood obesity is vital because it is near impossible to get children to lose weight and maintain it. A healthy diet and an active lifestyle should start from the pre-conception time itself and be continued through all stages of childhood.

Keywords: India, childhood, overweight, obesity, causes, consequences

1. Introduction

Non-communicable diseases are the biggest public health challenge of this century, and childhood obesity is an important part of this. Its rates have tripled in the US over the past 30 years. Today, 17% of US adolescents and 16% of children between 2 and 11 years are obese with prevalence being highest among Black and Hispanic children and adolescents [1]. Childhood obesity was so far thought to be a problem of the developed world, but it is increasingly being reported from middle- and low-income countries, especially from urban areas [2]. Obesity in children is not as easy to quantify as in adults. Body mass index is not an accurate measure of obesity in children. It is important to recognise childhood obesity and manage it, because if untreated, it can result in obesity in adulthood with all its attendant metabolic complications. Childhood obesity also has a deep psychosocial impact and is consistently associated with lower scholastic achievements. Weight once gained is difficult to lose, and hence prevention is important. This assumes greater significance with regards to children as compared to adults, because they are more susceptible to the constant bombardment by advertisements for energy-dense food [3]. Immuring them from an obesogenic environment is a priority and a challenge. A number of innovative programmes to tackle childhood obesity have been tried in different countries, and each one of them has important lessons for public health specialists and health policy makers. The WHO's Commission for Ending Childhood Obesity opines that this problem requires, 'a whole-government approach in which policies across all sectors systematically take health into account, avoid harmful health impacts, and thus improve population health and health equity' [4]. The magnitude of the problem, causative factors, complications of childhood obesity and some solutions will be discussed.

2. Prevalence

2.1 Global prevalence

Obesity in school children is today an uncomfortable reality. The global prevalence of obesity has doubled between 1990 and 2015. Worryingly, the rate of increase in obesity in children is higher than that in adults in many countries [5]. Globally, about 10% of school children in the 5–17 age groups are obese or overweight [5]. The prevalence varies from 30% in America to less than 2% in sub-Saharan Africa. In just three decades, the number of school-going children and adolescents with obesity has increased by 10-fold, from 11 million to 124 million (2016 estimates). In addition to this, another 216 million children were estimated to be overweight though not obese in 2016 [6]. The International Association for the Study of Obesity (IASO) and International Obesity Task Force (IOTF) reckon that 200 million school children worldwide are either overweight or obese [7]. The problem probably starts early in childhood. A 2010 report estimated that 42 million children under the age of 5 were overweight and of these, 35 million lived in developing countries. While the prevalence of childhood obesity may be plateauing in some developed countries, it is showing a steep rise in developing countries of Asia and Africa. Within Asia, China has the highest number (15 million) followed by India (14 million) [4]. Even within nations, certain subgroups like children of migrants and indigenous populations are at greatest risk of obesity [8].

The NCDRisC study pooled data for 2416 population-based studies. This included data of 31.5 million children and adolescents aged 5–19 years. The mean BMI in 1975 was 17.2 and 16.8 kg/m^2 for girls and boys, respectively. It was lowest in South-East Asia and East Africa, and highest in Polynesia, Micronesia and English-speaking regions. The age-standardised mean BMI for children and adolescents increased all over the world from 1975 to 2016. The increase was 0.32 kg/m^2 per decade for girls and 0.40 kg/m^2 per decade for boys. The mean BMI for girls and boys in 2016 was 18.6 and 18.5 kg/m^2, respectively. The age-standardised mean BMI in 2016 was still lowest in South-East Asia and east Africa and highest in Polynesia and Micronesia. It was 16.9 and 17.9 kg/m^2 for girls and boys respectively South -East Asia and Africa and 23.1 and 22.4 kg/m^2 for girls and boys respectively in Polynesia and Micronesia. The regions with the largest absolute numbers of obese children and adolescents were East Asia, the Middle-east, North Africa, South Asia and English-speaking regions. It is predicted that if post-2000 trends continue, then by 2022, the number of obese children will outstrip those with moderate and severe underweight [3].

Peltzer reported that the prevalence of overweight/obesity in school children aged 13–15 years in seven ASEAN countries (excluding Brunei) was 9.9% [9]. The highest prevalence of overweight/obesity in all eight ASEAN countries was in Brunei Darussalam (36.1%), followed by Malaysia (23.7%). It was lowest in Myanmar (3.4%) and Cambodia (3.7%) [10]. Pengpid and Peltzer also studied the prevalence and factors affecting obesity in children in six Pacific island countries of

Oceania. Among the 10,424 children in the age group of 13–16 years, the prevalence of overweight and obesity was 24.3 and 6.1%, respectively. The researchers used a BMI of >30 kg/m^2 to define obesity and defined overweight as a BMI between 25 and 29.9 kg/m^2. Therefore, their estimate may not be quite accurate [11].

2.2 Indian prevalence

India is caught in a nutrition paradox where stunting and underweight coexist with overweight and obesity in children. National Family Health Survey-4 (2015–2016) reported the prevalence of stunting, wasting and underweight in children <5 years to be 38%, 21% and 36%, respectively. In this survey, overweight was defined as weight for height being more than 2 SD above the median of the reference population. By this definition, 2% of Indian children under the age of 5 were overweight. Unfortunately, data of older children are not forthcoming from this survey [12]. The prevalence of overweight/obesity among adolescent Indian children rose from 9.8% in 2006 to 11.7% in 2009 [13]. Lobstein and Jackson-Leach computed that there will be 17 million obese children in India by 2025 [14]. This trend is reported from all over India, both in urban and rural areas. Prevalence of overweight/obesity in children in Delhi increased from 16% in 2002 to 24% in 2006 [15]. A study done in the urban areas of Udupi in South India, found prevalence of overweight and obesity in school children to be 10.8 and 6.2%, respectively [16]. Another study from Central India found 3.1% (95% CI 2.5–3.8) of children between 10 and 17 years to be overweight and 1.2% (95% CI 0.8–1.8) to be obese and overall 4.3% were overweight/obese [17]. From Surat, in Western India, Gamit et al. reported the prevalence of overweight and obesity to be 10.2 and 6%, respectively [18]. In Kanpur, the prevalence of overweight and obesity were 4 and 2%, respectively. The authors attributed this low prevalence, when compared to other studies from North India, to local dietary habits [19]. A systematic review conducted by Gupta et al., reported that prevalence of overweight, among 5–19 years children, ranged between 6.1 and 25.2%, while that of obesity ranged between 3.6 and 11.7% [20] Khadilkar et al., in 2010, estimated the combined prevalence of overweight and obesity to be 19.6% as per IOTF classification, while this was 27% according to WHO definitions [21]. Among adolescence, between 10 and 17 years, the percentage was 22.3 (as per IOTF cut off) and 29.8% (as per WHO cut off), and these age groups should be considered most vulnerable for adiposity [22]. The estimates will swing widely till all investigators adopt standard criteria for measurement of overweight and obesity.

3. Factors causing obesity in school children

Obesity is a result of imbalance between calorie intake and energy output. This may seem a facile explanation, but in reality it is due to a complex interplay of many factors. Biological factors can lead to childhood obesity through 'mismatch' and 'developmental' pathways [4].

3.1 Genetic factors

Obesity is probably polygenic in inheritance. BMI may be 25–40% inheritable. But, like for hypertension and diabetes, behavioural and environmental factors play a big role. Genetics may just account for less than 5% of all cases of childhood obesity [23]. Maternal undernutrition or malnutrition and placental insufficiency lead to epigenetic changes that put these children at greater risk for developing overweight and obesity when exposed to energy-dense foods and sedentary lifestyles when compared to children born of mothers with adequate nutrition. Maternal obesity or hyperglycaemia can also cause epigenetic changes, which predispose the children to increased deposition of fat tissue. Recent studies reveal that paternal obesity can also have an adverse effect on the offspring through epigenetic effects [4].

3.2 Individual factors

3.2.1 Gender

The GDB Collaborators Group did not find any gender difference in prevalence of obesity in children <20 years. In countries with high-medium and high SDIs, the prevalence was higher in boys than in girls with the trend reversing in late adolescence [5]. The NCDRisC study also reported that gender disparity had narrowed considerably all over the world by 2016. They reported a flattening of the curve for both sexes in North-western Europe, high-income English-speaking countries and Asia-Pacific regions. The plateauing was also seen for boys in South-western Europe and girls in Central and Andean Latin America. In contrast, a rise in BMI was noted for both sexes in East and South Asia and for boys in South-east Asia. The prevalence of obesity was highest in Polynesia and Micronesia in both sexes being 25.4% in girls and 22.4% in boys. This was followed by the high-income English-speaking countries. Obesity prevalence was between 1 and 2% in Cambodia, Burkina Faso, Vietnam, Ethiopia, India, Madagascar, Republic of Congo, Japan, Nepal, Niger and Chad. The number of girls with obesity increased from 5 million in 1975 to 50 million in 2016. For boys, the numbers are 6 million and 74 million, respectively [3]. However, other studies do report differences. The prevalence of overweight/obesity in children and adolescents is more in boys than in girls in developed countries (23.8 and 22.6%, respectively). In developing countries, it is lesser in boys than in girls (12.9 and 13.4%, respectively) [24].

Studies from different parts of India also show that it is more common in boys than in girls. Ramachandran et al. reported the prevalence of overweight to be 17% in boys and 15.8% in girls in the age group 13–18 years from Chennai [25]. In the study from Udupi in South India, the prevalence of overweight and obese were 11.0 and 7.1%, respectively, in boys and 10.6 and 5.4%, respectively, in girls [16]. Researchers from Wardha, in Central India, reported the prevalence of overweight/obesity to be 4.4% in boys and 4.3% in girls [17]. In Pune, in Western India, the prevalence of overweight in children in the age group 9–16 years was 27.5% for boys and 20.9% for girls [26]. In Surat, the prevalence of overweight and obesity in boys was 12.4 and 8.2%, respectively, and in girls it was 7.2 and 2.7%, respectively [18]. Kapil et al. reported the prevalence of obesity in children aged 10–16 years in Delhi to be 8.0% for boys and 6.0% for girls [27]. Chhatwal et al. also found higher prevalence of obesity among boys than girls. They attributed it to the cultural advantages that boys enjoy in India. They get larger helpings of food at home, snack more as they have greater freedom to go out and also participate negligibly in doing household chores. The gender disparity was highest in the most affluent socio-economic groups. Among children going to the affluent school, the prevalence of overweight was 25% in boys and 16.6% in girls ($p = 0.001$). The prevalence of obesity was 19.9 and 13.3%, respectively ($p = 0.003$). The prevalence was similar among boys and girls in the lower-income schools. They also found that only at the age of 15 years was prevalence of obesity/overweight more in girls than boys. This is explained by the pubertal hormonal surge and growth spurt that occurs earlier in girls than in boys [28]. These findings are reiterated in the systematic review of 28 studies by

Ranjani et al. who found that overweight and obesity were slightly more common in adolescent boys than girls in India [2].

3.2.2 Age

There is a distinct age pattern in childhood obesity. In their longitudinal study on 8544 children, Whitaker et al. reported that the prevalence of obesity was 13% at 9 years and dropped to 9% at 14 years and then increased again [29]. The GDB Collaborators Group also reported that the prevalence of obesity decreased with age till 14 years and then increased [5]. In the American NHANES 1999–2000 survey, the prevalence of overweight/obesity did not vary much in the age groups of 6–11 and 12–19 years (15.3 and 15.5%, respectively) [30]. The findings by Chhatwal et al. in Ludhiana mirrored Whitaker's study. Prevalence of obesity declined from 18.5% at 9 years to 7.6% at 14 year-end then again spiked at 15 years to 12.1% [28]. Ranjani et al. found that prevalence of obesity in under-fives was less than 2% across India. In children >5 years, it varied from 2 to 8%. Overweight rates were about 2× higher and were higher in North and East India than in South India. Among adolescents, the overall prevalence of overweight and obesity ranged between 3 and 24.7% and 1.5–28% respectively [2].

3.2.3 Dietary factors

With globalisation, the dietary mores of Indian children has also started changing rapidly. Gulati et al. found that a majority of children surveyed in four urban centres preferred to eat out; they felt that home food was 'old-fashioned'. Almost half of them also had their evening meals while watching television [31, 32]. Adolescents associate 'junk food' with independence and convenience and consider health food options odd [33].

In the Udupi study, there was no statistical correlation between frequent consumption of carbonated drinks and being overweight/obese [16]. But in Oceania, Pengpid and Peltzer found that consumption of >1 carbonated drink per day increased OR for obesity by 1.32 (95% CI 1.09–1.61, $p < 0.01$) [11].

A drastic behavioural change is seen in Indian children in senior secondary schools. Those interested in taking competitive examinations stop physical activity totally and adopt a sedentary lifestyle. They enjoy eating packaged food items to relieve stress. These are usually energy-dense high fat, sugar and salt (HFSS) foods. Both nocturnal snacking and consumption of HFSS foods in the breaks between study sessions can lead to significant weight gain. Snacks rich in refined sugars and fats are habit forming and children get addicted to their flavours and tastes. This perspective is supported by a growing body of neuroscience researchers who have demonstrated that the chronic consumption of energy-dense foods brings about changes in the brain's reward pathways that are central to the development and maintenance of habits. While it is difficult to precisely define 'eating behaviour', such habits are associated with pleasure centre in the brain (neural reward circuitries)—characterised by symptoms such as loss of control while eating, over consumption and/or binge eating, continued consumption of high calorie foods despite the knowledge of its negative consequences and inability to cut down despite the desire to do so [34, 35]. The vicious cycle of obesity in school children is shown in **Figure 1**.

The reinforcing value of food is higher among obese children than among children with normal weight. In general, bland foods are not eaten in excess; whereas, highly palatable foods are often consumed even after an individual's energy requirements have been covered. Some children fall prey to vicious cycle of impulsive

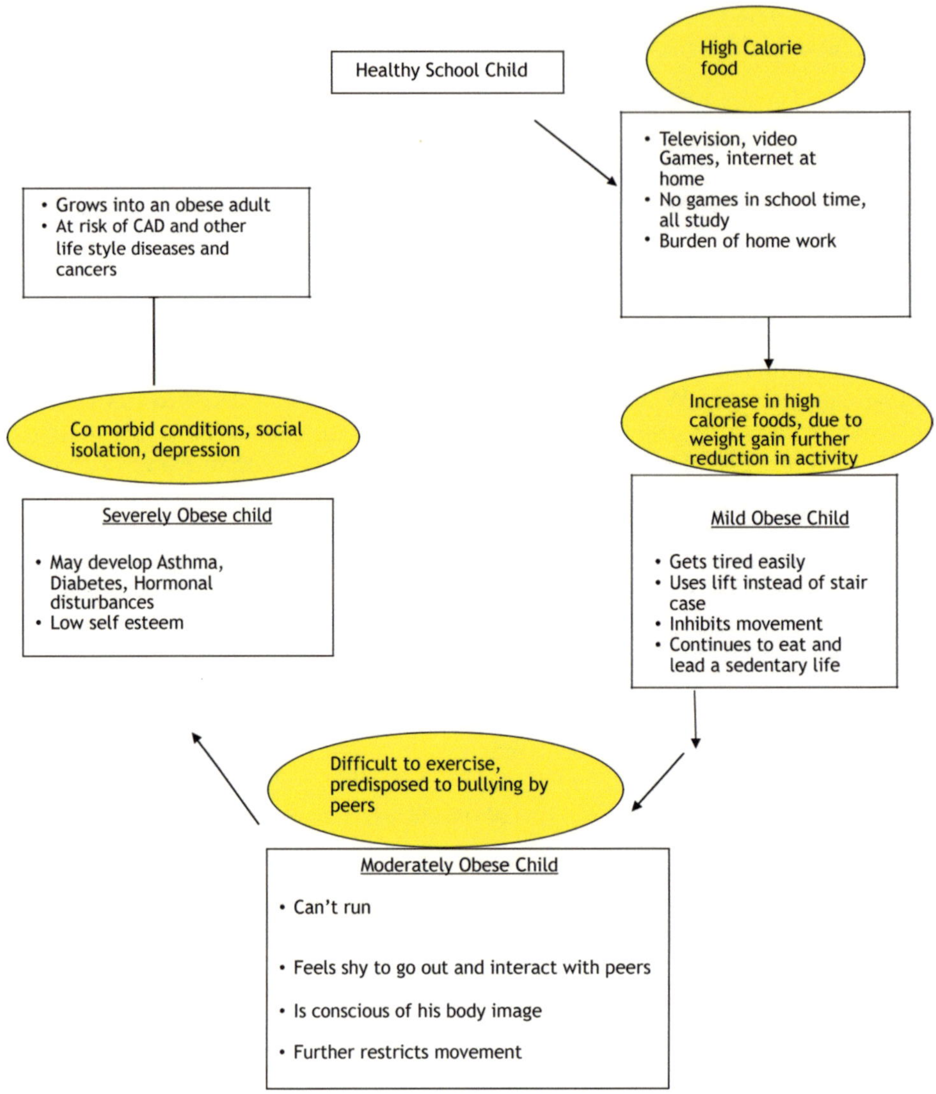

Figure 1.
Vicious cycle of obesity in school children.

eating. Highly impulsive children often do not think about the reactions or their consequences. Besides overeating, these children seem to be vulnerable to food triggers like the smell and taste of the food. It has been suggested that poor control of neural centres related to impulsivity and/or addiction could foster impaired control of food intake leading to overeating and subsequent obesity. Adaptive decision-making and the ability to delay gratification may positively influence eating behaviour, particularly in an energy-rich food environment, where conscious control of energy intake is essential for the maintenance of healthy body weight [36].

3.2.4 Physical activity

The Wardha study showed a good correlation between physical inactivity and childhood obesity. On univariate analysis, the odds ratio (OR) of obesity in school children was 2.064 if they played outdoors for less than 30 min a day. Step-down multiple logistic regression analysis showed OR for the same children to be 2.133 (95% CI: 1.373–3.301) [17]. In the study from Oceania, sedentary behaviour defined as sitting for ≥3 h/d increased the odds of being overweight/obese OR1.17 (95% CI 1.03–1.34, $p < 0.05$) [11]. More frequent participations in sports correlated well with greater accretion of fat free mass. This finding was independent of ethnicity, individual, family, community and socio-economic factors. Walking or cycling to school also resulted in a lower fat mass index [37]. Kunwar et al. studied the prevalence of obesity in school children in a military station in North-Eastern India and concluded that the prevalence of obesity in garrison schools was lower due to the greater emphasis laid on games and physical activity [38].

3.2.5 TV watching

Sedentary lifestyle is associated with higher adiposity. Every additional hour of TV-time per day increases the prevalence of obesity in children by 2% [23]. Govindan et al. found that watching TV for >2 h/d was significantly associated with obesity (boys OR 1.19, $p < 0.01$, girls OR1.19, $p < 0.01$) [39]. The National Institutes of Health, US also consider TV-time of >2 h as a definite risk for obesity [40]. TV watching (passive screen time) is unhealthier than active screen time (computer and video games) [41]. Hours of TV watching also directly correlate with increased intake of foods frequently advertised on TV like sweets, sweetened beverages, cookies, chocolates, sweetened cereals and salted snacks [42]. This habit of watching TV or playing games on mobile phones starts at an earlier age. During preschool period, most mothers have a tendency to feed children by distracting them. They let them watch cartoons on television or play games on mobile phones. This makes their job of feeding easier as the children do not resist feeding. In the process, they tend to overeat, being too distracted to signal the feeders that they are full. This tendency to overfeed themselves continues into adolescence also.

3.2.6 Psychosocial factors

Pengpid and Peltzer looked for impact of loneliness, lack of close friends, anxiety and worrying, suicidal ideation and bullying on occurrence of overweight/obesity in school-going children in Oceania. The OR for being overweight with lack of close friends was 0.72 (95% CI 0.56–0.92, $p < 0.01$) and with suicidal ideation OR was 1.42 (95% CI 1.21–1.66, $p < 0.001$). The association with other factors was not significant on multivariate regression analysis [11]. The lifetime risk for anxiety disorders is higher for obese adolescents in comparison to non-obese ones [43]. There is a bi-directional relationship between eating disorders and depression making both difficult to treat [44].

3.2.7 Familial factors

The family has a significant role to play in the development of childhood obesity. The influence starts even before the child is born. The first reported causal association of intra-uterine undernutrition resulting in obesity in the offspring later in life was from the observation of children born to women who were pregnant during the Dutch famine [45]. Intra-uterine malnutrition may lead to a higher susceptibility to excess weight gain due to increased fat stores, short stature and a preference for foods high in fats [46]. This is the 'mismatch' effect alluded to earlier. A phenomenon known as 'mirror imaging' between the mother and her baby is observed in India. The baby's birth size is predicted by the mother's size before pregnancy. Despite this, birth weight has been found to be a poor indicator of adiposity in the foetus. In Caucasian populations, birth weight is related to lean mass rather than to fat mass; whereas, in India, babies have more fat mass as compared to Europoid babies at every ponderal index. Babies with both low- and high-birth weights have a high risk of obesity in later life in India [47].

Maternal and paternal heights are independent predictors of childhood obesity. The highest adiposity is seen in children who exceed mid-parental height. Parental height may serve as a composite indicator of genetic factors, nutrition and growth during childhood [47, 48]. Many studies in India have shown that the mother's BMI correlates with the child's weight. This may be due to genetic factors and environmental factors such as shared diets and eating habits [31, 49]. Raskind et al. found that every overweight child had an overweight mother. The combination of overweight mother and child formed 11% of their study population which was one of the highest in Asian countries [50]. Rebecca Kuriyan studied the role of familial and sibling factors on abdominal adiposity in children in an urban location in South India. Multiple regression models showed that overweight status of father or mother was associated with the younger sibling having abdominal obesity (OR = 1.45 and 1.81, respectively). If both parents were overweight, the OR for the younger sibling having abdominal obesity was 1.63 (95% CI: 1.33–2.99). If the older sibling had abdominal obesity, then the OR for the younger sibling to have the same was 3.22 (95% CI: 2.30–4.50). When siblings were of the same sex, the odds were higher (OR 3.55, 95% CI 2.24–5.65) than if the siblings were of different sexes (OR 2.73, 95% CI: 1.67–4.46). The association was stronger among male sibling pairs (OR 4.18, 95% CI: 2.21–7.93) than female sibling pairs (OR 2.85, 95% CI 1.42–5.72). All the above findings were statistically significant ($p < 0.01$). These effects are probably due to behaviour modelling among siblings and this is strongest in same sex siblings. The younger child is likely to follow the elder sibling in a number of behavioural traits like academic engagement, smoking, alcohol use, substance abuse and sexual behaviour [48]. Not only are dietary habits of children modelled on those of their parents and peers, but they also pick up food preferences, intake and willingness to try new foods from them. The key to good dietary preferences is the availability and repeated exposure to a variety of healthy foods. Authoritative feeding refers to parents who determine what foods are offered and then allowing children to choose. This leads to a positive attitude to healthy eating. However, authoritarian restriction of 'junk foods' works in the opposite way. It increases the children's desire for these foods and leads to weight gain. It is also known that families that eat together consume healthier foods. There is a greater tendency to consume fast foods in single parent families or where both parents work. Eating out regularly and 'TV dinners' are both associated with higher intake of dietary fats [51, 52].

Peer support at school, supervision of studies by parents, parental connect with children and bonding have all been studied. Pengpid and Peltzer founds that odds for overweight/obesity correlated with peer support at school (OR1.28, 95%CI 1.08–1.53, $p < 0.01$), parental support (OR 1.33, 95%CI 1.13–1.58, $p < 0.001$) and parental bonding (OR 1.31, 05%CI 1.12–1.54, $p < 0.001$) [11].

3.2.8 Socio-economic factors

There are many commonalities in socio-economic factors associated with childhood obesity from studies across India. Urban background has the strongest association. Familial economic status, educational levels of parents and job profile of parents are other important factors. The type of school that children study in also is an important determinant. Strangely, data on religious denominations is conflicting.

Urbanisation is the strongest risk factor for obesity in India. Obesity is three times commoner in cities as compared to rural areas. Development of good roads and satellite television have blurred the divide between cities and villages. Youth migrating from villages to metros to study and work take back urban food habits and norms back to their villages. Thus, Indian villages are getting urbanised in their habits. This phenomenon is referred to as rubanisation or urbanisation in situ [47]. Bharathi et al. reported that the OR for obesity in school children from urban areas as compared to rural areas was 3.046 (95% CI: 1.662–5.582) [17]. Rapid urbanisation has led to 'McDonaldisation' of society in terms of an increase in the culture of eating out and eating fast foods. An important contributory factor to this change has been increasing financial independence of women, who are now spending less time in their kitchens. Such households often pack energy-dense convenient food in school tuck boxes and also offer the same as snacks between meals. This results in excess consumption of calories by the children and leads to fat gain.

Higher socio-economic status is another risk factor. The GDB Collaborator Group found prevalence of obesity to be higher in countries with higher socio-demographic index (SDI). A relative increase of 20% was found in the prevalence of obesity in children of both sexes between 1980 and 2015 in low SDI countries. The increase was greatest in countries with middle SDI [5]. An American study compared school children from two neighbouring communities, the first with a median household income of US$ 28610 and the second with US$ 46299. The prevalence of obesity was 22.2 and 12.6%, respectively ($p = 0.01$) [53]. Chhatwal et al. found a direct correlation between socio-economic status and overweight/obesity in children from three different schools in Ludhiana, Punjab. Prevalence of obesity was 15.5% in children from socio-economic class I (highest income group), 2.7% in children from class IV and 0% in children from class V (lowest income group.) [28]. Eagle et al. observed that as the average American household income decreased, frequency of consumption of fried food and TV or video time/week increased. Consumption of vegetables and moderate/vigorous physical exercise also proportionately decreased [54].

Kaur et al. reported three times higher number of overweight children (15.3%) and obese children (6.8%) in high-income schools as compared to children in lower-income schools [55]. Prevalence of overweight/obesity in children aged 14–17 years from urban Delhi was 29% in private schools and 11.3% in government-funded schools [15]. In Udupi, the percentage of children with BMI in overweight/obese range were 6.9%, 10.9% and 31.2% for government, aided and unaided/private schools, respectively ($p < 0.001$) [16]. Ramachandran et al. reported an overweight/obesity prevalence of 4.5% in low-income schools and 22% in better-off schools in Chennai [25]. Another interesting factor related to schools is the provision of free lunches or mid-day meals (in India). Govindan et al. reported that regular consumption of school lunches was associated with obesity in both boys and girls (boys OR 1.29, 95% CI 1.01–1.64, $p = 0.04$, and girls OR 1.27, 95%CI 1.00–1.62, $p = 0.05$) [39].

The effect of religion on childhood obesity is varied. In Udupi, the odds of overweight/obesity in children from Muslim or Christian homes was significantly higher (for Muslims the AOR was 2.26, and for Christians it was 1.60) in comparison to children from Hindu homes [16]. The authors attributed this to a focus on vegetables in the Hindu diet and a lack of meat [16]. In Wardha, however, the OR for obesity was 1.730 ($p = 0.036$) for Hindu children when compared to children from other communities [17]. Here, it probably was influenced by greater affluence of Hindus in comparison to Muslims and Christians.

Myths related to obesity in school children	Reality
Fat children are healthy, as they are not undernourished	Fat children are not healthy inside. About 28% of fat children have syndrome X. They have a risk for chronic lifestyle diseases
With age, children will gain height and loose fat	Majority of obese children become obese adults
So what, if a child is obese! Obesity is a problem of adults and not of children	Fat children are at risk of developing early diabetes. Girls may develop polycystic ovarian syndrome
Heart disease starts at old age	Hardening and blockage of the arteries starts at 11 years in boys and 15 years in girls
Children do not develop high blood pressure or high cholesterol	Many children will have high blood pressure and low HDL-cholesterol
Children should eat, drink and be merry. Childhood will not return	Children should enjoy being active as such energy will not come again later
Children by nature are physically active	Time on TV, Internet and studies leaves little time for play. Many do not participate in sports activity in mandatory sports periods in schools.
Observing a child to be fat is considered inauspicious	Obesity in children should be viewed with concern

Table 1.
Some common myths in India society related to obesity in school children.

4. Community/society level factors

Structural elements like road, transportation, structure of buildings, playgrounds, parks and public spaces influence obesity in children. Research conducted over the past decades provides increasing evidence that there is a direct correlation between easy access to supermarkets laden with cheap and readily available HFSS food and sweetened carbonated drinks and obesity in children. Increased concretisation and loss of public spaces and parks in cities have led to decrease opportunities for sports and a more sedentary lifestyle. Many poorer neighbourhoods are considered unsafe for children because of drug pedlars and predatory adults. Parents prefer to keep their children indoors. Even when they have to go out or attend school, the parents drop them by car. Walking or cycling to school often considered a healthy activity is thus lost [23].

Children are bombarded by commercials of confectionary, chocolates, sweetened cereals and fizzy drinks on TV, billboards and magazines. Celebrity endorsements are a big influence on children. Nothing can be more telling than endorsement of a fizzy drink by a cricketing or football legend. Most cultures also use sweets and food as inducements for good behaviour or rewards. This further reinforces the habit of HFSS food intake.

Some common food myths related to children are shown in **Table 1**.

5. Consequences of obesity in school children

At least 30% of obesity begins in childhood and 50–80% obese children become obese adults [17]. Obesity is linked to greater and earlier mortality. The GDB collaborator Group found that the lowest overall risk of death was in the BMI range of 20–25 kg/m^2 [5]. As in adult metabolic syndrome, hyperinsulinemia is a key to most of the complication of childhood obesity also. Some of the consequences of childhood obesity are enumerated in **Table 2**.

Physical	Psychological	Social
Respiratory and sleep problems Insulin resistance High blood pressure Dyslipidemia Musculoskeletal problems Gall stones Fatty liver	Low self-esteem, increased depressive symptoms and unhealthy dietary practices	Low participation in social activities Lack of social support due to less interaction with peers

Table 2.
Hazards of obesity in school children.

5.1 Hyperinsulinemia

There is an early leaning towards adult South-Asian phenotype in children, probably starting in neonatal period. Hyperinsulinemia and its attendant metabolic perturbations are more common in Asian neonates than in Caucasian ones [56]. Kuriyan and colleagues studied the waist circumference of Indian urban middle-class children between the ages of 6–16 years and found that their waist circumference was more than that of age- and sex-matched British children [57]. About one-third of the urban-Asian children have insulin resistance. The odds for hyperinsulinemia in one study were OR 4.7 (95% CI 2.4–9.4) in overweight children, OR 6.4 (95% CI 3.2–12.9) with high percentage body fat, OR 3.7 (95% CI 1.9–7.3) with high waist circumference, OR 6.8 (95% CI 3.3–13.9) with high waist hip ratio and OR 4.5 (95% CI 1.8–11.3) for sum of four skin-fold thicknesses (Sigma 4SF). Multiple logistic regression analysis showed that percentage body fat and Sigma 4SF were independent predictors of hyperinsulinemia with ORs being 3.2 and 4.5, respectively [58]. This being so, the risk of chubby children becoming obese adults is real.

5.2 Paediatric metabolic syndrome

In parallel with increasing prevalence of childhood obesity, the prevalence of paediatric metabolic syndrome, hypertension and type 2 diabetes mellitus are also increasing. Insulin resistance has been clearly been implicated in pathogenesis of hypertension, coronary artery disease and polycystic ovarian syndrome [59]. A study from Shimla in Himachal Pradesh showed prevalence of metabolic syndrome in school children to be 3.3% with odds of having metabolic syndrome being significantly linked to male sex, higher family monthly income, sedentary lifestyle and snacking in the evening [60]. The prevalence of metabolic syndrome in a study by Singh et al. in Chandigarh was 4.2%, and they did not find any difference between the sexes [61].

5.3 Childhood diabetes

The rise in prevalence of childhood obesity has mirrored the rise in prevalence of type 2 diabetes among children. For a long time, only type I diabetes was associated with childhood. The myth was shattered in 1979, when type 2 diabetes was described in children of Pima Indians. Type 2 diabetes accounts for 80% of childhood diabetes in Japan. The prevalence of type 2 diabetes in Japanese children rose from 0.2 to 7.3 per 100,000 children between 1976 and 1995 [62]. Ehtisham et al. observed that prevalence of type 2 diabetes in white UK children was significantly less than that in South-Asian children (0.10/100,000 vs. 1.42/100,000, $p < 0.001$). According to them, the relative risk for type 2 diabetes in an Asian child compared to a white child in UK was 13.7-fold. Family history of diabetes, prevalence of obesity in the family, female preponderance and pubertal onset were some of the other significant associations that they noted apart from the ethnic clustering [63]. Ripamonti et al. found the prevalence of impaired glucose tolerance (IGT) to be 11% among the 398 obese Italian children studied [64]. Wabitsch et al. studied 520 obese children in Germany, and noted the prevalence of IGT and type 2 DM to be 2.1 and 1.5%, respectively [65]. Vijayalakshmi Bhatia observed that type 2 DM accounted for 10% of diabetes detected in children between the ages of 10–18 [66]. A higher BMI, and increased truncal and abdominal fat were important determinants of hyperglycaemia and insulin resistance [67, 68]. The GDB Collaborators Group found diabetes to be the second commonest cause of BMI-related deaths and DALY. It accounted for 9.5% of all deaths at a BMI of $\geq$30 kg/m^2 and 4.5% occurred at a BMI of <30 kg/m^2 [5].

5.4 Dyslipidaemia

Nearly 17% of obese adolescent American youth have abnormal non-HDL-cholesterol. Class III obesity is associated with high total cholesterol (19%), low HDL-cholesterol ($\leq$19%) and high triglycerides (29%) [69]. The commonly observed pattern of dyslipidaemia in obesity is one with increased triglycerides (TG), decreased HDL-cholesterol (HDL-C) and high normal or mildly raised LDL-cholesterol (LDL-C). The NHANES data indicate that in the US 42.9% of children with BMI >95th percentile have this pattern of dyslipidaemia [70]. Obesity is consistently associated with low HDL-cholesterol values [71]. In obese children and adolescents, there is a positive correlation between BMI and levels of VLDL and LDL-cholesterols [72]. The Princeton follow-up study conducted family lipid surveys between 1973 and 1978. Of all the children surveyed, 808 agreed to be a part of a CVD survey when contacted in 1998 and 19 live subjects reported CVD events. These events occurred at a mean age of 37.1+ 4.9 years. BMI and TG levels in childhood correlated significantly with occurrence of CVD events ($p = 0.012$ and 0.0001, respectively) [73].

5.5 Hypertension

Childhood obesity is associated with future development of hypertension. In fact, elevated BMI even in infancy is associated with high BP later [74, 75]. Risk of hypertension is two-fold with obesity and four-fold with severe obesity [76]. The prevalence of hypertension in children in the US varies from 3 to 5%, but it rises to about 25% in children with obesity [77]. Yadav et al. found the prevalence of pre-hypertension and hypertension to be 1.14 and 2.57%, respectively, among school children in the age group of 10–16 years in Kanpur, North India. Among overweight children 6.25% were pre-hypertensive and 12.5% were hypertensive and among obese children, the figures were 14.28% and 42.5%, respectively. The association in both cases was statistically significant [19]. Vedavathy and Sangamesh studied prevalence of hypertension in school children between the ages of 11–19 in Bangalore. Pre-hypertension and stage I hypertension were found in 3.6% of the students. The prevalence was significantly higher in children with BMI >23 kg/m^2. Family history of hypertension and obesity were significantly associated with pre-hypertension and stage I hypertension in the children ($p < 0.001$) [78]. An epidemiological survey of school children in Delhi found the prevalence of hypertension (systolic, diastolic or both) to be 11.9% in boys and 11.4% in girls.

There was a positive correlation between hypertension and BMI [79]. In another study from North India, Gupta et al. surveyed 3851 children between the ages of 5 and 15 and found that 292 were obese. The prevalence of hypertension was 0.34% among the obese children and 0.16% among the non-obese children [80]. In another study from Ludhiana, where 5000 children in the age group of 5–17 years were studied, the prevalence of hypertension in obese children was 3.5% and among normal ones 0.23% [81]. Hypertension in obese children results from an interplay of numerous factors which include, increased intravascular volume, increased cardiac output, increased sympathetic tone, increased steroid production, increased sodium intake and increased sodium retention and hyperinsulinemia. Among adolescents, hormonal changes and biological maturation are additional contributory factors [82, 83]. By the time hypertension is diagnosed in childhood, 20–40% have left ventricular hypertrophy. This correlates with high carotid intimal-media thickness (cIMT), which is a known predictor of heart-failure in childhood [77].

5.6 Cardiovascular disease

In relation to high BMI, cardiovascular disease (CVD) was the leading cause for death and disability-adjusted life-years (DALY). It accounted for 2.7 million deaths and 66.3 million DALY. Among the obese, 41% of deaths and 34% of DALY were due to CVD [5]. Current adolescent overweight prevalence is estimated to increase future adult obesity by 5–15% by 2035, and this will result in an additional 100,000 CVD cases [84]. Cardiovascular disease associated with obesity is usually secondary to hypertension (already discussed above) and atherosclerosis. Atherogenesis is mainly due to sub-intimal deposition of LDL-cholesterol particles. The combined atherogenicity of childhood obesity is an ideal scenario for this to occur. High circulating levels of small LDL-cholesterol particles and decreased clearance of the same by LDL receptors increases risk of their entrapment in the sub endothelial matrix. Further, low levels of HDL-cholesterol limit reversal of cholesterol transport. An objective measure of the damaging potential of atherogenicity of combined dyslipidaemia in childhood is the carotid intimal-media thickness (cIMT). The Young Finns study followed up children from childhood for 21 years. Children with combined dyslipidaemia had significant cIMT compared to normo-lipidaemic controls even after adjusting for other factors [85]. The Childhood Cardiovascular Cohort (i3C) was a 23.4 years follow-up of 2893 children aged 12–18 years across three continents. i3C data showed a strong correlation between childhood obesity, hypertension and dyslipidaemia with high cIMT in adulthood. Obesity increased the risk for high cIMT 3.7 (2.0–7.0)-fold and hypertension by 1.9 (1.3–2.9)-fold [86]. Another study showed that 90% of children with high cIMT also had left ventricular hypertrophy [87]. Obesity has been associated with a 50% increase in heart-failure incidence among young adults (18–34 years) from 1987 to 2006 in the US [88]. The frequency of stroke and renal failure are also higher in young adults with history of childhood obesity [89, 90]. In a recent study published in JAMA, positive associations were observed between consumption of artificially sweetened soft drinks and death due to circulatory diseases (>2 drinks/day vs. <1 glass per month; HR 1.52; 95%CI 1.30–1.78, $p = 0.001$) [91].

Sub-clinical vascular inflammation may also be a contributory factor to development of CVD. In Indian adolescents, raised C-reactive protein (CRP) levels are seen in 13% of all subjects, 22% of overweight and 25% of obese ones. CRP levels have a strong association with percentage body fat, WHR, waist circumference and triceps skin-fold thickness [92].

5.7 Non-alcoholic fatty liver disease (NAFLD)

Non-alcoholic disease is a component of metabolic syndrome. It is being increasingly recognised since abdominal ultrasonography has become a common diagnostic tool. The overall prevalence of NAFLD in children is about 10%, which includes a prevalence of 17% in teenagers and 40–70% in obese children. Steatosis *per se* is benign and self-limiting but it can progress to non-alcoholic steatohepatitis (NASH) in 3–5% of patients [93]. In the US, about 12–24% of the children are obese and 10–25% of these have elevated serum transaminases. That means that 1–4% of children, in the US, are obese and have deranged transaminases and are at risk for NAFLD [94]. A more accurate estimation comes from an autopsy study done in San Diego. Steatosis was found in 9.6% of children between 2 and 19 years of age and in 38% of obese children autopsied between 1993 and 2003 [95]. Prevalence of NAFLD in obese children in China is estimated to be between 20 and 77% [96]. The latest theory on pathogenesis of NAFLD is a 'multi-hit' one where there is an interplay of numerous factors like hepatic fat accumulation, insulin resistance, oxidative stress due to genetic and epigenetic factors, unfavourable lifestyles, gut microbiota, gut-liver axis dysfunction, and trace element deficiency and fluctuations [97, 98]. The best predictors for NASH in obese individuals with no evidence of other liver disease are elevations of AST or ALT to >200 IU/L, or any elevation of AST (>46 IU/L) and ALT (>35 IU/L) for greater than 6 months. These criteria identified 100% cases of NASH in a small study [99]. If detected early, hepatic steatosis is reversible. Weight loss is the most effective treatment. A 10% reduction in weight can normalise AST, ALT values and decrease ultrasound evidence of fatty liver on 30 months follow-up [100]. Compliance to weight loss and lifestyle changes is poor, especially in children. A number of medical and surgical therapies are emerging. Medical approaches include micronutrient supplementation (Vit E, Vit D, PUFAs, choline), probiotics, anti-obesity medication, metformin, cysteamine, antioxidants, obeticholic acid, growth hormone, lipid-lowering agents and hormones like adiponectin, resistin and TNF alpha. Surgical approach is mainly bariatric surgery [93]. These therapeutic measures could serve as boosters for the weight loss and lifestyle programmes which are difficult to sustain on their own.

5.8 Other disorders

5.8.1 Endocrine

Adipocytes secrete hormones which have paracrine and exocrine actions. The common abnormalities noted include increased production of steroid hormones, decreased progesterone secretion in females and decreased testosterone secretion in males. There is also a strong association between obesity and occurrence of polycystic ovarian syndrome. A study from Bombay looked at the prevalence of PCOS among 600 girls in the age group of 15–19 years from under privileged backgrounds. The prevalence of PCOS by Rotterdam criteria was 22.5%. PCOS was more common in obese than non-obese girls ($p = 0.002$) [101]. In comparison to Caucasians, Asian girls develop PCOS at an earlier age, are more symptomatic and have more fasting hyperinsulinemia and lower insulin sensitivity [102].

5.8.2 Orthopaedic

The most serious orthopaedic disability associated with childhood obesity is slipped capital epiphysis of the femur. Blount disease is another disorder that has a strong association. About 50–80% of children with Blount disease are obese. Minor problems like flat feet, knock knees and frequent ankle sprains are also more common [83].

5.8.3 Psychosocial

Obesity is described as 'one of the most stigmatising and least socially acceptable conditions of childhood'. [103]. Not surprisingly, low self-esteem and poor body image adversely impacting scholastic performance are common in obese children. They are bullied and excluded from group activities, especially sports and games, because they are slower and less agile. They get marginalised and withdraw from society. This makes them more sedentary and also predisposes them to eating disorders which further worsen their obesity [104].

6. Interventions to tackle obesity in school children

The plateauing of BMI of children and adolescents in high-income countries may be due specific initiatives by governments, community groups, schools and individuals and increased public awareness about the hazards of childhood obesity. Findings from the i3C study identified obesity, hypertension and dyslipidaemia as the three key modifiable factors in childhood that result in high cIMT in adulthood. All can be addressed effectively by lifestyle modification and medication. Obesity is easily apparent but difficult to treat on a sustained basis due to a variety of reasons. Hypertension and dyslipidaemia are more difficult to identify due to confusing cut-offs and multiple guidelines. Lifestyle modification is easy to suggest but difficult to implement. Care-givers and parents lack sufficient knowledge about dietary modifications and exercise programmes to advise children. Depression, low self-esteem, lack of peer and parental support and rebellious nature of adolescents make implementation of lifestyle changes difficult. Thus, a multi-modal approach to childhood obesity is required. Even modest loss of weight can lead to significant reduction in TG levels and increase in HDL-C levels. Even without weight loss, regular exercise training can have the same effect on serum lipids [105].

The WHO has included tackling childhood obesity as one of its priority areas. It has suggested a three-pronged strategy: reducing the risk of obesity by addressing critical elements in the life course, tackling obesogenic environment and norms and lastly treating obese children to improve their current and future health.

There is enough evidence to support the fact that undernutrition during pregnancy, excessive weight gain during pregnancy, hyperglycaemia during pregnancy and smoking and exposure to other toxins increase the risk of obesity in the child during infancy and childhood. Even obesity in fathers can increase risk of obesity in the child through epigenetic factors. Ensuring good health during pregnancy and a safe delivery are both important for the child's health. The WHO guidelines include dietary advice to prospective parents before conception and during pregnancy, avoidance of smoking, alcohol and other toxins. Early detection of gestational diabetes and hypertension, monitoring and managing gestational weight gain are other important measures suggested. Ensuring that the baby is exclusively breast-fed during the first 6 months of life and that breast feeding is continued even after complementary feeding is started are important to prevent malnutrition and deposition of excess fat in the baby. The magnitude of the gap between policy and implementation can be gauged from the Indian NFHS 2015–2016 data which show that despite recommendations for exclusive breast feeding up to an age of 6 months, only 55% of Indian infants were actually exclusively breast-fed. Many children in this age group were given other foods like plain water (18%), other milk (11%) and complementary foods (10%). Breast feeding can be encouraged by educational programmes for pregnant women, legislation and regulations to provide feeding rooms and time for breast feeding in work places, and by giving new mothers maternity leave. Nations should implement the International Code of Marketing of Breast-milk Substitutes and other World Health Assembly resolutions to promote breast feeding. During infancy and childhood, parents and care-givers should be given guidance and support to encourage consumption of a variety of healthy foods, avoidance of sugar-sweetened milks and juices and energy-dense nutrient-poor foods. Enforcing regulations on marketing of complementary foods and beverages and subsidising healthy foods are other measures [5, 12].

Further, there should be government regulations on the types of foods and beverages that can be served in school meals. Provision of safe potable drinking water in schools is another basic requirement. Teaching children and parents about healthy eating and having an active lifestyle should be an integral part of school curriculum at all stages. Cookery class in schools is another way of teaching both children and parents about healthy food options. Making time in school schedules for play-time, encouraging sports by providing space and facilities both at schools and in communities will enable children to be physically active. A mandatory physical education programme is another good option. The government's role also includes enforcing ban of sale of HFSS foods and sweetened drinks in schools and around school premises.

Regular health check-ups and growth monitoring should also be an integral part of school life. Children who are overweight or obese should have easy access to treatment including psychotherapy, medications for hypertension, diabetes and dyslipidaemia and even bariatric surgery in extreme cases. Treatment of children should include parents or care-givers. This will provide the much needed emotional and psychological support these children will require to lose weight and change their lifestyles. Multi-specialty teams are required for a successful child-health programme. Successful programmes to tackle childhood obesity usually involve parents, teachers, community members, non-governmental organisations and private players. Some of the more successful international programmes are listed below:

1. Focus on school health education and changing lifestyle:

    a. Project Healthy Schools: This is a project set up by University of Michigan in collaboration with middle schools, community organisations and donors. It aims to educate and encourage children to eat healthy and lead healthy lives. The programme comprises of 10 health education activity modules that focus on eating more fruits and vegetables, consuming less sweetened drinks and sugary foods, eating slowly and eating less fatty food, being more active every day and spending less time in front of the screen [106].

2. Promoting better dietary choices:

    a. Pick a tick initiative: This was started in 1989 by the Australian National Heart Foundation. Healthy food packets could be distinguished from others by presence of a symbol along with the nutrition panel. Apart from helping people select healthy foods, the programme also championed vigorously against excessive salt intake [107].

b. Ensemble-prévenons-l'obésité-des-enfants (EPODE): This literally translates as: 'Together Let's Prevent Childhood Obesity'. This was a community initiative in which intervention were done in 10 French towns in France for children aged 5–12 who were overweight or at risk of weight gain. The approach was 'positive, concrete and stepwise' learning process with no stigmatisation of any culture, food habits, overweight and obesity. It targeted sales of healthy foods in schools, advertisements with respect to food and drinks on TV, internet and schools, mandatory nutritional information on nutrition label, subsidy on healthy foods through agricultural reforms and training for health professionals so that they were able to recognise and diagnose obesity risks in infancy, childhood and adolescence [108].

c. Healthy weight, Healthy lives: An initiative in England to tackle childhood obesity and hence later reduce obesity in adults. It was launched by the government in 2008. The various initiatives in this programme were promoting healthy growth and development of children, promoting healthier food choices, encouraging a more active lifestyle, incentivising good health and offering personalised help and support [109].

3. Promoting a more active lifestyle:

a. US White House Task Force on childhood obesity: This task force gave support to parents, adherence to limits on screen time and quality child care settings with nutritious food and ample opportunity for young children to be physically active. It also emphasised labels on food so that parents can make healthy food choices, improved school environment and lowered price of healthy foods. It improved access to safe parks, playgrounds and indoor and outdoor recreational facilities for children.

b. Tri-Policy initiative: This was done in Canada by creating a supportive environment to increase physical activity in children, early action to detect risk of overweight and obesity and promote availability and accessibility of nutritious foods and decrease the marketing of foods and beverages high in fat, sugar and/or sodium to children.

4. Government policy initiatives

a. New South Wales initiative in Australia: It focused on restoring the energy balance for the population, with a specific focus on children, young people, and their families by reducing the factors that give rise to an 'obesogenic' environment. It emphasised coordination between governments initiatives to tackle obesity along with industry and non-profit organisations.

b. Regulations regarding food advertisements: Brazil prohibits advertisements which are intended to influence children or adolescents to consume HFSS foods. Ireland has strictly banned using celebrities, icons and personalities to promote food products which target children. Norway prevents food advertisements on channels for children under 18 and South TV permits advertising for specific food categories only before, during and after programmes shown between 5 and 7 pm.

6.1 Actions taken in India to reduce childhood obesity in school children

Food Safety and Standards Authority of India (FSSAI) proposed a ban on sale of HFSS foods in school canteens in 2016. It also suggested categorisation of food items as 'green' or healthy foods constituting 80% of the food items, 'red' or common HFSS foods that should not be made available in schools; and 'yellow' category foods that should be eaten sparingly and could be made available in small portions and less frequently. In response to this, Maharashtra state government issued a notification instructing schools to stop serving HFSS food in their canteens. However, the same has not been implemented in other states. The Central Board of Secondary Education (CBSE) has also issued an advisory to all its affiliated schools to ensure that no HFSS food items are available in school canteens and within 20 m of their premises.

Ministry of Health and Family Welfare launched the School Health Programme in 2008 under the National Rural Health Mission (NRHM). The programme also aims to address physical and mental health needs of the children through nutritional interventions, yoga and counselling.

Food Safety and Standards Act, 2006 has provisions to prohibit advertisements that are misleading. These are monitored by the Advertisement Standards Council of India (ASCI). However, the advisories on misleading advertisements are not being strictly implemented. Kaushal et al. reported that the prevalence of misleading advertisements is about 60% [110]. A majority (90%) of these were for HFSS foods. The common methods of non-compliance included promotion of a food item with free gifts (57%), using celebrity endorsement on the food packaging (19%), making false claims (14%) and appealing with cartoons (10%). Apart from restrictions on food advertisements, we also need to strengthen nutrition labelling laws, and educate both parents and children about interpreting nutrient labelling. In India, food packages already have a labelling for vegetarian and non-vegetarian products. HFSS could also be labelled using colour codes as suggested above.

Family and parental guidance play an important role in preventing children from becoming obese. Family involvement can be pivotal in increasing physical activity, healthy eating patterns and decreasing sedentary time. Educating families and stakeholders about healthy eating pattern will help in cutting down on junk food in home and school, and increase healthy eating, thereby decreasing the risk of developing obesity.

Community level programs like CHETNA (Childrens' Health Education Through Nutrition and Health Awareness) and MARG (Medical education for children/adolescents for realistic prevention of obesity and diabetes and for healthy living) are a beginning. These programmes focus on building nutritional awareness and promoting increased physical activity, through pamphlets, lectures skits and group activities targeting both parents and children. They now cover 500,000 children in 15 towns/cities in North India [15]. Since children spend a significant amount of their day in schools, activities involving their peers in schools are smart ways of getting them interested. The government has recently introduced fitness test for all school children and compulsory physical activity during school hours. A 'Fit India' campaign has been announced by the prime-minister and a number of sports and film celebrities are part of the campaign. But much more needs to be done.

7. Conclusion

Obesity in Indian school children is a cause of concern. To tackle this menace, a sustained multi-pronged approach is required, where all stake holders join hands.

The strategy starts at the pre-conception time, continues during pregnancy, infancy and childhood. Apart from promoting healthy eating and an active lifestyle, it also includes active case finding among overweight and obese children and aggressive management of diabetes, hypertension and dyslipidaemia apart from weight loss. Legislations targeting infant feeds, HFSS, artificially sweetened soft drinks, nutrient labelling and food advertisements are important. Government have to be serious about implementing these legislations and they should also formulate imaginative programmes to target childhood nutrition and lifestyle.

Author details

Vangal Krishnaswamy Sashindran[1*] and Puja Dudeja[2]

1 Principal Medical Officer, HQ Central Air Command, Prayagraj, India

2 Colonel (Pensions), Office of Director General Armed Forces, New Delhi, India

*Address all correspondence to: vksashindran@gmail.com

References

[1] Ogden CL, Carroll MD, Curtin LR, Lamb MM, Flegal KM. Prevalence of high body mass index in US children and adolescents, 2007-2008. JAMA. 2010;**303**:242-249

[2] Ranjani H, Mehreen TS, Pradeepa R, Anjana RM, Garg R, Anand K, et al. Epidemiology of childhood overweight & obesity in India: A systematic review. The Indian Journal of Medical Research. 2016;**143**(2):160

[3] NCD Risk Factor Collaboration (NCD-RisC). Worldwide trends in body-mass index, underweight, overweight, and obesity from 1975 to 2016: A pooled analysis of 2416 population-based measurements studies in 128.9 million children, adolescents, and adults. The Lancet. 2017;**390**:2627-2642

[4] Report of the Commission on ending childhood obesity. World Health Organization, Geneva. 2016

[5] The GBD. Obesity collaborators. Health effects of overweight and obesity in 195 countries over 25 years. The New England Journal of Medicine. 2015, 2017;**377**:13-27

[6] NCD Risk Factor Collaboration (NCD-Ris C). Worldwide trends in body-mass index, underweight, overweight, and obesity from 1975 to 2016: A pooled analysis of 2416 population-based measurement studies in 128·9 million children, adolescents, and adults. Lancet. 2017;**390**:2627-2642

[7] World Health Organisation, World Obesity Federation (2018). Taking Action on Childhood Obesity WHO

[8] Taveras EM, Gillman MW, Kleinman K, Rich-Edwards JW, Rifas-Shiman SL. Racial/ethnic differences in early-life risk factors for childhood obesity. Pediatrics. 2010;**125**:686-695

[9] Pengpid S, Peltzer K. Overweight, obesity and associated factors among 13-15 years old students in the Association of South-East Nations member countries, 2007-2014. The Southeast Asian Journal of Tropical Medicine and Public Health. 2016;**47**(2):250-262

[10] Peltzer K, Pengpid S. Leisure time physical inactivity and sedentary behaviour and lifestyle correlates among students aged 13-15 in the association of Southeast Asian nations (ASEAN) member states, 2007-2013. International Journal of Environmental Research and Public Health. 2016;**13**(2):217

[11] Pengpid S, Peltzer K. Overweight and obesity and associated factors among school-aged adolescents in six Pacific island countries in Oceania. International Journal of Environmental Research and Public Health. 2015;**12**:14505-14518. DOI: 10.3390/ijerph12114505

[12] National Family Health Survey-4(2015-16). International Institute of Population Sciences. Mumbai

[13] Gupta DK, Shah P, Misra A, Bharadwaj S, Gulati S, Gupta N, et al. Secular trends in prevalence of overweight and obesity from 2006 to 2009 in urban asian Indian adolescents aged 14-17 years. PLoS One. 2011;**6**(2):e17221

[14] Lobstein T, Jackson-Leach R. Planning for the worst: Estimates of obesity and comorbidities in school-age children in 2025. Pediatric Obesity. 2016;**11**(5):321-325

[15] Bharadwaj S, Misra A, Khurana L, Gulati S, Shah P, Vikram NK. Childhood

obesity in Asian Indians: A burgeoning cause of insulin resistance, diabetes and sub-clinical inflammation. Asia Pacific Journal of Clinical Nutrition. 2008;**17**(S1):172-175

[16] Gautam S, Jeong H. Childhood obesity and its associated factors among school children in Udipi, Karnataka, India. Journal of Lifestyle Medicine. 2019;**9**(1):27-35

[17] Bharati DR, Deshmukh PR, Garg BS. Correlates of overweight and obesity among school going children of Wardha city, Central India. The Indian Journal of Medical Research. 2008;**127**:539-543

[18] Gamit SS, Moitra M, Verma MR. Prevalence of obesity and overweight in school going adolescents of Surat city, Gujarat, India. International Journal of Medical Science and Public Health. 2015;**4**(1):42-47

[19] Yadav KS, Yadav MB, Yadav C. Prevalence of overweight, obesity and hypertension among school going children in district Kanpur, Uttar Pradesh, India: A longitudinal study. International Journal of Contemporary Pediatrics. 2019;**6**(1):159-162

[20] Gupta N, Goel K, Shah P, Misra A. Childhood obesity in developing countries: Epidemiology, determinants, and prevention. Endocrine Reviews. 2012;**33**(1):48-70

[21] Khadilkar VV, Khadilkar AV. Revised Indian academy of pediatrics 2015 growth charts for height, weight and body mass index for 5-18-year-old Indian children. Indian Journal of Endocrinology and Metabolism. 2015;**19**(4):470

[22] Pillai RN. Modelling Studies for a 'Whole of Society (wos)' Framework to Monitor Cardio-Metabolic Risk Among Children (6 to 18 years). Ph.D. Dissertation. Universita' Degli Studi Di Verona. 2018. Available from: http://www.inclentrust.org/inclen/wp-content/uploads/6_D2_Rakesh-Pillai_Thesis_03_Mar_18.pdf [Accessed: 10 June 2019]

[23] Anderson PM, Butcher KE. Childhood obesity: Trends and potential causes. The Future of Children. 2006;**16**:19-45

[24] Ng M, Fleming T, Robinson M, Thomson B, Graetz N, Margono C, et al. Global, regional, and national prevalence of overweight and obesity in children and adults during 1980-2013: A systematic analysis for the global burden of disease study 2013. Lancet. 2014;**384**:766-781

[25] Ramachandran A, Snehalatha C, Vinitha R, Thayyil M, Kumar CK, Sheeba L, et al. Prevalence of overweight in urban Indian adolescent school children. Diabetes Research and Clinical Practice. 2002;**57**(3):185-190

[26] Rao S, Kanade A, Kelkar R. Blood pressure among overweight adolescents from urban school children in Pune, India. European Journal of Clinical Nutrition. 2007;**61**:633-641

[27] Kapil U, Pathak P, Singh P, Dwivedi SN, Bhasin S. Prevalence of obesity among affluent adolescent school children in Delhi. Indian Pediatrics. 2002;**39**(5):449-452

[28] Chhatwal J, Vema M, Riar SK. Obesity among pre-adolescent and adolescents of a developing country (India). Asia Pacific Journal of Clinical Nutrition. 2004;**13**(3):231-235

[29] Whitaker RC, Wright JA, Pepe MS, Seidel KD, Dietz WH. Predicting obesity in young adulthood from childhood and parental obesity. The New England Journal of Medicine. 1997;**337**(13):869-873

[30] Ogden CL, Flegal KM, Carroll MD, Johnson CL. Prevalence and trends

in overweight among US children and adolescents 1999-2000. JAMA. 2002;**288**:1728-1732

[31] Gulati S, Misra A, Colles SL, Kondal D, Gupta N, Goel K, et al. Dietary intakes and familial correlates of overweight/obesity: A four-cities study in India. Annals of Nutrition and Metabolism. 2013;**62**(4):279-290. [PubMed: 23689065]

[32] Center for Disease Control and Prevention. Contributing Factors. 2010. Available from: http://www.cdc.gov//obesity/childhood/contributing_factors.html. [Accessed: 01 July 2014]

[33] Chapman G, Maclean H. "Junk food" and "healthy food": Meanings of food in adolescent women's culture. Journal of Nutrition Education and Behavior. 1993;**25**:108-113

[34] Vucetic Z, Reyes TM. Central dopaminergic circuitry controlling food intake and reward: Implications for the regulation of obesity. Wiley Interdisciplinary Reviews: Systems Biology and Medicine. 2010;**2**:577-594

[35] Stice E, Yoket S, Bohon C, Martin N, Stolen A. Reward circuitry responsively to food predicts future increases in body ass: Moderating effects of DRD2 and DRD4. NeuroImage. 2010;**50**(4):1618-1625

[36] Stice E, Spoor S, Ng J, Zald DH. Relation of obesity to consummatory and anticipatory food reward. Physiology & Behaviour. 2009;**97**(5):551-560

[37] Bosch LSMM, Wells JCK, Lum S, Reid AM. Associations of extracurricular physical activity patterns and body composition components in multi-ethnic population of UK children(the size and lung function in children study): A multi-level modelling analysis. BMC Public Health. 2019;**19**:573

[38] Kunwar R, Minhas S, Mangla V. Is obesity a problem among school children? Indian Journal of Public Health. 2018;**62**:153-155

[39] Govindan M, Gurm R, Mohan S, et al. Gender differences in physiologic markers and health behaviors associated with childhood obesity. Pediatrics. 2013;**132**:468-474

[40] National Institutes of Health; US National Library of Medicine. Screen Time and Children. Available at: https://medlineplus.gov/ency/patientinstructions/000355.htm [Accessed: 22 June 2016]

[41] Vuong B, Rogers R, Corriveau N, et al. Passive screen time associated with unhealthy dietary consumption and physiological characteristics: A closer look at childhood behaviors. Journal of the American College of Cardiology. 2014;**63**:A1292

[42] Story M, Neumark-stainzer D, French S. Individual and environmental influences on adolescent eating behaviours. Journal of the American Dietetic Association. 2002;**102**:S40-S51. [PubMed: 11902388]

[43] Britz B, Siegfried W, Ziegler A, Lamertz C, Herpertz-Dahlmann BM, Remschmidt H, et al. Rates of psychiatric disorders in a clinical study group of adolescents with extreme obesity and in obese adolescents ascertained via a population based study. International Journal of Obesity and Related Metabolic Disorders. 2000;**24**:1707-1714. [PubMed: 11126229]

[44] Rawana JS, Morgan AS, Nguyen H, Craig SG. The relation between eating- and weight-related disturbances and depression in adolescence: A review. Clinical Child and Family Psychology Review. 2010;**13**:213-230.[PubMed: 20632207]

[45] Ravelli GP, Stein ZA, Susser MW. Obesity in young men after famine exposure in utero and early infancy. The New England Journal of Medicine. 1976;**295**:349-353

[46] Bateson P, Gluckman P, Hanson M. The biology of developmental plasticity and the predictive adaptive response hypothesis. Journal of Physiology. 2014;**592**(11):2357-2368. [PubMed: 24882817]

[47] Yajnik CS. Obesity epidemic in India: Intrauterine origins? Proceedings of the Nutrition Society. 2004;**63**:387-396

[48] Kuriyan R, Rodgers N, Thomas T, Aravind J, Subramanian SV, Kurpad AV. The role of familial and sibling factors on abdominal adiposity: A study of south Indian urban children. Asia Pacific Journal of Clinical Nutrition. 2018;**27**(4):869-874

[49] Gupta S, Kapoor S. Gender differences in familial aggregation of adiposity traits in Aggarwal Baniya families. Eurasian Journal of Anthropology. 2011;**2**(2):85-95

[50] Raskind IG, Patil's SS, Haardorfer R, Cunningham SA. Unhealthy weight in Indian families: The role of the family environment in the context of the nutrition transition. Population Research and Policy Review. 2018;**37**(2):157-180

[51] Sahoo K, Sahoo B, Choudhury AK, Sofi NY, Kumar R, Bhadoria AS. Childhood obesity: Causes and consequences. Journal of Family Medicine and Primary Care. 2015;**4**(2):187-192

[52] Moens E, Braet C, Bosmans G, Rosseel Y. Unfavourable family characteristics and their associations with childhood obesity: A cross-sectional study. European Eating Disorders Review. 2009;**17**:315-323. [PubMed: 19452495]

[53] Jackson EA, Eagle T, Leidal A, et al. Childhood obesity: A comparison of health habits of middle-school students from two communities. Clinical Epidemiology. 2009;**1**:133-139

[54] Eagle TF, Sheetz A, Gurm R, Woodward AC, Kline-Rogers E, Leibowitz R, et al. Understanding childhood obesity in America: Linkages between household income, community resources, and children's behaviors. American Heart Journal. 2012;**163**:836-843

[55] Kaur S, Sachdev HP, Dwivedi SN, Lakshmy R, Kapil U. Prevalence of overweight and obesity amongst school children in Delhi, India. Asia Pacific Journal of Clinical Nutrition. 2008;**17**(4):592-596

[56] Yajnik CS, Lubree HG, Rege SS, Naik SS, Deshpande JA, Deshpande SS, et al. Adiposity and hyperinsulinemia in Indians are present at birth. The Journal of Clinical Endocrinology and Metabolism. 2002;**87**:5575-5580

[57] Kuriyan R, Thomas T, Lokesh DP, Sheth NR, Mahendra A, Joy R, et al. Waist circumference and waist for height percentiles in urban south Indian children aged 3-16 years. Indian Pediatrics. 2011;**48**:765-771

[58] Misra A, Vikram NK, Arya S, Pandey RM, Dhingra V, Chatterjee A, et al. High prevalence of insulin resistance in post-pubertal Asian Indian children is associated with adverse truncal body fat patterning, abdominal adiposity and excess body fat. International Journal of Obesity and Related Metabolic Disorders. 2004;**28**:1217-1226

[59] World Health Organization, Department of Non-Communicable Disease Surveillance. Definition,

Diagnosis and Classification of Diabetes Mellitus and its Complications. Report of a WHO Consultation. Part 1: Diagnosis and Classification of Diabetes Mellitus. Geneva: World Health Organization. 1999

[60] Gupta A, Sachdeva A, Mahajan N, Gupta A, Sareen N, Pandey RM, et al. Prevalence of paediatric metabolic syndrome and associated risk factors among school-age children of 10-16 years living in district Shimla, Himachal Pradesh, India. Indian Journal of Endocrinology and Metabolism. 2018;**22**(3):373-378

[61] Singh R, Bhansali A, Sialy R, Aggarwal A. Prevalence of metabolic syndrome in adolescents from a north Indian population. Diabetic Medicine. 2007;**24**(2):195-199

[62] Kitagawa T, Owada M, Urakami T, et al. Increased incidence of non-insulin dependent diabetes mellitus among Japanese schoolchildren correlates with an increased intake of animal protein and fat. Clinical Pediatrics (Phila). 1998;**37**:111-115

[63] Ehtisham S, Hattersley AT, Dunger DB, Barrett TG. First UK survey of paediatric type 2 diabetes and MODY. Archives of Disease in Childhood. 2004;**89**:526-529

[64] Ripamonti G, De Medici C, Guzzaloni G, Morn G, Ardizzi A, Morabito F. Impaired glucose tolerance in obesity in children and adolescents. Journal of Physiology and Biochemistry. 2003;**59**:217-223

[65] Wabitsch M, Hauner H, Hertramf M, Muche R, Hay B, et al. Type II diabetes mellitus and impaired glucose regulation in Caucasian children and adolescents with obesity living in Germany. International Journal of Obesity and Related Metabolic Disorders. 2004;**28**:307-313

[66] Bhatia V, National Task Force IAP. Childhood prevention of adult diseases: Insulin resistance and type 2 diabetes mellitus in childhood. Indian Pediatrics. 2004;**41**:443-457

[67] Abate N. Insulin resistance and obesity. The role of fat distribution. Diabetes Care. 1996;**19**:292-294

[68] Lundgren H. Adiposity and adipose tissue distribution in relation to incidence of diabetes in women. Results from prospective population study in Gothenburg, Sweden. International Journal of Obesity. 1989;**13**:413-423

[69] Skinner AC, Perrin EM, Moss LA, Skelton JA. Cardiometabolic risks and severity of obesity in children and young adults. The New England Journal of Medicine. 2015;**373**:1307-1317

[70] Centers for Disease Control and Prevention. Prevalence of abnormal lipid levels among youths --- United States, 1999-2006. MMWR. Morbidity and Mortality Weekly Report. 2010;**59**:29-33

[71] Anderson KM, Wilson PW, Garrison RJ, Castelli WP. Longitudinal and secular trends in lipoprotein cholesterol measurements in general population sample. The Framingham offspring study. Atherosclerosis. 1987;**68**:59-66

[72] Guida F, Guzzaloni G, Moreni G, Morabito F. Lipid profile, adiposity in children and adolescents. Minerva Pediatrica. 1989;**41**:449-458

[73] Morrison JA, Glueck CJ, Woo JG, Wang P. Risk factors for cardiovascular disease and type 2 diabetes retained from childhood to adulthood predict adult outcomes: The Princeton LRC follow up study. International Journal of Pediatric Endocrinology. 2012;**2012**(1):6-14

[74] Falkner B, Gidding SS, Ramirez-Garnica G, Wiltrout SA, West D, Rappaport EB. The relationship of body mass index and blood pressure in primary care pediatric patients. The Journal of Pediatrics. 2006;**148**(2):195-200 PMID:16492428

[75] Perng W, Rifas-Shiman SL, Kramer MS, et al. Early weight gain, linear growth, and mid-childhood blood pressure: A prospective study in project viva. Hypertension. 2016;**67**(2):301-308 PMID:26644238

[76] Parker ED, Sinaiko AR, Kharbanda EO, et al. Change in weight status and development of hypertension. Pediatrics. 2016;**137**(3):e20151662 PMID:26908707

[77] Flynn JT, Kaelber DC, Baker-Smith CM, Blowey D, Carroll AE, Daniels SR, et al. Clinical practice guideline for screening and management of high blood pressure in children and adolescents. Pediatrics. 2017;**140**:e20171904

[78] Vedavathy S. Sangamesh. Prevalence of hypertension in urban school going adolescents of Bangalore, India. International Journal of Contemporary Pediatrics. 2016 May;**3**(2):416-423

[79] Laroia D, Sharma M, Dwivedi V. Profile of blood pressure in normal school children. Indian Pediatrics. 1989;**26**:531-536

[80] Gupta AK, Ahmed AJ. Childhood obesity and hypertension. Indian Pediatrics. 1991;**28**:810-816

[81] Anand NK, Tandon L. Prevalence of hypertension in children. Indian Pediatrics. 1994;**49**:1065-1069

[82] Feld LG, Springale JE, Was WR. Special topics in pediatric hypertension. Seminars in Nephrology. 1998;**18**:295-303

[83] Kaur S, Kapil U, Singh P. Pattern of chronic diseases amongst adolescent obese children in developing countries. Current Science. 2005;**88**(7):1052-1056

[84] Bibbins-Domingo K, Coxson P, Pletcher MJ, Lightwood J, Goldman L. Adolescent overweight and future adult coronary heart disease. The New England Journal of Medicine. 2007;**357**:2371-2379

[85] Juonala M, Viikari JS, Ronnemaa T, Marniemi J, Jula A, Loo BM, et al. Associations of dyslipidemias from childhood to adulthood with carotid intima-media thickness, elasticity, and brachial flow-mediated dilatation in adulthood: The cardiovascular risk in young Finns study. Arteriosclerosis, Thrombosis, and Vascular Biology. 2008;**28**(5):1012-1017

[86] Koskinen J, Juonala M, Dwyer T, Venn A, Thomson R, Bazzano L, et al. Impact of lipid measurements in youth in addition to conventional clinic-based risk factors on predicting preclinical athero- sclerosis in adulthood: International childhood cardiovascular cohort consortium. Circulation. 2018;**137**:1246-1255. DOI: 10.1161/CIRCULATIONAHA.117.029726

[87] Sorof JM, Alexandrov AV, Cardwell G, Portman RJ. Carotid artery intimal- medial thickness and left ventricular hypertrophy in children with elevated blood pressure. Pediatrics. 2003;**111**:61-66

[88] Barasa A, Schaufelberger M, Lappas G, Swedberg K, Dellborg M, Rosengren A. Heart failure in young adults: 20-year trends in hospitalization, aetiology, and case fatality in Sweden. European Heart Journal. 2014;**35**:25-32

[89] Sultan S, Elkind MS. The growing problem of stroke among young adults. Current Cardiology Reports. 2013;**15**:421

[90] Vivante A, Golan E, Tzur D, Leiba A, Tirosh A, Skorecki K, et al. Body mass index in 1.2 million adolescents and risk for end-stage renal disease. Archives of Internal Medicine. 2012;**172**:1644-1650

[91] Mullee A, Romaguera D, Pearson-Stuttard J, Viallon V, Stephen M, et al. Association between soft drink consumption and mortality in 10 European countries. JAMA Internal Medicine. 2019;**03**:E1-E12. DOI: 10.1001/jamainternmed.2019.2478

[92] Arya S, Isharwal S, Misra A, Pandey RM, Rastogi K, Vikram NK, et al. C-reactive protein and dietary nutrients in urban Asian Indian adolescents and young adults. Nutrition. 2006;**22**:865-871

[93] Clemente MG, Mandato C, Poeta M, Vajro P. Pediatric non-alcoholic fatty liver disease: Recent solutions, unresolved issues, and future research directions. World Journal of Gastroenterology. 2016;**22**(36):8078-8093

[94] Mathur P, Das MK, Arora NK. Non-alcoholic fatty liver disease and childhood obesity. Indian Journal of Pediatrics. 2007;**74**(4):401-407

[95] Schwimmer JB, Deutsch R, Kahen T, Lavine JE, Stanley C, Behling C. Prevalence of fatty liver in children and adolescents. Pediatrics. 2006;**118**:1388-1393

[96] Chan DF, Li AM, Chu WC, Chan MH, Wong EM, Liu EK, et al. Hepatic steatosis in obese Chinese children. International Journal of Obesity and Related Metabolic Disorders. 2004;**28**:1257-1263

[97] Berardis S, Sokal E. Pediatric non-alcoholic fatty liver disease: An increasing public health issue. European Journal of Pediatrics. 2014;**173**:131-139 [PMID: 24068459]. DOI: 10.1007/s00431-013-2157-6

[98] Goyal NP, Schwimmer JB, et al. Clinics in Liver Disease. 2016;**20**:325-338 [PMID: 27063272]. DOI: 10.1016/j.cld.2015.10.003

[99] Lerret SM, Garcia-Rodriguez L, Skelton J, Biank V, Kilway D, Telega G. Predictors of non-alcoholic steatohepatitis in obese children. Gastroenterology Nursing. 2011;**34**(6):434-437

[100] Vajro P, Fontanella A, Perna C, Orso G, Tedescom VAD. Persistent hyperaminotransferasemia resolving after weight reduction in obese children. The Journal of Pediatrics. 1994;**125**:239-241

[101] Joshi B, Mukherjee S, Patil A, Purandare A, Chauhan S. Vaidya R.a cross-sectional study of polycystic ovarian syndrome among young adolescent and young girls in Mumbai, India. Indian Journal of Endocrinology and Metabolism. 2014;**18**(3):317-324

[102] Wijeyaratne CN, Balen AH, Barth JH, Belchetz PE. Clinical manifestations and insulin resistance (IR) in polycystic ovary syndrome (PCOS) among south Asians and Caucasians: Is there a difference? Clinical Endocrinology. 2002;**57**:343-350

[103] Schwimmer JB, Burwinkle TM, Varni JW. Health-related quality of life of severely obese children and adolescents. JAMA. 2003;**289**:1813-1819

[104] Budd GM, Hayman LL. Addressing the childhood obesity crisis. The American Journal of Maternal Child Nursing. 2008;**33**:113-117. [PubMed: 18327110]

[105] Cook S, Kavey R-EW. Dyslipidemia and pediatric obesity. Pediatric Clinics of North America. 2011;**58**(6):1363-1373

[106] Rogers R, Krallman R, Jackson EA, DuRussel-Weston J, Palma-Davis LV, de Visser R, et al. Top ten lessons learned from project healthy schools. The American Journal of Medicine. 2017;**130**:990.e1-990.e7

[107] Dalton CB. The National Heart Foundation Pick the tick program. The Medical Journal of Australia. 1993;**158**(8):577

[108] Borys JM, Richard P, Ruault du Plessis H, Harper P, Levy E. Tackling health inequalities and reducing obesity prevalence: The EPODE community approach. Annals of Nutrition & Metabolism. 2016;**68**(Suppl 2):35-38. DOI: 10.1159/000446223 Epub 2016 Jun 16

[109] Healthy Weight, Healthy Lives: A Cross-goverment strategy for England. PublicationsPolicyAndGuidance/DH_082378

[110] Kaushal N, Dudeja P. Food advertisements boon or bane: A prevalence study of misleading food advertisements in India. Journal of Childhood Obesity. 2017;**2**(4):17-19

Chapter 16

Innovations in Vector-Borne Disease Control in India

Susanta Kumar Ghosh and Chaitali Ghosh

Abstract

India is the second largest populous and democratic country in the world. Several geo-ecological settings are favorable for most of the vector borne diseases (VBDs) in the country. Malaria, Lymphatic Filariasis (LF), Japanese Encephalitis (JE), Dengue (DEN), Chikungunya (CHIK) and Kala-azar (KA) are major VBDs. Kyasanur Forest Disease (KFD), Plague and Chandipura virus (CHPV) infections have limited and localized foci, but needs attention. Crimean-Congo Hemorrhagic Fever (CCHF) and Zika are recent entries in India that also need to be handled on priority. National Vector Borne Disease Control Program (NVBDCP) is responsible for control and prevention of all these diseases. Malaria, LF, JE, DEN, CHIK and Zika are transmitted by different species of mosquitoes. KA and CHPV are transmitted by shadflies, while KFD, CCHF by ticks; plague by fleas. Scrub typhus (ST) responsible for acute encephalopathy syndrome (AES) is transmitted by *Leptotrombidium* mite species. It needs specific and strategic action plan in view of the diversified biodiversity. New innovations to strengthen the public health responses are the main intervention protocols. Already two diseases Guineaworm (*Dracunculiasis*) transmitted by different species of Cyclops, and polio have been successfully eradicated/eliminated from India. Such experience would be very helpful for the elimination of malaria, LF and KA, and all are on the elimination drive.

Keywords: vector-borne disease, malaria, lymphatic filariasis, Japanese encephalitis, Dengue, Chikungunya, kala-azar, Kyasanur forest disease, plague, Chandupura virus, Crimean-Congo hemorrhagic fever, Zika, elimination, surveillance, India

1. Introduction

India is a republic democratic and second most populous country in the world having a population of over 1.30 billion people in Asian continent entirely in the northern hemisphere. This is a country of great diversified ethnicities, religions, languages, cultures and food habits. One of the oldest civilizations in the world, Indo-Aryans (72%) of North India, Dravidians of South India (25%), Mongoloids (3%) and other minority populations constitute the ethnic groups. Dravidians are the original inhabitants of the country. The Indus Valley Civilization or the Harappan Civilization with a link to the Indo-Aryans migrated to the country at about 1800 BC. With this background, India has been a model country in many aspects. It is bounded by the Great Himalayas in the north, extends southwards covering Tropic of Cancer ultimately meets into the Indian Ocean between the Bay of Bengal on the east (east coast) and the Arabian Sea on the west (west coast). Both the coasts cover the Peninsular India and the Deccan Plateau. The mainland extends between Latitudes 8° 4′ and 37° 6′ North,

Longitudes 68° 7′ and 97° 25′ East and measures about 3214 km from North to South between the extreme Latitudes and about 2933 km from East to West between the extreme Longitudes. It has a land frontier of about 15,200 km. The total length of the coastline of the mainland, Lakshadweep Islands and Andaman & Nicobar Islands is 7516.6 km [1, 2].

There are several vector-borne diseases (VBDs) in India and most of them are transmitted by mosquitoes. These are malaria, LF, JE, DEN, CHIK and Zika. Sandfly-linked diseases are KA and CHPV, while KFD and CCHF by ticks, and ST by mites, while Plague by fleas mostly from rodent hosts. The vectors and the VBD control operations and preventions are implemented by the National Vector Borne Disease Control Program (NVBDCP) and National Centre for disease Control (NCDC) at national level. Many other national institutes under the aegis of Indian Council of Medical Research, Department of Biotechnology and Indian Council of Agricultural Research additionally support the program by doing research on these diseases. The research findings help in implementing the control of all VBDs. The respective state health departments implement the program following the guidelines provided by the NVBDCP. At present malaria, LF and KA are in the process of elimination; malaria by 2030 and the latter two diseases by 2020. A detailed action plan and proper implementation protocols are needed for achieving the goals.

2. Search methods

Searched MEDLINE (PubMed); CABS Abstracts; checked the reference lists of all studies identified by the search. Also performed Google Search on specific topics. Examined references listed in review articles and previously compiled bibliographies.

3. Mosquito-borne diseases

Mosquitoes are small flying insects that constitute the maximum species in the taxon of animal kingdom. They are considered as the deadliest animals in the world. As per the recent report, there are 3541 recorded number of mosquito species in the world distributed in 2 sub-families, 11 Tribes and 11 Genera. In India 404 species (11.4%), 50 Genera (44.6%) and 63 *Anopheles* species (13%) are recorded [3]. Several mosquito species are responsible for transmission of human diseases. In this chapter details of VBDs in India are discussed.

3.1 Malaria

Among all VBDs in India, malaria contributes the lion's share. India has contributed substantially on malaria research and strategies for its control, and is a signatory to the National Framework for Malaria Elimination (NFME) with an aim to eliminate this disease by 2030. Detailed information on malaria and its elimination process have been described earlier [4, 5]. Some recent information will be shared in this communication.

3.2 Lymphatic Filariasis

After malaria, human LF is the second most mosquito-borne disease in India, and among the tropical diseases, this disease stands after malaria and tuberculosis. LF is caused by the nematode parasites found in the lymphatic system, damage the system leading to deformities of body organs especially elephantiasis and hydrocoel, relentless disability causing social stigma. Globally three parasites *Wuchereria bancrofti*, *Brugia malayi* and *Brugia timori* are responsible for LF. In India *W. bancrofti* is the most predominant species (98%) while *Brugia malayi* (2%) is limited to the coastal belts in Kerala, Goa and also in Gujarat. *Culex quinquefasciatus* is the main vector of *W. bancrofti*, while *Mansonia annulifera* is the main vector species of *B. malayi* transmission [6].

In India, National Filaria Control Program (NFCP) was launched in 1955 with an aim to control the disease following vector control, treatment of filarial cases, and thus making the endemicity delimited. A district level survey in 2000 revealed that of the 289 districts, 257 were endemic for LF [7]. In 2004, elimination of LF program was launched in 255 districts of 16 states and 5 union territories. In the beginning, diethylcarbamazine (DEC) was introduced under the Mass Drug Administration (MDA) program, and in 2006 Albendazole was added with DEC with an aim to eliminate LF by 2015. A review in December 2015 showed that of the 255 districts 222 had reported microfilaria rate 1%, and in 53 districts MDA was withdrawn as halt in transmission was indicated. Transmission Assessment Survey (TAS) was qualified for 68 districts. The remaining districts were struggling to achieve the goal making the MDA twice in a year.

The World Health Organization (WHO) estimated that LF is found in 80 tropical and subtropical countries with 120 million infected cases, and with one billion people at risk, 947 million people are threatened, whereas 40 million people are disfigured by this infection [8]. Four countries India, Indonesia, Bangladesh (all Asian countries) and Nigeria (Africa) contribute about 70% of the LF infection in the world. In 2000, WHO launched Global Program to Eliminate Lymphatic Filariasis (GPELF). In 2012, the WHO neglected tropical diseases roadmap reconfirmed the target date for achieving elimination by 2020. India also reemphasized its commitment for GPELF [8].

In the 10th GPELF meeting in New Delhi, India in June 2018, government of India launched Accelerated Plan for Lymphatic Filariasis Elimination (APELF). A triple drug therapy or IDA (Ivermectin, DEC and Albendazole) along with community engagement and fortified salt with DEC has been planned for accelerating the LF elimination in India [9]. IDA has been rolled out successfully across four districts as a pilot project in India. These districts are Arwal in Bihar (20 December 2018), Simdega in Jharkhand (10 January 2019), Nagpur in Maharashtra (20 January 2019) and Varanasi in Uttar Pradesh (20 February 2019). A total of 8.07 million people out of 10.7 million vulnerable people (75.4%) were benefitted with the IDA medicines. The Government of India has decided to scale up IDA approach in all endemic districts on a 'Mission Mode' approach to eliminate LF by 2021. The APELF provides free morbidity management and disability prevention services through kits and corrective surgeries [10].

3.3 Japanese Encephalitis

Japanese Encephalitis (JE) is one of the mosquito-borne diseases in India that has remained a troublesome for public health professionals. JE is caused by JE virus (JEV) under *Flaviviridae* family primarily infects the brain. The disease is spread by *Culex* mosquitoes. Pigs especially piglets as multiplying host and egret birds are hosts for JEV. This disease was first reported in 1871 and currently prevalent in 24 countries in Southeast Asia and Western Pacific regions which is the rice growing area [11]. About 3 billion people under risk in this region with 68,000 symptomatic cases and 17,000 deaths every year, often appear in huge outbreaks following high mortality [12].

The first human case in India was reported from North Arcot district of Tamil Nadu in 1955. Subsequently it was reported in 1973 from Bankura and Burdwan districts in West Bengal. Currently this disease is present all over the country mostly in the Eastern states. In India *Culex vishnui* subgroup mosquitoes *Cx. tritaeniorhynchus, Cx. vishnui* and *Cx. pseudovishnui,* have been reported as major vectors of JE. Other species like *Cx. gelidus, Cx. epidesmus* have also been implicated in the transmission [13].

Though vector management is the main strategy for the control of JE, but due to many factors this remains to be the secondary option. However, use of long lasting insecticide nets (LLINs) both by humans and in pig sties has been very effective in Assam [14]. In India, the JEV is genotype III. The main containment is the use of SA 14-14-2 Chinese vaccine. But the coverage in endemic areas of Gorakhpur, Uttar Pradesh was very low at 42.3% [15]. The vaccine is covered in children under 15-year age. Now in 20 districts in the states of Assam, West Bengal and Uttar Pradesh, vaccination in adults aged between 15 and 65 has been recommended by NVBDCP since more number of adult JE cases were reported in these states [12]. A new Indian vaccine JENVAC—a single dose inactivated JE Vaccine has been developed. This Vero cell derived vaccine is prepared from an Indian strain (Kolar-821564XY) of the JEV [16].

3.4 Dengue, Chikungunya and Zika

Dengue, Chikungunya and more recently Zika epidemics are spreading throughout the world at a faster pace especially in the Americas. All these diseases are caused by arboviruses. Dengue and Zika are Flavivirus (Family *Flaviviridae*) while Chikungunya is Alphavirus under *Togoviridae* family. These diseases are primarily transmitted by two species of *Aedes* mosquitoes, *Ae. aegypti* and *Ae. albopictus*. Both are invasive and endemic species which can adapt with the local conditions, dispersed by their immaculate mechanism of their desiccation-tolerant eggs. Moreover, all these viral diseases are carried forward through the process of trans-ovarian transmission. This means when a mother mosquito infected with virus are stored in their gonads (reproductive organs), the viruses are carried forward to the next generation. In most situations, these infected eggs when carried with the breeding containers especially through tyres establish in a new area [17, 18].

Currently about 4 billion cases of dengue in more than 128 countries are reported. About 390 estimated cases of dengue are recorded globally. There are 4 serotypes present in dengue virus and a fifth serotype of DENV was detected from Malaysia [19]. In India, epidemics of dengue have been reported from 1990, and all the 4 serotypes are present. In 1780, first epidemiology of dengue was described in Madras (now Chennai), and first outbreak was reported in Calcutta (now Kolkata) in 1963 [20]. Now this disease is reported almost all over India. There is no effective treatment for dengue. Recently one vaccine for dengue has been developed, but it is effective only on seropositive cases. In 2019, Sri Lanka, Philippines and Bangladesh have declared emergency situations in these countries [21–23]. So the situation is very grave and needs immediate solutions.

Chikungunya additionally is causing public health problem in the country. This disease was first reported in Tanzania in 1952-53. From this location it has spread in most of tropical Africa and Asia. In India, a huge outbreak was reemerged in 2006 after its first report in 1973 [24]. Currently this disease is reported almost in every state along with dengue. There is no specific treatment for this disease since it is self-limiting. It is assumed that this disease does not cause mortality in India, but certain report may say otherwise. In Ahmadabad city, there were excess deaths during Chikungunya outbreak in 2006 [18].

Zika is a new disease that rocked the Latin American countries mainly in Brazil in 2015. As of July 2019, a total of 87 countries and territories have had evidence of autochthonous mosquito-borne transmission of Zika virus (ZIKV), distributed across four of the six WHO Regions (African Region, Region of the Americas, South-East Asia Region, and Western Pacific Region) [25]. As such this disease does not cause much clinical emergencies. In certain cases, neurological complications in adults and children with Guillain-Barré syndrome are associated with ZIKV. Its effect on fetuses in pregnant women is a matter of serious concern. The babies are born with microcephaly, preterm birth and miscarriage. In other word babies are born with small heads leading to several abnormalities. Several reports also indicated sexual route of transmission from asymptomatic carriers [26].

In India first report of Zika was reported in September 2018 from a 78 year-old women in Jaipur, Rajasthan. Immediately a rapid response team was formed and detailed investigations were made by the government of India. Massive surveillance all over India was initiated including in all international airports and ports as a part International Health Regulations. Special care was taken on pregnant women especially in the suspected areas. In 2018, 157 Zika cases have been detected, that included 63 pregnant women. All cases were confirmed by RT-PCR method. No cases of microcephaly or congenital Zika syndrome were reported. The government of India has established 34 laboratories for Zika surveillance and diagnosis to strengthen the especially established 'National Zika Action Plan' [27].

Recent news of 'First sexually transmitted dengue case confirmed in Spain' is a much disturbing matter and deep concern. This indicates that viral infections may affect gonad cells [28].

3.5 Sandfly transmitted diseases

3.5.1 Kala-azar

Kala-azar (KA) is considered the most devastating neglected tropical disease caused by the protozoan parasite *Leishmania*. There are over 20 species of *Leishmania* that is transmitted by over 90 species of Sandflies (*Phlebotomus* spp.). Generally, three forms of this disease are reported namely visceral leishmaniasis (VL), cutaneous leishmaniasis (CL) and mucocutaneous leishmaniasis (ML). This infection is mostly prevalent in the poorest people linked to malnutrition, poor living conditions and resources. Annually estimated new cases between 0.7 and 1 million and some 26,000–65,000 related deaths are reported in the world [29].

VL is commonly known as Kala-azar. The clinical cases may turn fatal if not treated in time. An estimated 50,000–90,000 new cases are reported annually, and most cases occur in Bangladesh, Brazil, China, Ethiopia, India, Kenya, Nepal, Somalia, South Sudan and Sudan. Post-Kala-azar dermal leishmaniasis (PKDL) is a complicated form of VL. It is also known as Post-Kala-azar dermatosis characterized by muscular, maculopapular and nodular rash on face, arm and upper part of the trunk. This is mostly found on patients recovered for VL [29].

The most common form of the disease is CL. It causes skin lesions leaving scar marks and stigma. It is estimated that 0.6–1 million new cases are reported from Afghanistan, Algeria, Brazil, Colombia, Islamic Republic of Iran, Iraq and the Syrian Arab Republic [29].

ML is responsible for a partial or total destruction of mucous membranes of the nose, mouth and throat. Over 90% of ML cases occur in Bolivia, Brazil, Ethiopia and Peru [29].

India is endemic for both VL and CL cases. PKDL cases are on the increasing trend. CL caused by *Leishmania major* and *L. tropica* mostly present in north-western states in India mainly in Rajasthan and Punjab. The worst area is Bikaner district of Rajasthan [30].

VL primarily caused by *L. donovani* was endemic in India especially in the eastern Uttar Pradesh, undivided Bihar and West Bengal. In fact, undivided Bengal is considered the oldest KA endemic area in the world. Drastic reduction of cases was reported due to application of DDT during malaria eradication program in the 1960s. In India, government of India initiated KA elimination program in endemic states in 1990–91. Approximately 130 million people in 611 blocks are at risk. Currently drastic reduction of cases is recorded in the elimination phase. Many joint initiatives have been undertaken with potential partners like Bill and Melinda Gates Foundation, KalaCore Consortium and government like institutions ICMR-Rajendra Memorial Research Institute (RMRI) and National Center for Disease Control (NCDC) and WHO to eliminate this disease by 2017. However, this is aimed at 2020 to eliminate this disease. The office of the Prime Minister (PMO) and the health department are monitoring the progress of the work [30].

For elimination of KA a national roadmap has been created and shared to all the states for implementation at village-level. Continuous supply of Liposomal Amphotericin B (AmBisome) injection has been ensured since single day single dose has improved treatment compliance. Regular supply of rapid diagnostic test kit is also ensured. Government of India will compensate INR 500 for KA and INR 2000 for PKDL cases as loss of wages. Besides this, INR 300 to the Accredited Social Health Activist (ASHA) or health staff for KA patient surveillance and treatment. Additionally, ASHAs are INR 200 for the indoor residual spray and also community engagement and mobilization [30].

Miltefosine (MF) (hexadecylphosphocholine), a lysophospholipid analog, was mainly developed as an anticancer drug and in 2011, WHO added MF as essential medicine. MF has been used for VL, but due to possible resistance this drug has been kept under hold. However, this is prescribed in PKDL cases [31].

3.5.2 Chandipura virus

Chandipura virus (CHPV) belongs to the genus Vesiculovirus, family *Rhabdoviridae*. This infection was discovered during an acute febrile outbreak in Nagpur, Maharashtra state, India from two febrile cases in 1965. The available information suggests that sandflies are the vectors for this virus while antibodies against this have been detected in a wide range of vertebrate animals. In recent years, CHPV has emerged as encephalitic pathogen. Many outbreaks especially in children have been documented from different areas of India; in 2004, 2005, 2007 and 2008 from Andhra Pradesh, in 2005, 2009 to 2012 from Gujarat and in Vidarbha region of Maharashtra during 2007 and 2009–12 [32].

During the outbreaks in Maharashtra CHPV has been isolated from pools of Sandflies. However, CHPV has also been isolated from human samples during 1971–72 in Nigeria, and hedgehogs (*Atelerix spiculus*) during entomological surveillance in Senegal, Africa during 1990–1996. Recently this virus was also detected from Bhutan and Nepal, and from wild toque macaques (*Macaca sinica*) at Polonnaruwa, Sri Lanka during 1993. This suggests its circulation in many tropical countries. All these factors indicate that Sandflies are the vector of CHPV [32].

In 2019, a 5-year old girl reported died due to CHPV infection in Gujarat. This is an indication that this virus is still remains to be a cause of concern [33].

3.6 Mite-transmitted diseases

3.6.1 Scrub typhus

Scrub typhus (ST)—a rickettsial infection is caused by the gram-negative obligate intracellular coccobacillus pathogen *Orientia tsutsugamushi*. Its transmission to humans is by the bite of larval stage (chigger) of *Leptotrombidium* mites under

Trombiculidae family. This disease is endemic in Southeast Asia and Southwest Pacific regions generally known as *tsutsugamushi* triangle [34].

In India, first cases of ST were reported from Himachal Pradesh and were prevalent between 1960s and 1970s in many states and union territories. However, subsequently this disease disappeared possibly due to the use of insecticides for vector control and also the wide use of antibiotics to febrile cases with Tetracyclines and Chloramphenicol. ST is responsible for one of the causes of acute encephalopathy syndrome (AES) especially in children. WHO recognizes this disease is most underdiagnosed and under-reporting febrile illness demanding hospitalization. Post-monsoon is the most favorable period of ST as most of the cases are reported during this time. It is reported that the ongoing AES outbreaks in Gorakhpur areas in Uttar Pradesh were due to ST along with JE [35]. This made the public health officials to shift the treatment schedule. Doxycycline is recommended, thus saved many children. Similar observations were also recorded in Odisha and Assam states. This recent experience necessitated to undergo routine diagnostic tests for ST where AES is the most prevalent. Thus this disease can be contained and lives of many children can be saved [35]. Recently ICMR-DHR has drawn a generalized guideline for scientific management of ST [36].

3.7 Tick borne diseases

3.7.1 Kyasanur Forest Disease

Kyasanur Forest Disease (KFD) or generally called monkey fever by the local people is a forest tick-borne virus serocomplex of the genus *Flavivirus*, family *Flaviviridae*. The disease causes fever, hemorrhage, and encephalitis and has a 3–10% case-fatality ratio. It is not contagious transmits to man through bite of hard ticks primarily *Haemaphysalis spinigera* and many other *Ixodid* spp. The nymphs are active feeding form of the immature stage of the tick. This species is mostly prevalent in forest and feed on a number of small mammals, rodents, shrews, insectivorous bats, squirrels, rats and even many birds maintain the natural enzootic cycle of the virus in the forest ecosystem. Two non-human primates, black-faced langurs (*Semnopithecus entellus*) and red-faced bonnet macaques monkeys (*Macaca radiata*) get the virus infection by tick bite and are susceptible to the infection. Man is the dead end host. Cattle are the main hosts play an important role in maintaining the tick population [37].

KFD virus (KFDV) was first detected in a moribund black-faced langurs (*Semnopithecus entellus*) in Kyasanur forest near Baragi village in Sagar taluk of Shivamogga distirct, Karnataka state (erstwhile Mysore state) in 1957. In the beginning KFDV was restricted to three taluks i.e. Sagar, Shikaripur and Sorab of Shivamogga district. Subsequently it spreaded to other areas of Karnataka namely Udipi, Uttara Kannada, Mangaluru, Dakshina Kannada, Chikmagalur and Chamarajanagar district, Bandipur Tiger Reserve Forest, Karnataka. Outbreaks were reported in Thirthahalli taluk, Shivamogga district in 2014 and Belagavi district in 2016 Karnataka state. In 2015, outbreaks also occurred in four villages Northeast Goa. During serological studies, presence of KFDV were found in other areas of India such as parts of the Saurashtra region in Gujarat State, forested regions west of Kolkata, West Bengal State, and the Andaman Islands [38].

The increase in number of new foci and cases indicates that ecobiological changes due to deforestation and use of new land for farming and cattle grazing could lead to spread of KFD virus to newer geographical areas [38].

KFDV has been found only in monkeys, humans, and *Haemaphysalis spinigera* ticks in the KFD-epidemic region of south India. This virus was initially suspected as a Russian spring-summer (RSS) complex of viruses. But KFDV is only reported from India. The other closely related to KFDV are Omsk hemorrhagic fever virus in Siberia, Alkhurma virus in Saudi Arabia and Nanjianyin virus in China [38].

3.7.2 Crimean-Congo hemorrhagic fever

Crimean-Congo haemorrhagic fever (CCHF) is a zoonotic viral hemorrhagic infection and the virus (CCHFV) belongs to the genus *Nairovirus* under the family *Bunyaviridae*. CCHF was recognized for the first time in 1944, in the West Crimean region of the former Soviet Union, during a large outbreak, and the virus was subsequently isolated in 1956 from a human case. The average case-fatality rate is 30–50%; this varies between 5 and 80% in various outbreaks. The disease is endemic in Asia, Africa, East Europe, and the Middle East countries, that include Iran, southern Russia, the Balkans, Turkey, Pakistan, China, Iraq, the United Arabic Emirates, Oman, Kuwait, and Saudi Arabia. Considered as an occupational disease, CCHFV is transmitted by the bite of infected ticks or through direct contact with the infected blood and tissues of animals as well as nosocomial infections. *Hyalomma marginatum* and *Ixodid* spp. of ticks are the main vectors of CCHFV [38, 39].

The existence of CCHF in India was first confirmed in 2011 in Gujarat state from a nosocomial source. This case started with an index case having a history of tick bites with a close contact with animals. Another nosocomial infection was recorded in June 2012 from Ahmadabad city ended with two fatalities. In 2013, a non-nosocomial CCHF outbreak in Amreli district, as well as positive *Hyalomma* tick, animal and human samples in various areas of Gujarat state, suggested that the virus is widespread in Gujarat state, India [40]. In September 2019, a high alert was sounded after two suspected siblings of CCHF surfaced in Jodhpur, Rajasthan state. On enquiry, it was found that their father was undergoing treatment for CCHFV in a hospital in Ahmadabad. All recovered from the infection [41].

The disease also transmitted man to man via nosocomial source. Once a man gets infected, the disease is transferred to other close family members who accompanied the infected individual to the hospital, lived in the same house, and attended the funeral of a person who had died due to CCHFV, or came in contact with infected body fluids. The normal route is through a bite from an infected tick. CCHFV circulates in nature in the enzootic route of 'tick-vertebrate-tick' cycle [38].

3.8 Flea-transmitted diseases

3.8.1 Plague

Plague is one of oldest vector-borne diseases known to mankind. It is a zoonotic disease that means an animal disease that can spread to humans—caused by a Gram-negative bacteria *Yersinia pestis*. It is transmitted to humans through the bite of infected fleas that live among rodents such as rats, squirrels, chipmunks, wood rats, prairie dogs, and rabbits. Usually epidemics of human plague are followed by rodent epizootics or rat fall in domestic and peri-domestic settings. There are three forms of the infection; (i) bubonic plague primarily affects the lymph nodes; (ii) septicemic plague affects the bloodstream and can be contracted by handling infected animals; (iii) pneumonic plague affects the lungs and can spread from person to person, though rarely, through contaminated air droplets [42].

Plague was mentioned in Bhagvata Purana (155–600 BC), as a disease. This disease also known as 'Black Death' in the fourteenth century panendemic was responsible for a major public health problem throughout India till the mid twentieth century AD. The epidemic was started in the year 1895–1896, and reached its peak in 1907. During the two decades between 1898 and 1928 there were over 12 million deaths in undivided India. The mortality rate due to plague was calculated to be 1.8 per 100,000 populations between 1949 and 1958. Since then mortality had declined and reached zero level during 1967. The reason for drastic decline was attributed to the use of DDT mainly introduced during National Malaria Eradication Program, and also use of streptomycin and sulfanomide. In the subsequent years between 1959 and 1966 there was a resurgence of plague in the South Indian sates of Tamil Nadu, Andhra Pradesh, and Karnataka. This may be due to discontinuation of DDT in the national program. Following this, in 1994, a bubonic plague outbreak at Mamla village, Beed district, Maharashtra and a pneumonic plague outbreak in Surat, Gujarat were recorded. This costs heavy revenue due travels restrictions at national and international levels. In 2002, a localized outbreak of pneumonic plague occurred in Hatkoti, Shimla district, Himachal Pradesh, and a bubonic plague outbreak occurred in Dangud village, Uttarkashi district, Uttarakhand in 2004 [42].

Xenopsylla cheopis—the flea species the main vector of plague is believed to be originated from the valley of Nile. It is distributed throughout the world. *Xe. astia*is restricted in its distribution to the oriental region and in India it is widely distributed in peri-domestic and wild situations. *Xe. brasiliensis*, originally distributed from Africa was a very common species in domestic and peri-domestic settings in Peninsular India. However, currently this species is not abundant in India. In India, of the 128 species of rodents belonging to 46 genera 8 are considered to be the zoonotic reservoirs of various diseases. Domestic rats especially *Rattus rattus* and peri-domestic *Rattus norvegicus* are the most common hosts of these vector fleas. The sylvatic cycle of plague is maintained among the wild rodent hosts. It has been observed that most rodent species propagate their populations during the bamboo flowering seasons that occur once in every 10–12 years. Hence, proper prior preventive arrangements must be undertaken to prevent rodent-linked diseases and also huge damage to crops [42].

4. Discussion

India is a vast country with several geo-ecological diversities on ethnicities, languages, socio-cultural, and political settings. Most of the vector borne diseases in India or elsewhere are governed by the local environmental factors. In the present situation, climate change is a big threat to the entire world. There are unprecedented uncertainties in disease prediction resulting some unrelated outbreaks do occur in the present situation. To encounter this situation, a robust public health response mechanism must be in place in every state. On this direction, Integrated Disease Surveillance Program (IDSP) is in place to take immediate action to contain any outbreaks including VBDs.

In the present situation, malaria, LF and KA are under the process of elimination. Already two timelines of elimination for LF and KA have been extended, and now aiming to eliminate the two diseases by 2020. As per the present information, it may not be possible to achieve this goal by 2020. However, several efforts such as inclusion of ivermectin for ELF and strengthening of case detection and enhancement of incentives for each CL and PKDL for KA are highly encouraging. In case of malaria elimination, several initiatives have been taken. One such is Malaria Elimination Research Alliance—India (MERA—India). This will address the immediate research needs that will support the national program. Today the major issues are how to tackle the outdoor transmission, role of asymptomatic in malaria transmission especially in the high burden tribal areas where the real malaria problem exists. A robust smart surveillance system with application of artificial intelligence and mechanical learning must be introduced for better program implementation with correct prediction. Studies on vector behavior and responses of existing drugs to the malarial parasites and insecticides to the local vectors especially *Anopheles culicifacies* in most rural areas; *An. fluviatilis* and *An. minimus* in hilly terrain areas; *An. dirus* in forest areas especially in Northeast India. Resistance of synthetic pyrethroids (SPs) to most vector species is a matter of concern, because these are used in LLINs and no other molecules are available to replace them. In this direction recent study on use of atovaquone adding on glass substrate led to the killing of *P. falciparum* parasites in blood-fed *Anopheles* mosquitoes. This can be applied on LLINs along with SPs for better results. Other sporontocidal antimalarial drug Tefenoquine can also be used [43]. A special action may be taken for *An. stephensi*—the main urban malaria vector. This invasive species is rapidly making its footprints with the fast urbanization process. Already reports indicate that it has invaded Sri Lanka and some African countries [44, 45]. This is indicative of strong implementation of International Health Regulation act.

NVBDCP is the nodal agency for all vector borne diseases in India. Dengue, Chikungunya and more recently Zika are all transmitted by the two species of *Aedes* mosquitoes namely *Ae. aegypti* and *Ae. albopictus*. These two species are also highly invasive and endemic—the former is more associated with domestic and peri-domestic environments; while the later in the forest-fringed areas. Efforts to control the vector population using the genetic engineering tools are encouraging, but needs correct and specific genetic analysis of the target species as the recent report in Brazil deems strategic introspection [46].

Cattle including pigs play an important role in maintaining the enzootic cycle of most of VBDs. In recent years, diseases transmitted by ticks and mites are on the rise. This may be attributed to more man and animal contacts. Due to population pressure man is encroaching new areas especially in the forest ecosystem. It has been observed that cattle are the main host for ticks and mites to maintain their population. It is, thus, important to grow cattle population under controlled conditions with the help of local veterinary department. Open grazing of such cattle in the affected areas must be prevented so as to boost the enzootic transmission of KFD, CCHF and ST types of diseases. ST was diagnosed as the main AES problem in Gorakhpur, UP especially in the children. Treatment with doxycline contained the outbreak of AES besides other additional containment measures [34].

Similarly, sandflies also depend on cattle for maintenance of their own population in the endemic areas of KA and CHPV. Pigs also grown in most wet areas since these are easy source of income generation especially in the poorer section of the society. This is not an organized sector. Steps must be taken so as to make proper sty and protected with LLINs by which pig-mosquito contact can be minimized [14]. Recently genetically engineered high protein-rich pink pigs have been produced that can convert into pin-revolution. In this way JE transmission can be prevented [47].

Cow dung is a good source of organic manure traditionally practiced in India for ages. It has been observed that cows are reared for milk and manure purpose almost in each village household of rural India. But in most of tribal areas a very few household rears cattle making a very low human and cattle ratio. This may be one of the potential factors resulting high human blood index in the main vector *An. fluviatilis* [48]. So promotion of cattle in all the tribal areas must be on priority. On the other hand, community-level cow dung-based biogas plant must be encouraged in each village. In this way, good quality manure and self-sustained biogas can make the rural community self-reliant. Moreover huge carbon emission from the cattle produce can be prevented and thus carbon-related green-house effects can be curtailed.

Irrigation system is intimately associated with VBDs. Most mosquito-borne diseases can be controlled if integrated irrigation can regulate the water supply preventing mosquito breeding and also water conservation. Application of blue green algae in rice field can significantly reduce the mosquito population especially *Culex* species responsible for JE [49].

India is now heading for many good initiatives aiming for better livelihood under which *Swachh Bharat Abhiyan* (Clean India Movement), providing housing to poor people, free from Open Defecation (OD) are gaining some results. Providing toilets to each village under OD program has two benefits. First, avoiding soil contamination for which anti-micobial resistance can be managed. Second, outdoor malaria transmission can be prevented especially among women community who generally go for OD in groups in the evening hours when malaria vectors take advantage of such situations. Thus, use of LLINs becomes less effective in such village settings. But construction of water storing tank in each toilet must be mosquito proofed, otherwise *Aedes*-related diseases may be introduced in new areas [4].

It has been observed that in most urban cities there are defects in architectural design for building constructions where making a box on each parapet attracts water collection when the outlet pipe is blocked. This becomes potential breeding ground for *Aedes* and *An. stephensi* mosquitoes. This design must be abandoned to avoid creating unnecessary artificial breeding grounds for potential vector mosquitoes [50].

In most water starving areas where local people store water in open cemented or plastic tanks support *Aedes* breeding. Such tanks must be replaced with mosquito-proof water storing tanks to avoid mosquito breeding [51].

India has a strong primary health care system. The primary health management begins from the Sub-center (SC) where local people report for any disease. This needs to be empowered for better health seeking behavior. Recently a health reform program *Ayushman Bharat* (long life for India) has been introduced in India. It has two arms; coverage of health insurance for poorest 500 million people up to $ 7000 (INR 500,000) of care per year, regardless of preexisting conditions, and reinvestment in primary care. These SCs have been converted into 'Health and Wellness Centers' to deliver comprehensive primary health care [52].

In 2018, the Uttar Pradesh (UP) government initiated a unique DASTAK campaign in association with UNICEF (United Nations Children's Fund) to control JE and other AES causing VBDs. The entire state machinery visited door-to-door campaign in 38 districts affected by JE and AES. It has been planned in every village of state's 75 districts to create awareness about communicable diseases. In this large-scale campaign, many state departments such as health, primary education, rural development will work together to spread awareness about diseases through mass media communication. The campaign will ensure availability of clean drinking water, promote sanitation drive, ensure vaccination and prompt treatment of diseases. Such program must be launched in every state because most VBDs are present throughout the country [53].

India is a democratic country where local working administration is governed by the elected members generally called *Panchayat Raj Institution*. It is the duty of the local health department to empower these members to take correct decisions and implementation of all health-related programs. However, social movement needs to strengthen the community engagement for achieving better health goals.

Already India has the required experience for eradication/elimination of Guinea worm and polio. This experience will help in better implementation of the VBDs under elimination process. However, the recent report by WHO has warned that malaria elimination is not possible in near future. This means malaria elimination is not possible by 2030. But India must take proper steps to eliminate malaria by 2030 [54].

5. Conclusion

As mentioned it is evident that there are needs of innovations in containing VBDs in India. In the present situation, there are many opportunities in India that must be put into actions to find solutions in containing VBDs. It is not at all good that two diseases LF and KA have failed to keep their elimination targets. That means there were some serious lapses in planning the elimination concept. The new target to eliminate both these diseases has been earmarked to 2020 and 2021, respectively. But the current situations do not seem to achieve this goal [55, 56]. However, renewed efforts should be made to fulfill the goal. On the other hand, dengue and other VBDs are posing a serious threat to the public health professionals. It has been observed that most of the VBDs are linked to epizootic environment. Hence, organized and organic farming should be given priority to reduce the man and vector contact. There are many government programs aiming to uplifting of general improvement of social status of the community. This will surely impact on the VBDs. Hence, it is the duty of all to accelerate the implementation of all programs related to VBDs and make India free from all Neglected Tropical Diseases (NTDs) to fulfill the Sustainable Development Goals (SDGs).

Conflict of interest

The authors declare no conflict of interest.

Author details

Susanta Kumar Ghosh[1*] and Chaitali Ghosh[2]

1 ICMR-National Institute of Malaria Research, Bengaluru, India

2 Tata Institute for Genetics and Society, Bengaluru, India

*Address all correspondence to: ghoshnimr@gmail.com

References

[1] Profile—Know India: National portal of India. Available from: https://knowindia.gov.in/profile/

[2] India—Demographic trends | Britannica.com. Available from: https://www.britannica.com/place/India/Demographic-trends

[3] Tyagi BK, Munirathinam A, Venkatesh A. A catalogue of Indian mosquitoes. International Journal of Mosquito Research. 2015;**2**(2):50-97

[4] Ghosh SK, Rahi M. Malaria elimination in India—The way forward. Journal of Vector Borne Diseases. 2019;**56**:32-40

[5] Ghosh SK, Ghosh C. New ways of tackling malaria. In: Claborn D editor. Current Topics in the Epidemiology of Vector-Borne Diseases. 2019. ISBN 978-1-83880-022-2. (in press)

[6] WHO. Report of a Consultative Meeting, lymphatic Filariasis Infection and Disease Control Strategies. TDR/CTD/FIL/PENAN/1 1994. 1994. pp. 1-2

[7] Sebasan S, Palaniyandi M, Das PK, Michael E. Mapping of lymphatic filariasis in India. Annals of Tropical Medicine and Parasitology. 2000;**94**:591-606

[8] Lymphatic filariasis. Available from: https://www.who.int/news-room/fact-sheets/detail/lymphatic-filariasis

[9] India adopts new strategy to accelerate Lymphatic Filariasis elimination. Available from: https://health.economictimes.indiatimes.com/news/diagnostics/india-adopts-new-strategy-to-accelerate-lymphatic-filariasis-elimination/64574044

[10] Dr Harsh Vardhan Announces Scale-up of Triple-drug Therapy to Achieve the Elimination of Lymphatic Filariasis by 2021. Available from: https://pib.gov.in/PressReleasePage.aspx?PRID=1589596

[11] WHO. Japanese Encephalitis. Fact Sheet No 386, December 2015. Available from: https://web.archive.org/web/20170713162555; http://www.who.int/mediacentre/factsheets/fs386/en/

[12] Kulkarni R, Sapkal GN, Kaushal H, Mourya DT. Japanese Encephalitis: A brief review on Indian perspectives. The Open Virology Journal. 2018;**12**(Suppl-2, M8):121-130

[13] Kumari R, Joshi PL. A review of Japanese encephalitis in Uttar Pradesh, India. WHO South-East Asia Journal of Public Health. 2012;**1**:374-395

[14] Dutta P, Khan SA, Khan AM, Borah J, Sarmah CK, Mahanta J. The effect of insecticide-treated mosquito nets (ITMNs) on Japanese Encephalitisvirus seroconversion in pigs and humans. American Journal of Tropical Medicine and Hygiene. 2011;**84**:466-472

[15] Murhekar MV, Oak C, Ranjan P, Kanagasabai K, Shinde S, Pandey AK, et al. Coverage and missed opportunity for Japanese encephalitis vaccine, Gorakhpur division, Uttar Pradesh, India, 2015: Implications for Japanese encephalitis control. Indian Journal of Medical Research. 2017;**145**:63-69

[16] About Jen Vac. Available from: https://www.bharatbiotech.com/jenvac.html

[17] WHO. Dengue Changing Epidemiology. Available from: http://www.searo.who.int/india/topics/dengue/dengue_factsheet.pdf

[18] Cecilia D. Current status of dengue and chikungunya in India. WHO

South-East Asia Journal of Public Health. 2014;**3**(1):22-27

[19] Murhekar M, Joshua V, Kanagasabai K, Shete V, Ravi M, Ramachandran R, et al. Epidemiology of dengue fever in India, based on laboratory surveillance data, 2014-2017. International Journal of Infectious Diseases. 2019. DOI: 10.1016/j.ijid.2019.01.004

[20] Ganeshkumar P, Murhekar MV, Poornima V, Saravanakumar V, Sukumaran K, Anandaselvasankar A, et al. Dengue infection in India: A systematic review and meta analysis. PLoS Neglected Tropical Diseases. 2018;**12**(7):e0006618

[21] More than 200,000 infected with dengue in Sri Lanka. Available from: https://gulfnews.com/amp/world/asia/more-than-200000-infected-with-dengue-in-sri-lanka-1.1564998600673?_twitter_impression=true

[22] Philippines declares a national dengue epidemic after 622 deaths. Available from: https://edition.cnn.com/2019/08/07/health/philippines-dengue-epidemic-intl-hnk/index.html

[23] 40 dead in Bangladesh due to dengue outbreak. Available from: https://www.indiatoday.in/world/story/40-dead-in-bangladesh-due-to-dengue-outbreak-1581919-2019-08-18

[24] Murhekar M, Kanagasabai K, Shete V, Joshua V, Ravi M, Kirubakaran BK, et al. Epidemiology of chikungunya based on laboratory surveillance data—India, 2016-2018. Transactions of the Royal Society of Tropical Medicine and Hygiene. 2019;**113**:259-262

[25] ZIKA Epidemiology Update. Available from: https://www.who.int/emergencies/diseases/zika/zika-epidemiology-update-july-2019.pdf

[26] WHO. Zika Virus Infection: India. Available from: https://www.who.int/emergencies/diseases/zika/india-november-2018/en/

[27] Clinical Guidance for Healthcare Providers for Prevention of Sexual Transmission of Zika Virus. Available from: https://www.cdc.gov/zika/hc-providers/clinical-guidance/sexualtransmission.html

[28] First sexually transmitted dengue case confirmed in Spain. Available from: https://www.telegraph.co.uk/news/2019/11/08/first-sexually-transmitted-dengue-case-confirmed-spain/

[29] Leishmaniasis. Available from: https://www.who.int/en/news-room/fact-sheets/detail/leishmaniasis

[30] Leishmaniasis India. Available from: https://www.who.int/leishmaniasis/burden/Leishmaniasis_India/en/

[31] Khanra S, Sarraf NR, Anjan K, Das AK, Roy S, Manna M. Miltefosine resistant field isolate from Indian Kala-Azar patient shows similar phenotype in experimental infection. Scientific Reports. 2017;**7**:10330. DOI: 10.1038/s41598-017-09720-1

[32] Sapkal GN, Sawant PM, Mourya DT. Chandipura viral encephalitis: A brief review. The Open Virology Journal. 2018;**12**:44-51

[33] 5-year-old Girl Dies of Chandipura virus in Gujarat. Available from: https://www.indiatoday.in/india/story/5-year-old-girl-dies-of-chandipura-virus-in-gujarat-1570198-2019-07-17

[34] Chunchanur SK. Scrub typhus in India—An impending threat! Annals of Clinical Immunology and Microbiology. 2018;**1**:Article No. 1003

[35] Bal M, Mohanta MP, Sahu S, Dwibedi B, Pati S, Ranjit M. Profile of pediatric scrub typhus in Odisha, India (2019). Indian Pediatrics. 2019;**56**:304-306

[36] Rahi M, Gupte MD, Bhargava A, Varghese GM, Arora R. DHR-ICMR guidelines for diagnosis and management of rickettsial diseases in India. Indian Journal of Medical Research. 2015;**141**:417-422

[37] Munivenkatappa A, Sahay RR, Yadav PD, Viswanathan R, Mourya DT. Clinical & epidemiological significance of Kyasanur forest disease. Indian Journal of Medical Research. 2018;**148**:145-150

[38] Mourya DT, Yadav PD, Patil DY. Highly infectious tick-borne viral diseases: Kyasanur forest disease and Crimean–Congo haemorrhagic fever in India. WHO South-East Asia Journal of Public Health. 2014;**3**(1):8-21

[39] Shahbazi N, Sahar Firouz K, Karimi M, Mostafavi E. Seroepidemiological survey of Crimean-Congo haemorrhagic fever among high-risk groups in the west of Iran. Journal of Vector Borne Diseases. 2019;**56**:174-177

[40] Mourya DT, Yadav PD, Gurav YK, Pardeshi PG, Shete AM, Jain R, et al. Crimean Congo hemorrhagic fever serosurvey in humans for identifying highrisk populations and high-risk areas in the endemic state of Gujarat, India. BMC Infectious Diseases. 2019;**19**:104

[41] Rajasthan on Alert After Suspected Cases of Congo Fever Surface in Jodhpur. Available from: https://www.indiatoday.in/india/story/rajasthan-alert-suspected-cases-congo-fever-surface-jodhpur-1595139-2019-09-03

[42] Biswas S. Plague in India: A review. Journal of Communicable Diseases. 2018;**50**:60-75

[43] Burrows J, Fidock DA, Miller RS, Rees S. Blocking *Plasmodium* development in mosquitoes: A powerful new approach for expanding malaria control efforts. American Journal of Tropical Medicine and Hygiene. 2019;**101**:734-735

[44] Dharmasiri AGG, Yashan Perera AY, Harishchandra J, Herath H, Aravindan KH, Jayasooriya TR, et al. First record of *Anopheles stephensi* in Sri Lanka: A potential challenge for prevention of malaria reintroduction. Malaria Journal. 2017;**16**:326

[45] Takken W, Lindsay S. Increased threat of urban malaria from *Anopheles stephensi* mosquitoes, Africa. Emerging Infectious Diseases. 2019;**25**(7):1431-1433

[46] Evans BR, Kotsakiozi P, Costa-da-Silva AL, Ioshino RS, Garziera L, Pedrosa MC, et al. Transgenic *Aedes aegypti* mosquitoes transfer genes into a natural population. Scientific Reports. 2019;**9**:3047. DOI: 10.1038/s41598-019-49660-6

[47] A 'Pink Revolution' Quietly Takes Shape in Maharasthra. Available from: https://www.thehindu.com/business/Industry/pink-revolution/article26168901.ece

[48] Sahu SS, Gunasekaran K, Krishnamoorthy N, Vanamail P, Mathivanan A, Manonmani A, et al. Bionomics of *Anopheles fluviatilis* and *Anopheles culicifacies* (Diptera: Culicidae) in relation to malaria transmission in East-Central India. Journal of Medical Entomology. 2017;**54**:821-830

[49] Victor TJ, Reuben R. Effects of organic and inorganic fertilisers on mosquito populations in rice fields of southern India. Medical and Veterinary Entomology. 2000;**14**(4):361-368

[50] Dev V, Ghosh SK. *Anopheles* (*Cellia*) stephensi Liston 1901, the vector of urban malaria—An imminent threat to malaria elimination in India. Proceedings of the National Academy of Science, India Section B: Biological Sciences.

[51] Ghosh SK, Chakravarthy P, Panch Sandhya R, Pushpalata K, Tiwari SN,

Ojha VP, et al. Comparative efficacy of two Poeciliid fish in indoor cement tanks against chikungunya vector *Aedes aegypti* in villages in Karnataka, India. BMC Public Health. 2011;**11**:599

[52] Das S, Jha AK. Getting coverage right for 500 million Indians. New England Journal of Medicine. 2019;**380**:2287-2289

[53] UP Launches DASTAK Campaign to Eradicate AES & JE. Available from: https://currentaffairs.gktoday.in/launches-dastak-campaign-eradicate-aes-je-07201970459.html

[54] 'Malaria Will Not Be Eradicated in Near Future' Warns WHO. Available from: https://www.theguardian.com/world/2019/aug/23/malaria-will-not-be-eradicated-in-near-future-warns-who

[55] The Epidemic You Don't Know About. Available from: https://timesofindia.indiatimes.com/india/the-epidemic-you-dont-know-about/articleshow/61680295.cms

[56] Rijal S, Sundar S, Mondal D, Das P, Alvar J, Boelaert M. Eliminating visceral leishmaniasis in South Asia: The road ahead. BMJ. 2019;**364**:k5224